Lose Weight,
Live Healthy

OTHER WORKS BY THE AUTHOR

Maximize Your Body Potential: Lifetime Skills for Successful Weight Management,
Third Edition (2003)

Binge No More: Your Guide to Overcoming Disordered Eating (1999)

The New Maximize Your Body Potential (1997)

What Your Doctor Can't Tell You about Cosmetic Surgery (1995)

Now That You've Lost It (1992)

*Maximize Your Body Potential** (1986)

Taking Charge of Your Weight and Well-being (1978)

*Winner of an award from the American Medical Writers Association.

Lose Weight,
Live Healthy

A Complete Guide to Designing Your Own Weight Loss Program

JOYCE D. NASH, PH.D.

BULL PUBLISHING COMPANY
BOULDER, COLORADO

Bull Publishing Company
P.O. Box 1377
Boulder, CO 80306
(800) 676-2855
(303) 545-6354 (fax)
www.bullpub.com

Library of Congress Cataloging-in-Publication Data

Nash, Joyce D.
Lose weight, live healthy: a complete guide to designing your own weight loss program / Joyce D. Nash
p. cm.
ISBN 978-1-933503-61-5
1. Weight loss. 2. Exercise. 3. Motivation (Psychology). I. Title.
RM222.2N347 2011
613.2'5—dc22
2011006949

ISBN: 978-1-933503-61-5

Distributed in the United States by:
Independent Publishers Group, 814 North Franklin Street, Chicago, IL 60610

Publisher: James Bull
Interior Design and Production: Dianne Nelson and Laura Kedro, Shadow Canyon Graphics
Cover Design: Lightbourne, Inc.
Developmental Editor: Erin Mulligan

Manufactured in the United States of America

First Edition
10 9 8 7 6 5 4 3 2 1

ABOUT THE AUTHOR

JOYCE D. NASH, PH.D., is a clinical psychologist in private practice in Menlo Park, CA, specializing in the treatment of eating disorders and anxiety disorders. She holds two Ph.D.s—one in clinical psychology from the Pacific Graduate School of Psychology in Palo Alto, CA, and one in communication from Stanford University. She also completed postdoctoral work at the Stanford University School of Medicine, during which time she founded the Diet and Weight Control Clinic at Stanford. Dr. Nash has authored nine books on behavioral medicine subjects and weight-related topics. For more information about Dr. Nash, visit her website at www.joycenashphd.com. For more information about *Lose Weight, Live Healthy* and the associated blog, go to www.loseweightlivehealthyguide.com.

CONTENTS

INTRODUCTION

RECENTLY THE NEWS FEATURED A STORY OF A MAN who was asked to leave his airplane seat because he was too big to fit into it comfortably. It was his habit to buy two adjacent seats, but on this occasion, he had purchased the last available seat. He was angry about the airline's policy, but other passengers were relieved at his ejection. Obesity is all around us in America. A popular TV program, "The Biggest Loser," shows obese people competing for prize money—and dubious fame—by losing the most weight. A number of magazines regularly include stories about ordinary people who have been successful at losing weight, detailing their process and giving advice. And celebrity news magazines frequently carry feature articles of celebrities who have gained or lost a lot of weight and relate their struggles with food obsessions and eating. Kirstie Alley, who has sometimes weighed well over 100 pounds above healthy weight, had a reality show on TV exhibiting her struggle with weight. Dr. Oz and other television hosts campaign against obesity with programs meant to inform—and sometimes embarrass. Michelle Obama has taken up the cause of childhood obesity. The flow of diet books and other books on how to lose weight continues apace. Weight loss surgery is increasingly accepted as a last resort for severe obesity. And the news media highlight the increasing obesity rates. Making a permanent change in lifestyle is difficult but necessary to succeed in losing weight, but despite the hype, few have succeeded in making this conversion. A new approach is needed for achieving success.

BEHAVIOR CHANGE

Lose Weight, Live Healthy: A Complete Guide to Designing Your Own Weight Loss Program differs in several ways from other books on weight management and healthy lifestyle. First, it emphasizes evidence-based behavior change strategies, including self-monitoring for diet and exercise, goal setting, environmental management, use of reward, cognitive change, problem solving, interpersonal coping skills, and relapse prevention. It also addresses the challenges to changing from rarely discussed perspectives—for example, emergence from the invisibility of being obese and sex after weight loss. It integrates mindfulness-based and acceptance-based therapy principles with proven successful concepts for weight reduction and lifestyle change. In addition, it includes tips for using the latest technology—smartphone apps and the Internet—to achieve success.

Behavior therapy has evolved in recent years. A new emphasis on mindfulness and values, which is an adjunct to basic behavioral principles, contributes to Acceptance and Commitment Therapy (ACT, pronounced as a single word). This book introduces concepts from ACT therapy, an approach to mindfulness and well-being developed and articulated by Dr. Steven Hayes at the University of Nevada–Reno and his associates. ACT encourages us to define personal values and develop guiding principles that can provide us with direction for our behavior and actions, and to accept our thoughts and feelings instead of fighting them. The aim of ACT is to allow us to create a rich, full, and meaningful life while accepting the pain that inevitably comes with living.

TECHNOLOGY

A feature that makes *Lose Weight, Live Healthy* unique in its field is the inclusion of information on using technology to help with lifestyle change. The Internet, smartphone apps, and other new communication technologies (e.g., blogs, videos, iPods, iPads, podcasts) have experienced rapid growth, especially over the past decade. Over 75 percent of American adults in 2007 reported using the Internet, and 79 percent of those reported obtaining health information online.

The Internet and smartphones are increasingly able to provide information and therapy programs and applications that target weight loss, weight management, physical activity, and other lifestyle changes (e.g., quitting smoking, managing insulin medication, managing hypertension, engaging in meditation). Many of these applications now incorporate behavioral therapy principles and, in many cases, facilitate personal contact—social support—with others who are engaged in a similar change effort.

Lose Weight, Live Healthy provides the comprehensive information you need to design your own weight loss and healthy lifestyle program, supplemented by recommendations for using Internet programs and smartphone applications.

WHAT TO EXPECT IN *LOSE WEIGHT, LIVE HEALTHY*

Chapter 1, Understanding the Relationship between Weight and Health, provides essential information on how weight impacts health. If you are undecided about undertaking a lifestyle change, you may be persuaded by the evidence of the health risks posed by overweight and obesity discussed in this chapter. Definitions of overweight and obesity are provided, as well as a means of assessing your body mass index (BMI). The chapter also discusses the causes of weight problems, and the effect that obesity has on your mental and physical health.

Of course, motivation for change is always a problem. In Chapter 2, Getting and Staying Motivated, you will discover which of the stages of change you are currently in, and how to get more motivated by doing a cost–benefit analysis of your reasons for changing or not changing. Ways of getting social support are addressed. An important part of this chapter is a discussion of values—the foundation for successful lifestyle change and one of the core processes of ACT.

Chapter 3, Changing Behavior, lays the groundwork for making positive changes. It discusses the ABC model of thinking and behavior, and teaches you how to intervene in a behavior pattern. Included in this chapter are basic behavior change strategies such as self-monitoring, environmental management, and use of rewards for encouraging new habits and behaviors. Mindfulness and acceptance are also important topics in this chapter.

Chapter 4, Eating for Health, provides up-to-date information on nutrition, including tools you need to make positive food choices. Using a food exchange system is an easy way to group foods together based on calories and nutritional value. Information about glycemic load and glycemic index are especially helpful for diabetics or those who are at risk for diabetes. If you think you are a "sugarholic," this chapter will help you address your addiction to sugar. Also discussed is the fullness factor—a way of evaluating foods on the basis of how full you feel upon eating them.

Chapter 5, Getting Started with Exercise, will help you overcome barriers to exercise and ease into an exercise program that works for you. To start or revitalize a fitness program, check out this chapter. You can learn how to choose a gym or a personal trainer. If you simply need to get moving, the section on increasing activities of daily living will help you do just that.

Thinking, also known as cognition, includes self-talk, attitudes, beliefs, assumptions, and interpretations. Chapter 6, Managing Thinking and Self-Talk, addresses cognition in all its forms—conscious thoughts, underlying beliefs, and even tricks your mind can play on you. Some kinds of self-talk help you achieve goals, while other kinds of self-talk hinder you from getting what you say you want. This chapter provides specific examples of helping and hindering self-talk.

Yes, we all talk to ourselves. In fact, there is always an inner dialogue going on between different parts of our selves. Chapter 7, Challenging Your "Inner Voices," will help you learn to recognize the different subpersonalities that we all have, and choose which ones are best to listen to. You can strengthen your own healthy voice and learn to not indulge those parts of you that prefer unhealthy alternative behaviors.

Stress is often a trigger for emotional eating. Learning to use distress tolerance and emotion regulation skills is critical. So is becoming more appropriately assertive and managing interpersonal conflict. These behavioral skills are presented in Chapter 8, Addressing Stress. This chapter discusses both problem-focused and emotion-focused coping, and teaches more effective strategies for addressing stress.

As many as 50 percent of obese people struggle with binge eating. Chapter 9, Stopping the Binge Cycle, helps you learn how to intervene in and prevent binge eating. You will learn how to interrupt the tension building phase of the cycle and find alternatives to using binge eating to deal with painful emotions.

Backsliding—a succession of small slips—is usually a part of any change effort. The key is to recover from small slips or lapses before they become total relapse and a return to old habits. Chapter 10, Dealing with Backsliding, helps you identify high-risk situations and plan for coping better with them. Typical high-risk situations involve social occasions, emotions, and transition times—the time between finishing one task and starting another.

Every lifestyle change comes with challenges—some of which are not anticipated. Chapter 11, Overcoming Challenges to Change, addresses how to handle compliments, cope with the expectations of others, face sex again, dress for change, and deal with a changing body image. Other challenges involve loss of the invisibility and the unsettling emotions that accompany regaining some weight.

For the severely obese, weight loss surgery may be the final option for attaining a healthier lifestyle. Chapter 12, Considering Weight Loss Surgery, helps you understand how bariatric surgery leads to weight loss and what the basic surgery options are. After surgery, challenges continue—how to avoid cheating, what to do if there is excess skin left after the initial operation, and what it means to transition to a new lifestyle.

Throughout the text of the book, tips are provided for using smartphone apps and the Internet to expand your knowledge and increase your chances for success. For example, several apps that are highly regarded for weight loss include **SparkPeople**, **LoseIt**, and **Calorie-Counter**. Other apps help with a variety of related issues, such as meditation (**White Noise**), stress management (**Breath Pacer**), yoga (**Yoga STRETCH**), and hiking (**Trails**). Of course there is seemingly infinite information on the Internet on all sorts of topics. But how do you know what to trust and how to avoid websites designed to sell you something, including wrong information? Surfing the Net can waste a lot of time. In *Lose Weight, Live Healthy*, the author has vetted the sites for you. You can expect to find good and reliable information at the Internet programs recommended in this book.

SUGGESTIONS FOR USING THIS BOOK

Lose Weight, Live Healthy is designed as either a standalone book, or to be used with adjunctive Internet programs and smartphone apps. It can be used with or without a counselor or therapist. It is not necessary to be a "techie" to use this book. The reader who does not want to use technology can get much help from this book without accessing the Internet or using a smartphone. The choice is up to the reader.

Conceivably health professionals may wish to use this book in their work with clients, either as a standalone or in conjunction with technology. At the end of the book there are suggestions for health professionals who wish to do this, along with a brief review of the literature on using technology for weight management.

ACKNOWLEDGMENTS

As with most books, many people have contributed behind the scenes, not the least of whom was my editor, Erin Mulligan, who helped me through several iterations of editing and provided many helpful edits and suggestions. Dianne Nelson, the final editor of the book, did yeoman work in polishing the final text, and I thank her for her efforts. Thanks go to Alex Morris and his associates, too, for bringing this book into being. My thanks go also to Elyse Robin, R.D., who reviewed the information in the chapter on nutrition. Help with the exercise chapter was provided by Scott Norton, a personal trainer and founder of Axis Personal Training, in Menlo Park, California, and to Tien Tran, my personal trainer, and founder of Transform Fitness, also in Menlo Park, California. Valuable input for the chapter on weight loss surgery was given by Laura Matteucci, RN, director of the Mills Peninsula Bariatric Surgery Program in Burlingame, California. I extend my thanks as well to Evelyn Tribole, R.D., and Elyse Resch, R.D., authors of the excellent book *Intuitive Eating*, for their help in adapting the 10 important points in their book for publication in this one. I also appreciate the work of Steve Hayes, Ph.D., and his associates, who developed Acceptance and Commitment Therapy (ACT). Last, but certainly not least, I owe a great deal of thanks to Jim Bull, of Bull Publishing Company, for his confidence in my work.

COMMENTS

All the people described in this book are composites of real individuals, but their stories and descriptions have been disguised. Any similarities to actual persons are merely coincidence.

To participate in a blog on healthy living, go to **www.loseweightlivehealthyguide.com**. If you find a smartphone app that you like, please tell me about it. You can reach me at **info. drnash@comcast.net**. Also, look for tips and information on my Facebook Page and become a fan; go to **www.facebook.com/loseweightlivehealthy**.

— *Joyce D. Nash, Ph.D.*

CHAPTER ONE

Understanding the Relationship Between Weight and Health

*Nita was considerably overweight. Her young daughter Gaby was, too. Nita worked two jobs trying to make ends meet; often it was easier to pick up dinner at the local Mc-Donalds than to try to cook at home. Nita disliked the taste of diet drinks and preferred drinking Classic Coke. Gaby went to a nearby grade school, which provided lunches; typical choices included corn dogs, chicken nuggets, chips, cookies, apples, and sweet drink options. Nita worried that Gaby had to walk back and forth to school, even though it was only a few blocks, because the neighborhood was known to be unsafe. She insisted that Gaby stay inside to play or do her homework. Gaby didn't have many friends at school, anyway—she was teased about her weight, and about her mother's weight. Nita's doctor told her that her blood pressure was high, as was her cholesterol, and that she needed to lose weight. Nita had tried diets before, but none worked. Recently, Nita had purchased an iPhone. She installed **SparkPeople**, a free application, or "app," to help her with weight loss. It provided access to support groups and information that helped her start a weight loss and healthy eating effort; she found the blogs and stories especially helpful. Nita also found help for budgeting and planning at **www.betterbudgeting.com**. As Nita began to change the way she shopped and cooked, her actions helped Gaby change her unhealthy habits as well.*

The Epidemic of Obesity

Given that more than 60 percent of U.S. adults are overweight or obese, and that many health care professionals recommend weight loss to reduce the risk of obesity and type 2 diabetes, finding ways to make weight loss, weight maintenance, and physical activity programs more widely accessible is a national health priority. Obesity is at epidemic proportions in the United States—indeed, in most Westernized countries. Since the mid-seventies, the prevalence of overweight and obesity has increased sharply in both adults and children. Data from two NHANES[1] surveys covering more than two decades show that among adults aged 20–74 years the prevalence of obesity increased from 15.0 percent (in the 1976–1980 survey) to 32.9 percent (in the 2003–2004 survey).[2] Today, two in every three adults aged 20 and over is overweight or obese, and one in every three children is. One of four adults meets the criterion for obesity—having a body mass index (BMI) of 30 or greater. Excess body fat increases the risk of many diseases, as well as of premature death. Of course, weight is just one measure of health. People who are slimmer but don't exercise or eat nutritious foods aren't necessarily healthy just because they don't appear overweight. Excess body fat can be a killer for both those who are obese as well as for some who appear to be of average weight.

TIP Over the past decade, the Internet, smartphones, and other new communication technologies (e.g., personal digital assistants [PDAs], iPods, iPhones, podcasts, blogs, chat rooms, interactive video and television, computer-aided instruction) have experienced rapid growth as potential tools against a variety of health-related problems. Thousands of applications and programs now exist that provide health and fitness information, a means of monitoring food intake and activity levels, and feedback on reaching weight and exercise goals; many include options such as calorie counters, weight tracking, pedometers, and blood pressure monitors. Technology is beginning to provide help for those who are caught in the epidemic of obesity. For more information on the epidemic of obesity, visit **www.obesityinamerica.org** and **www.cdc.gov/obesity/**.

What Is a Healthy Weight?

A healthy weight is the weight your body naturally settles into when you consistently eat a varied and nutritious diet of moderate caloric intake appropriate to your age, gender, and body type and when you are physically active on a regular basis so that calories in and out balance. A body mass index (BMI) chart or equation is used by some people to determine a healthy weight range. This works for most people, though not for a select few elite athletes, such as football players, who may appear overweight according to the chart when in fact they simply have a lot of muscle, which weighs more than fat. Similarly, a marathon runner, bicycle racer, or ice skater may register at the lower end of the BMI scale because he or she has long, lean muscles and a high proportion of lean body mass. Thus, in rare cases, the BMI chart is not a good approximation of body fat. Similarly, it is not considered a good single measure of healthy weight for children, pregnant women, or the sick or elderly, the latter of whom have in most cases lost muscle mass as well as bone density.

At the same time, persons who, according to the BMI chart, are in the upper regions of the "healthy" weight range may need to consider losing some weight if they have two or more factors indicating risk for heart disease (e.g., a person with high levels of low-density lipoprotein cholesterol or LDL—one type of lipid or fat that circulates in the blood—and who also has high blood pressure) or if they don't get much exercise. And people who have other diseases associated with a high weight, such as coronary artery disease, type 2 diabetes, or sleep apnea may also be advised to lose weight even if their BMI is within the recommended healthy range (BMI 19.5–24.9).

A new concern is "normal weight obesity," or NWO.[3] This is characterized by having a BMI in the healthy weight range but with a large percentage of body fat—more than 30 percent for women and 20 percent for men. This condition carries risks similar to being overweight or obese. Such people appear to be at an acceptable weight but tend to have less muscle mass and lighter bones; this is often true of older people in particular. The remedy is to do a combination of aerobic exercise and strength or resistance training exercise to build up muscle mass and strengthen bones.

Despite the existence of a number of different methods for measuring levels of body fat in individuals, there is no agreement about how to decide how much body fat is detrimental to health, or therefore about precisely when weight loss should be recommended.[4,5] Still, it is safe to say that a truly healthy weight is one that minimizes risk of weight-related diseases, that is realistic for your body and heredity, and that can be comfortably maintained by healthy choices and habits, including regular exercise. If in doubt, check with your physician. Even those whose jobs require a lot of activity and who don't appear overweight may have risk factors for disease that are undiagnosed or may appear to be thin but actually have a high percentage of body fat.

Other factors such as inactivity and smoking must be considered when assessing what is a healthy weight. Smoking contributes to lower weight but increases the risk of disease and premature death. BMI alone should not be used to determine an "ideal" body weight range, but it is a good guide for beginning to assess disease risk. Other body measures that correlate with health are waist circumference and waist-to-hip ratio, both of which have been shown to be related to higher risk of coronary heart disease. Experts agree that BMI together with waist girth and waist-to-hip ratio are important initial screens for unhealthy body weight.

TIP

A good source for general health information on the Internet is **WebMD.com**. It also is available in an app for the iPhone and other smartphones. **WebMD Mobile** is an app that allows access to a fairly extensive medical database online. There are three basic ways to search for information: Symptoms, Treatments, and First Aid.

Defining Overweight and Obesity

Overweight and obesity are both labels for ranges of weight that are greater than what is generally considered healthy or that have been shown to correlate with the risk of certain diseases and other health problems. Although there are some exceptions, as noted in the previous section, for most adults BMI is a reliable indicator of body fatness and is one measure commonly used to assess whether body weight is healthy.

BODY MASS INDEX

Body mass index, a statistical measure of the relationship between a person's weight and height, is useful when generalizing about groups of people. Healthcare professionals use BMI to classify people as underweight, healthy weight, overweight, and obese. Although BMI correlates well with the amount of body fat, it does not directly measure body fat. As a result, it is no more than one possible indicator and is not necessarily accurate when applied to a particular individual. In addition to body fat, it is also necessary to take into account race, gender, and age. For example, compared to whites, Asians tend to have lower BMIs but higher percentages of body fat.[6] Women have more fat under the skin than men, who have greater muscle mass than women of the same weight. Elder adults tend to weigh less than middle-aged adults, usually because they have lost muscle mass.

There are various formulae[7] for determining body mass index, but the easiest way is to look it up in the table that gives weight ranges for BMI. To check your BMI, refer to Table 1.1 or use the formula given in the endnotes for this chapter.

TIP   You can install the **BMI Calculator** free app on your iPhone. There are also multiple free BMI charts available on the Internet. For one that takes into account gender, go to: **www.halls.md/body-mass-index/av.htm**.

Although the cutoff points for weight ranges of BMI are somewhat arbitrary, for adults a healthy weight is generally defined as having a BMI of 19.5–24.9. Overweight is defined as having a body mass index of 25.0–29.9, and obesity as having a body mass index of 30.0 or more. Those with a BMI of 40.0–49.9 are designated as severely obese (i.e., having serious health risk), and those with a BMI above 50 are termed morbidly obese. A BMI less than 19.5 is underweight, and a BMI of 17.5 or less is one criterion used to diagnose anorexia nervosa. Generally speaking, younger people should be closer to the lower end of the recommended healthy weight range, while older adults may be in the upper ranges of healthy BMI weights.

Table 1.1
BMI

BMI	Underweight				Healthy Weight							Overweight						Obesity		
	17	17.5	18	18.5	19	20	21	22	23	24	24.9	25	26	27	28	29	29.9	30	35	40
4'10"	81	84	86	89	91	96	101	105	110	115	119	120	124	129	134	139	143	144	168	192
4'11"	84	87	89	92	94	99	104	109	114	119	123	124	129	134	139	144	148	149	173	198
5'	87	90	92	95	97	102	108	113	118	123	128	128	133	138	143	149	153	154	179	205
5'1"	90	93	95	98	101	106	111	117	122	127	132	132	138	143	148	154	158	159	185	212
5'2"	93	96	98	101	104	109	115	120	126	131	136	137	142	148	153	159	164	164	191	219
5'3"	96	99	102	105	107	113	119	124	130	136	141	141	147	153	158	164	169	169	198	226
5'4"	99	102	105	108	111	117	122	128	134	140	145	146	152	157	163	169	174	175	204	233
5'5"	102	105	108	111	114	120	126	132	138	144	150	150	156	162	168	174	180	180	210	241
5'6"	105	108	112	115	118	124	130	136	143	149	154	155	161	167	174	180	185	186	217	248
5'7"	109	112	115	118	121	128	134	141	147	153	159	160	166	173	179	185	191	192	224	256
5'8"	112	115	118	122	125	132	138	145	151	158	164	165	171	178	184	191	197	197	230	263
5'9"	115	119	122	125	129	136	142	149	156	163	169	169	176	183	190	197	203	203	237	271
5'10"	119	122	126	129	133	139	146	153	160	167	174	174	181	188	195	202	209	209	244	279
5'11"	122	126	129	133	136	143	151	158	165	172	179	179	187	194	201	208	215	215	251	287
6'	125	129	133	137	140	148	155	162	170	177	184	184	192	199	207	214	221	221	258	295
6'1"	129	133	137	140	144	152	159	167	174	182	189	190	197	205	212	220	227	228	265	303
6'2"	132	136	140	144	148	156	164	171	179	187	194	195	203	210	218	226	223	234	273	312
6'3"	136	140	144	148	152	160	168	176	184	192	199	200	208	216	224	232	239	240	280	320
6'4"	140	144	148	152	156	164	173	181	189	197	205	206	214	222	230	238	246	247	288	329

Assessing Body Composition

While BMI is easy to use and is a far better method for assessing healthy weight than using a scale, there are number of other methods for estimating body composition, including skin-fold thickness measurement, hydrodensitometry (underwater weighing), bioelectrical impedance assessment (BIA), and dual-energy X-ray absorptiometry (DEXA). Each of these procedures has advantages and disadvantages, and all have some margin of error. Regardless of the method used, 10–25 percent body fat is generally considered healthy in an adult man, and 18–32 percent in an adult woman. Fat percentages above these levels are unhealthy.

TIP   For more information on calculating body composition, visit **www. annecollins.com/body-fat-calculators.htm**.

SKIN-FOLD THICKNESS

In *skin-fold thickness measurement* an instrument called a caliper is used to measure the thickness of fat at one or more sites on the body. This is one of the most commonly used ways for assessing body fat. However, it is more prone to error than other methods, in part because it requires skill on the part of the person doing the measuring and also because it depends on the number and location of sites measured. If the calipers are not accurate, the readings will be false. If fewer locations are measured, there is greater chance for error. Furthermore, skin-fold thickness does not measure interstitial body fat (fat within and between muscles and organs). Skin-fold thickness measurement is based on the assumption that the subcutaneous adipose layer (i.e., the layer of fat just under the skin) reflects total body fat, but this association varies with age, gender, and race.

UNDERWATER WEIGHING

Underwater weighing, also called hydrodensitometry, is based on the principle that fat tissue is less dense than muscle and bone. The process involves a specially constructed water tank in which the individual is submerged while exhaling all the air in his or her lungs. Until recently, this method has been considered the reference standard for body composition studies, and the most accurate method for measuring body composition. However, measurements are often difficult to obtain because the process requires special equipment and many people have difficulty exhaling all of their breath underwater.

BIOELECTRICAL IMPEDANCE ANALYSIS

Bioelectrical impedance analysis (BIA) is done by passing a small, harmless electrical current through the body and measuring electrical resistance. The underlying principle is that lean body mass conducts electricity better than body fat. Taken together with height and weight, the resistance measurement yields an estimate of the percent of body fat. Results can vary based on how much water is in the body and where the electrodes are placed. To obtain the most precise reading, the person being tested should fast for four hours and lie down for several minutes prior to testing. (This is why most bathroom scales that measure body fat are not very accurate, even though they do send a small current through the feet to assess body fat.) BIA may not be accurate in very obese individuals, and it is not useful for tracking short-term changes in body fat brought about by diet or exercise.

DUAL ENERGY X-RAY ABSORPTIOMETRY

Dual energy X-ray absorptiometry, also called *DEX or DEXA,* is emerging as the new reference standard for body composition studies, replacing underwater weighing. However, like BIA, this method can be affected by how much water is contained in body tissues at the time of measurement (dehydration will affect its accuracy). It is also unclear how this method can be used for assessing body composition except through repeated measurements that would show changes. For now, DEXA remains a method used more by scientists and medical professionals than for common assessment of body composition.[8]

Health Measurements

The "beer belly" (also called the "pot belly" or "Buddha belly") is a visible manifestation of abdominal fat and has been recognized as the type of fat most associated with the highest health risks (as compared with fat located elsewhere in the body). The primary reason abdominal fat is unhealthy is that it is metabolically active, producing hormones and chemicals that harm the cardiovascular and other body systems. When waist size shrinks, levels of interleukin-6 (an inflammatory chemical produced by fat and certain other tissues) also decrease. Even if you aren't a lot overweight but you carry excess weight in your trunk, and you have other weight-related factors such as high blood pressure or high cholesterol, it is best to reduce your abdominal fat in order to decrease your risk of coronary heart disease and diabetes.

The purpose of determining waist and hip girth is to gain a measure of the amount of abdominal fat (also known as visceral fat). A flexible tape measure is all that is needed to assess waist circumference and hip circumference or girth. The waist measurement is taken at the narrowest waist level, or if this is not apparent, at the midpoint between the lowest rib and the top of the hip bone. The tape should not be pulled too tight or left too loose. The hip girth measurement is taken over minimal clothing or when nude, at the level of the greatest protrusion of the buttock muscles. When such measurements are taken, the gluteal muscles should be relaxed and not tensed. A person should stand with feet slightly apart when the hips are measured.

TIP **SparkPeople** allows you to track body measurements such as waist and hips. It also includes wellness measures such as stress level, quality of sleep, and health measurements such as blood pressure and blood sugar. This Internet program is a little more difficult to use than some others because it is so detailed, and it has lots of ads that allow the site to operate for free. But the opportunity to link up with others who are also trying to lose weight is a big plus. Check it out at **www.sparkpeople.com**.

WAIST GIRTH MEASUREMENT

The National Institutes of Health contends that risk for developing diseases increases greatly for women with a waist girth measurement of 35 inches or more and for men with a measurement of 40 inches or more. Table 1.2 gives risk levels for waist or abdominal girth. Those in the high or very high risk levels should consider undertaking a serious weight loss endeavor.

Table 1.2 WAIST OR ABDOMINAL GIRTH IN INCHES BY RISK LEVEL		
Risk	**Men**	**Women**[9]
Very High	>47	>43.5
High	39.5–47	35.5–43
Low	31.5–39	28.5–35
Very Low	<31.5	<28.5

WAIST-TO-HIP RATIO

The ratio of waist circumference to hip circumference is related to the risk of coronary heart disease. To assess waist-to-hip ratio, simply divide the waist measurement by the hip girth.

Table 1.3 shows levels of waist-to-hip ratios for men and women. Men with a waist-to-hip ratio of greater than .95 or women above .85 have unacceptable levels of risk.

Table 1.3 LEVELS OF RISK FOR WAIST-TO-HIP RATIO		
Risk	Men	Women[9]
Extreme	>1.00	>.90
High	.95–1.00	.85–.90
Average	.90–.95	.80–.85

Children, Teens, and Weight

Adults aren't the only ones getting fatter. Overweight is a serious health concern for children and adolescents. Data from the two NHANES surveys mentioned above (1976–1980 and 2003–2004) show that the prevalence of overweight has been increasing in children and teens as well as in adults. The data for these periods show that for children aged 2–5 years, the prevalence of overweight and obesity increased from 5.0 percent in the earlier study to 13.9 percent in the later study. For those aged 6–11 years, the prevalence increased from 6.5 percent to 18.8 percent. And for those aged 12–19 years, the prevalence increased from 5.0 percent to 17.4 percent.[10] Altogether, a staggering 32 percent of all children carry more pounds than they should.

Obese boys and girls are starting to develop the illnesses that used to be associated only with adults in their forties and beyond—diabetes, heart disease, gallstones, and liver disease. Overweight and obese children and teens are increasingly being diagnosed with type 2 diabetes[11] (originally termed adult-onset diabetes), as well as hypertension. Overweight and obese kids are also at greater risk for heart attacks and stroke. These diseases were unheard of among young people just a few decades ago. Overall, 90 percent of overweight kids have at least one avoidable risk factor for heart disease. What's more, large kids are more likely to be teased and bullied by peers, are more likely to suffer more social stigma and ostracism, and are at greater risk for depression.

A chart of body mass index adjusted for children and adolescents is recommended by the Centers for Disease Control (CDC) and the American Association of Pediatrics (AAP) for initial screening for overweight or underweight in children beginning at age 2.[12] The CDC defines as overweight those children with a BMI at or above the 85th percentile for weight in relation to height for their age; obesity is defined as weight at the 95th percentile or higher. BMI helps identify children at risk for health problems such as type 2 diabetes and high blood pressure, but it is only a rough measure, and is not the only measure recommended for use. Other assessments such as skin-fold thickness and evaluations of diet, physical activity level, and family history are also considered in assessing health risk.

TIP For more information on assessing excess weight in children, go to **www.cdc.gov/healthyweight/assessing/BMI/childrens_BMI**.

Dynamics of Body Fat

To understand the damage that obesity can do, it is helpful to have an understanding of the dynamics of fat, but keep in mind that experts do not completely understand everything about fat. The accepted wisdom is that people are all born with a fixed number of fat cells, and gaining or losing weight is simply a matter of filling or emptying these cells. But things now appear to be more complicated than that. As weight increases beyond "normal," the number of fat cells also increases. Presumably fat cells, including these additional ones, can never be lost—and the more fat cells a person has, the harder it is to lose weight.

And fat cells don't just sit there and do nothing—at least not the ones deep inside the body. While fat stores just under the skin are relatively benign, deeper visceral fat inside the body can surround and even suffuse vital organs such as the liver. Visceral fat cells also secrete hormones and cytokines (proteins that affect the immune system), which regulate the way cellular fuel is maintained and managed in the body. As food calories are absorbed, the pancreas secretes insulin, which prompts the liver to convert sugars into fat. Fat cells then release leptin, a hormone that tells the body that it has received enough calories. (Hormones are chemical messengers that regulate body processes.) In essence, leptin puts the brakes on eating, when you eat healthy amounts of food, by making you feel satisfied. Eating too many calories keeps insulin levels high and eventually leads to insulin resistance and, in due time, to type 2 diabetes. In the meantime, the disruption in these feedback mechanisms causes the brain and body to feel constantly hungry.

Additionally alarming to doctors is the impact of excess weight on the liver. This organ orchestrates the breakdown and distribution of fats and sugars from the diet. When too many calories from fat or sugar come in, the liver starts to keep some of the excess for itself, causing the development of a liver streaked with fat—that is, a fatty liver. Many overweight children already show abnormal levels of liver enzymes, and one-third suffer from liver damage. The remedy is for these children to get active and keep calorie input in line with what's burned off in activity. For children, as with adults, the bottom line is to eat moderately and get plenty of exercise.

Causes of Overweight and Obesity

Many factors play a role in the development and maintenance of weight problems including genes and heredity, hormones, environment, culture, gender, age, differences in metabolism, poor diet, emotional eating, and lack of exercise.

GENES AND HEREDITY

Genes play a part in how your body balances calories and energy. Children whose parents are obese are at greater risk of becoming overweight or obese. A family history of obesity increases the chances of becoming obese by about 25–30 percent. A child who is obese in childhood is all but certain to become an obese adult. But heredity alone does not doom a person to becoming overweight or obese; genes merely create a susceptibility to gaining weight. Behavior and other factors combine to make that vulnerability a reality.

A person can influence the amount of body fat he or she has with a good diet and regular exercise. It is not possible to change genetic makeup by willpower any more than it is possible to make yourself taller or shorter by wishing. But people can and do still achieve healthy weight goals—even those who have a family history of obesity. A person whose family is overweight or obese must commit to a lifestyle that includes regular exercise and healthier eating in order to achieve and maintain a healthy weight.

HORMONES

The endocrine system is made up of glands that secrete hormones into the bloodstream. (Recall that hormones are chemicals that regulate body processes.) The endocrine system works with the nervous system and the immune system to help the body cope with different events and stresses. Excesses or deficits of hormones can lead to obesity. A number of hormones are involved in obesity; some of the important ones include leptin, estrogen, ghrelin, and insulin.

Leptin, the Fat Hormone

The hormone leptin is produced by fat cells and is secreted into the bloodstream from body fat stores or adipose tissue. In healthy bodies, leptin reduces appetite by acting on specific centers of the brain to lessen the urge to eat. It also seems to control how the body manages its store of body fat. Since leptin is produced by body fat, leptin levels tend to be higher in obese people than in people of normal weight. A key issue currently being researched is why obese people are obese in spite of having higher than usual levels of this appetite-reducing hormone. In other words, why do heavier people have higher than average levels of leptin yet still eat more than they should? One theory is that obese people aren't as sensitive to the effects of leptin—thus, leptin is not effectively controlling appetite for them.

This theory has arisen from the various studies that have shown that blood leptin levels drop after people undertake low-calorie diets. Dramatically reduced leptin levels that result from strict low-calorie diets are believed to upset the balance in the body and in fact increase, rather than decrease, appetite and slow metabolism. This may be one factor in explaining why crash dieters usually regain their lost weight and is another argument in favor of combining exercise with calorie control to reach a healthy weight. It argues for slow, steady weight loss from making lifestyle changes instead of engaging in quick-weight-loss, fad diets.

Estrogen, the Female Hormone

As noted earlier in the chapter, body fat distribution plays an important role in the development of obesity-related conditions such as heart disease, high blood pressure, stroke, type 2 diabetes, gallbladder disease, breathing problems, certain cancers, and some forms of arthritis. Abdominal fat poses a greater risk factor for disease than fat stored in the buttocks, hips, and thighs. Estrogen, one of the female reproductive hormones (made by the ovaries and responsible for prompting ovulation every menstrual cycle) helps to determine body fat distribution. Women of childbearing age tend to store fat in the lower body and have a "pear shape," while men and postmenopausal women tend to store fat around the abdomen and upper back and are "apple shaped." Postmenopausal women with reduced estrogen often tend to store excess weight in the breasts as well as the abdomen, contributing further to the apple shape. Postmenopausal women on estrogen supplements don't accumulate fat around the abdomen, but are more likely to add fat around the thighs and hips. In terms of health, pear shapes are preferable to apple shapes.

Ghrelin, the Hunger Hormone

Ghrelin is a growth hormone found in the stomach lining as well as other places in the body. It is responsible for stimulating the appetite before eating. In laboratory tests, humans who are injected with ghrelin report an increase in hunger. In addition, research demonstrates that ghrelin suppresses the utilization of fat in adipose tissue. (Adipose tissue is where the body stores fat.) In essence, ghrelin appears to be at least partially responsible for letting the body know when it is hungry and for keeping the brain and body informed about the energy balance in the body. Those who are obese may be acutely sensitive to ghrelin and thus experience more hunger than people who are not overweight. Interestingly, those who undergo certain types of weight loss surgery may experience a drop in ghrelin and feel less hungry.

Insulin, the Metabolism Hormone

Insulin is a key hormone in metabolism; its levels rise as levels of body fat increase. Obese people often have chronically high insulin levels and as a result are resistant or insensitive to the hormone. This puts them at risk for developing type 2 diabetes. It is well established that tissues such as muscle and fat can become insulin-resistant. Research provides evidence that insulin receptors in the brain help control food intake and body weight. It is possible that insulin resistance and leptin resistance act together to increase hunger and thus contribute to obesity and type 2 diabetes.

How Behavior Influences Hormones

Obese people have hormone levels that encourage the accumulation of body fat. But they also engage in behaviors such as overeating and not exercising that over time "reset" the processes that regulate appetite and body fat distribution; thus they are physiologically more inclined to gain weight or to maintain a higher weight. The body is always trying to maintain balance, so it resists any short-term disruptions such as crash dieting. However, there is evidence to suggest that long-term behavior changes, such as healthy eating and regular exercise, can retrain the body to shed excess body fat and keep it off.

ECONOMICS AND ENVIRONMENT

Obesity discriminates by race and environment. According to the CDC's figures, 30.7 percent of white American children are overweight or obese, compared with 34.9 percent of black children and 38 percent of Mexican American children. But race is hard to separate from income level and geography. Children who live in families below the poverty line—less than $22,050 for a family of four as of 2009—are more likely to be overweight or obese than kids in families that earn at least four times that amount (over $80,000). Compared to urban kids, rural kids tend to be more obese. Children living in the South traditionally eat a diet heavy in fried foods—and have the highest levels of obesity in America.

Socioeconomic factors play a big role in obesity trends. A high rate of obesity in children is often associated with low-income neighborhoods with a close proximity to fast food restaurants, lack of playgrounds, and the need to stay indoors for safety. Candy and packaged snacks are prominently displayed in many stores in lower-income neighborhoods where kids can walk in and buy candy, soda, and chips. Children who frequent these stores often choose sugary soft drinks instead of plain water as a result of product placement. Fast food is also typically cheap, and easy to access.

Research shows that families that eat together in a relaxed, fun manner and who take time to plan and prepare meals together have a lower risk of obesity.[13] Families who have lower incomes may find it more challenging to organize regular mealtimes and budget for healthy meal preparation. Both parents may be working and have different schedules from the children, which can make it difficult for families to eat together and to spend time together in a relaxed way at mealtime. Eating may occur with the television turned on, which distracts from a family experience.

Fear of personal harm can keep adults and children from exercising out of doors in certain neighborhoods. Gyms cost money, and those with a low income may not be able to afford a gym membership. Having exercise equipment at home can be a solution for those who are better off, but even then, too often such equipment gets ignored, and regular exercising does not happen. How to get regular exercise is discussed further in Chapter 5, Getting Started with Exercise.

The home, work, and social environments all affect food choices. Having high-calorie food readily available in the home makes a person vulnerable to eating excess calories and developing obesity. Busy work schedules may argue for buying and eating processed, frozen, or fast foods, all of which are often high in fat and calories. Fresh foods such as fruits and vegetables cost money, and budget constraints may contribute to the choice of cheaper and more fattening foods such as fast foods. Co-workers who bring food to the office daily, who celebrate birthdays with extra sweets, or who serve doughnuts or other food at meetings make it more difficult to say "no" to extra eating. Friends or family whose main entertainment is cooking big meals or dining out make it harder to choose wisely. Working in or from the home with the refrigerator ever present is another hazard for overeating.

CULTURE

Hunger is not always the cause of overeating. Numerous cultural factors influence the choices you make about what and how much you eat. You learn to cook, and to eat, the way you were brought up. Food preferences and choices are learned early in life. Fried foods, foods using lard, and heavy sauces characterize some cuisines. Social events and family rituals are often centered on meals that are large as well as high in fat and calories. In today's high-stress, high-achieving culture, it is often perceived as easier to go to a restaurant or buy takeout or processed foods than to cook a healthy meal at home from scratch. Even though many people have gotten the message to reduce fat in their diets, many believe they can eat as much as they want if only the food is labeled low-fat or nonfat. As a result, they still take in too many calories to maintain healthy weight. Children are still rewarded with sweets for behaving well, and adults still treat themselves with food, using almost any excuse to do so.

GENDER

Muscle uses more energy than body fat does. Men have more muscle than women and are heavier to begin with; as a result, at rest men burn 10–20 percent more calories than women do. For this reason, a woman who eats about the same amount of calories as the average man is more likely to be overweight or obese than the man. What's more, men often have an easier time losing weight. A good analogy is a car with a big engine versus one with a four- or six-cylinder engine. The bigger the engine, the more gas a car consumes. Men have bigger engines than women, so they can consume more calories without gaining weight.

AGE

Remember the way your body morphed at puberty? One day a girl is a beanpole, and the next an hourglass—a young man's shoulders and chest seem to grow broader almost overnight. Well, once a woman hits about 40, her shape starts shifting again.[14] Although premenopausal women gain fat in the lower body to nourish children, women whose reproductive years are drawing to a close gain fat in their upper bodies. The results can be larger breasts, the emergence of fat on the back, little fat pouches near the armpits that hang over the bra, and—of course—rolls around the middle.

As a person gets older, the amount of muscle in the body tends to decrease without exercise, and body fat accounts for a greater percentage of weight. (This decline is worse in people who haven't been doing muscle-building exercise.) Lower muscle mass leads to a decrease in metabolism and a resulting slowdown in calorie-burning with age. In this way, changes in muscle mass and metabolism reduce caloric needs as time goes on. If food intake is not decreased and exercise increased, weight is gained over time and with aging. On the other hand, muscle-building exercise such as weight-lifting can preserve or increase muscle mass despite aging. The message? Exercise your body to hedge your bets against accelerated aging.

METABOLISM

The body gets the energy it needs from food through metabolism—the chemical processes in the body's cells that convert the fuel from food into the energy needed to do everything from growing to thinking to moving. Some people have a fast metabolism and burn calories easily; others have a slow metabolism (actually, a more efficient system for extracting and storing calories) and may struggle with gaining weight and trying to lose it. Restricting calories slows down metabolism (i.e., makes the body's metabolism more efficient), making it harder to lose weight. This is because the body is naturally "wired" to resist significant changes in weight, especially over short periods of time.

Losing weight is difficult and requires sustained effort, especially for those who are obese. The failure to lose weight quickly can make you think that your body has a metabolic problem. In fact, less than 2 percent of all obesity is the result of metabolic problems such as thyroid or endocrine problems. (Your doctor is the only one who can assess if a metabolic problem is contributing to your weight.) The best way to boost metabolism is through exercise. Metabolic benefits from exercise can last up to 24 hours after exercising.

EMOTIONAL EATING

Food is often a source of solace or celebration. Painful emotions often lead to problem eating. If you feel blue, sad, lonely, or bored, you may turn to food. Some people refer to food as their "best friend" because it is easily available and it pushes troubles to the background. But even pleasant feelings can produce overeating. Most people celebrate social events with food, and feeling happy can lead to eating more than you'd like.

Many people use food to escape the pain and dissatisfaction inherent in everyday life. No one feels happy all the time, but some people feel unhappy or "blah" most of the time. The former is the normal state of things, but the latter state is likely to be a kind of chronic, low-level depression that some people come to accept as "normal." Accepting that life has its disappointments—an unsatisfactory job, ungrateful children, an emotionally detached partner, demanding parents, or whatever—and working with or around them is necessary for creating a satisfactory life. This means changing what can be changed and accepting what can't. We need to do what we can to influence a difficult situation, but if in the end little changes, then we must either learn to accept what is and make the best of it, or leave the situation. Too many people resort to food to salve emotions instead of acting according to their core values—e.g., making healthy choices, contributing appropriately to a happier family life, working toward financial stability, and being guided by other overarching life values.

Emotional eating behaviors can have roots in childhood. When a parent has issues with a child's eating or weight, that parent may set limits on eating or criticize the child's behavior. This often leads to the child's sneaking food and lying about eating. This problem can carry into adulthood, especially when weight continues to be an issue. Wanting to avoid criticism or even any discussion of weight, the now-adult child is likely to continue to lie or to get angry with or resent parents or other adults who disapprove. Past experience with a parent playing "food policeman" can set up an unhealthy psychological situation from which emotional eating often results. Many people in this situation talk of having an internal "rebel" that rejects any attempts to set limits on their eating, even self-imposed limits. The emotional connection between past humiliation and the need for more adaptive behavior in the present is the challenge to be met in such cases.

Alternatively, the person who is sensitive about her weight may become a people-pleaser in the hope of winning the approval and love of others who she hopes won't notice her weight. She cares for others and disregards her own needs, thereby gaining the satisfaction in life she craves. When she feels lonely, she eats; when she feels unappreciated, she resorts to food to fill the void.

Some people who have experienced an eating disorder such as anorexia or bulimia in their youth may find themselves struggling with overeating later in life. In all likelihood, their original issues with weight, shape, food, and body image were never adequately resolved even if their original disorder temporarily abated. When stress or some crisis in their current life occurs, they either fall back into old habits (e.g., restricting, bingeing, and purging) or follow the opposite path and overeat. In either case, food is being used to avoid the pains and unpleasantness that life presents.

Or, someone who was an athlete earlier in her life may find herself or himself later in life with a weight problem. What worked in the past to maintain weight no longer works. While the athlete probably never had to think much about managing weight or just did more exercise or cut back on calories when he or she needed to "make weight," the person now finds it harder to stay at a healthy weight. If the eater engages in compulsive eating, he or she further defeats finding a solution. It is necessary for such people to redefine their relationship with food and exercise (e.g., "this is what I usually eat," "this is what I rarely eat," "this is what I do in terms of physical activity"). Later chapters emphasize this need.

Other psychological factors that can produce emotional eating include how a person thinks about food and eating. A person may make excuses and rationalizations to give himself or herself permission to eat in unhealthy ways ("This has been such a stressful day; I deserve a treat" or "Well I've blown it, so why not keep eating?"). If you have difficulties being assertive, you may resort to food to stuff down painful feelings. Thinking of yourself as someone who can't resist food or who has a sweet tooth makes it harder to incorporate changes in lifestyle that are necessary for weight management success. "I'm a chocoholic" is a self-definition sure to make it harder to resist temptation. To overcome emotional eating and succeed in making a lifestyle change that leads to a healthy weight, you must redefine who you are and how you act in relation to food and exercise.

TIP A good source for information and links to other websites on emotional eating is **www.weightloss.about.com/od/emotionaleating1/emotional_ eating.htm**. Another interesting site that provides tips for overcoming emotional eating is **www.emotionaleatingsecrets.com**.

LACK OF EXERCISE

Overweight or obese people are usually less physically active overall than normal weight adults. And if people with weight problems do exercise, it usually ends up being inconsistent or inadequate in some way. (Those who are obese but do exercise regularly are few and far between;

they still maintain a higher weight, probably because they eat excess calories despite their high activity level.) Obese people often have difficulty moving around to get exercise. Additional weight can cause pain in the feet, ankles, and knees. It can also cause shortness of breath and bring on fatigue easily. In addition, self-consciousness may keep an obese person from going to the gym or exercising in other public places.

In general, opportunities for exercising, as well as motivation to do so, seem to be decreasing. Adults as well as children spend more time in front of the TV, playing video games, or using the computer, and less time getting out and moving. Exercising is often not a high priority for most overweight people, especially if they have busy schedules. This, despite promising research showing that regular exercise can significantly improve the quality of life of inactive, overweight, older women. Just exercising three to four times a week for at least six months provides these benefits; and the more exercise the better the benefits.[15]

HIGH-FAT AND HIGH-CALORIE FOOD CONSUMPTION

As is discussed in Chapter 4, Eating for Health, what we eat is important. Different kinds of food provide our bodies with different types of nutrients and different amounts of energy. Ounce for ounce, fat has more calories than carbohydrates (nine versus four, respectively). Foods high in sugar are often high in fat as well. Vegetables are complex carbohydrates that are high in fiber and cause the body to burn more calories during digestion than foods high in fat do. These are the "good" carbohydrates—they help to lower overall cholesterol in the blood. (Cholesterol is a blood lipid, or fat; in the right kind and the right amount [high-density or HDL cholesterol] it is needed by the body, but too much of the wrong type of cholesterol [low-density or LDL cholesterol] can have negative health effects.) The "bad" carbohydrates are the "white" ones—white bread, white rice, white pastas, foods made from white flour (even when "enriched"), and foods made from white sugar (in any of its forms), such as sugary soft drinks, juice drinks, and sweets. Bad carbohydrates contribute to weight gain. Increased consumption of sugary soda and fast food account for a large part of the additional calories consumed by most Americans. For many people, alcohol is also a source of excess calories.

Trans fats are manmade fats created by adding hydrogen to vegetable oil to make a more solid substance that extends shelf life and preserves taste. When you see the words "partially hydrogenated" or "shortening" on the label, these refer to trans fats. Saturated fats (found in animal products like red meat and butter) and trans fats actually raise the level of low-density (LDL) cholesterol, the "bad" cholesterol, in your blood, and decrease the level of high-density (HDL) cholesterol—the "good" cholesterol. Foods in which saturated and trans fats are typically found include crackers, candies, cookies, snack foods, baked goods, fried foods, and processed foods.

And of course it is not just what you eat, but how much you eat that affects your weight. Many people focus so much on avoiding "fat" calories and forget to monitor total calories. Portion size is always important, even if a food is low-fat or low-calorie—and especially if it is not. Restaurants serve large portions to attract customers, even though the "serving" normally provided is actually equal to multiple servings.

Why do we keep eating once our basic energy needs are met? Science has uncovered some important instigators of overeating.[16] Three food components in various combinations tantalize taste buds: fat, salt, and sugar. Think about a typical American chain restaurant meal. Start with tortilla chips—lots of fat and salt. (Try putting some chips on a paper napkin or in a paper bag and see what happens; the grease quickly seeps into the paper.) Add cheese dip for the chips; the ingredients are heavy cream (fat), and cheese (fat), plus some onion or spices. How about a bacon cheeseburger for your entree? Ground beef has a high fat content, bacon is fat and salt, cheese adds more fat, and finally the sauce is mostly fat and salt. And to drink—what about one of those flavored coffee drinks? A flavored frozen cappuccino drink such as a Frappuccino is made up of a coffee mix that might include sugar, whipped cream (fat and sugar), chocolate chips (fat and sugar), and some chocolate drizzle (sugar). Why do these foods win over our appetites rather than healthy and weight-reducing vegetables? Because they are mouth entertainment!

Humans eat, at least in part, for stimulation. The environment gives us lots of cues to eat. And food is entertainment in itself. The three ingredients just mentioned that drive consumption—fat, salt, and sugar—also stimulate the neurotransmitter dopamine in the brain, making us want to eat. Any combination of these "big three" produces a roller-coaster sensation of taste in the mouth that is very satisfying. The sight of food that has texture, color, temperature, and mouth-feel can trigger appetite when you are not really hungry. Just a photograph of good-looking food can do this alone, and the smell of fatty food cooking is very compelling even to people without overeating problems.

What to do about this? First, you need to develop a new way of eating that is your own definition of healthy—and happy—eating that keeps the three taste teasers in check. That means you should eat foods that contain any of these ingredients in moderation. What satisfies is personal, but a good strategy is to focus your eating on foods that occur in nature, like whole grains, beans, vegetables, and fruit, combined with lean protein and an appropriate amount of "good" fats—that is, monounsaturated fats such as canola oil and olive oil. It is best to avoid prepared foods as much as possible. It is also necessary to plan ahead to deal with temptations and to be on the alert for emotions that might make you more vulnerable to inappropriate eating and the use of food as a means of self-soothing. You need to define your own internal guidelines for what you eat (without making these into hard-and-fast rules).

Obesity and Physical Health

About 97 million adults in the United States are overweight or obese. Obesity and overweight contribute to increased risk of poor health, including heart disease, high blood pressure, high cholesterol, type 2 diabetes, insulin resistance, stroke, gallbladder disease, osteoarthritis, sleep apnea, and endometrial, breast, prostate, and colon cancers. Obese women are at risk for pregnancy complications, and obese people have a higher incidence of arthritis and joint problems.

CORONARY HEART DISEASE

Coronary heart disease (CHD) refers to ailments of the heart caused by a narrowing of the coronary arteries, which reduces the blood supply to the heart. In people with CHD, fatty substances—primarily cholesterol—and fibrous tissue accumulate on artery walls, forming raised tissue patches called plaques. If a plaque breaks loose and shuts off or reduces blood flow in an artery, the heart muscle or the brain is deprived of oxygen and nutrients, and a heart attack or stroke occurs.

Research[17,18,19,20] has found that those who had heart attacks and who were overweight but not obese typically had heart attacks up four to six years earlier than normal-weight people. Obese people had heart attacks nearly a decade earlier than their normal-weight counterparts. In a study by the Mayo Clinic that adjusted for other health conditions such as high blood pressure, high cholesterol, and diabetes, excess weight was still directly related to earlier heart attacks. Overweight patients had heart attacks on average 3.6 years earlier than normal-weight people, and obese people had heart attacks an average of 8.2 years earlier. What's more, there is only a one-in-two chance of surviving a heart attack. Higher body weights are also associated with increases in premature death from other causes as well.

A diet low in saturated fats and high in fiber, fruits, whole grains, and vegetables reduces cardiovascular risk. Likewise, regular exercise and avoiding smoking are necessary to protect your heart. Blood pressure tends to rise with age, so you may want to purchase a blood pressure cuff from a drugstore to check your blood pressure at home as you get older. Your physician should monitor your blood pressure and medications as necessary to manage hypertension. A diet low in salt is considered by many healthcare professionals to be a good idea.

The Heart Disease Risk Calculator app is now available for the iPhone and possibly other smartphones.

CANCER

Evidence is now in that fat cells produce hormones that contribute to the development of certain cancers, especially those of the breast, endometrium (uterine lining), prostate, and colon. As discussed earlier in the section on hormones in this chapter, the fat cells of overweight people are sometimes less sensitive to insulin, a hormone that regulates blood sugar. When fat cells are less sensitive to insulin, the body has to produce more insulin in order to remove sugar from the bloodstream. Extra insulin spurs cells to divide faster than they would otherwise, thereby increasing the chances of random mutations or glitches in a cell's life cycle. This can ultimately lead to the runaway cell growth seen in cancer.

Colon cancer is a particular risk since colon cells divide much more rapidly than other body cells and are thought to be especially sensitive to insulin. With weight gain, existing fat cells expand and additional ones are added to accommodate more stored energy. More or bigger fat cells work even harder to make the hormones that put the overweight or obese person at high health risk. One-third of cancer deaths each year are attributed to nutrition factors, including obesity. Eating more plant-based foods and less saturated fats and trans fats can reduce the risk of cancer.

TYPE 2 DIABETES

Diabetes affects nearly 24 million Americans. Three of every five people with type 2 diabetes have at least one complication of the disease, according to the *American Association of Clinical Endocrinologists*. Complications include cardiovascular disease, vision loss, kidney disease, or loss of limbs. Officially diabetes is the seventh-deadliest disease in the United States and is known to be an underreported contributing factor in deaths.

Diabetes is a disease in which the body does not produce or properly use insulin. Insulin helps your body convert sugar, starches, and other food into the energy needed for daily life. Type 2 diabetes, the type usually associated with obesity, primarily involves insulin insensitivity rather than lack of insulin production, as in type 1 diabetes, also known as juvenile diabetes. When insulin resistance occurs together with hypertension, high LDL and low HDL cholesterol, and certain other abnormalities, this is called metabolic syndrome, or Syndrome X. People classified as having this syndrome have a greater risk of premature death than those without it.

 TIP A number of websites provide information on managing diabetes; for example, check out **www.DiabetesType2Management.com**. Also, numerous smartphone applications, both free and for a fee, are also available for diabetics. Visit **www.MyDiabetesCentral.com** to see a list of these that includes reviews. Most of these apps allow the user to enter glucose, insulin, food, and exercise data. Another website of interest to diabetics is **www.DiabetesMine.com**—and Apple has an app out for the iPhone and the iPod called **DiabetesPilot**.

One out of four Americans aged 60 or older now has type 2 diabetes. Another 40 percent of those aged 40 to 70 are pre-diabetic—that is, their blood sugar levels are higher than normal but not quite high enough to be diabetic—and many do not know it. The link between weight and type 2 diabetes is clear: more than 80 percent of people with diabetes are overweight or obese. Now scientists know that fat cells, especially those in the visceral fat around the belly, send out signals to other cells in the body, which result in the cells functioning abnormally. Some of these signals produce low levels of chronic inflammation and interfere with the insulin receptors on cells. In the process, these fat cells raise the risk of heart disease and other illnesses such as cancer and stroke.

Trans fats in the diet are especially bad for diabetics, but a diet high in refined carbohydrates—sugar, corn syrup, white flour, white rice, white bread, some cereals, and even some supposedly whole-wheat breads—also increases risk. Sugar itself does not cause diabetes, but sweetened foods, especially liquid calories from sweetened beverages, are a major contributor to obesity and subsequently to type 2 diabetes. The bottom line is that it is best to stay away from sugary soft drinks, fruit juices (which are high in sugar), white bread, potatoes, white pasta, and sweets. Avoiding these products can help with weight loss and reduce the risk of developing type 2 diabetes. The good news is that risk can be reduced without a lot of weight loss. Of course, exercise is a necessity to lose weight and improve the health of diabetics as well.

If you already have diabetes, you know you need to be careful about what and when you eat, and that you need to monitor your blood glucose. People with diabetes need to eat a low-glycemic diet—avoiding refined carbohydrates and choosing foods that have a low impact on blood sugar levels. Chapter 4, Eating for Health, provides more information on a glycemic diet and offers advice on keeping a food record, measuring portions, tracking calories, and, of course, choosing foods wisely. Losing weight and keeping it off is the best way to cope with diabetes.

DEMENTIA

Obesity is also associated with dementia. A meta-analysis study of research (a summary or overview of research outcomes that assesses the degree of effect of those outcomes) from 1995 to 2005 found that obesity and high cholesterol increased the risk of dementia and associated illnesses such as Alzheimer's-type dementia.[21] This review suggested that obesity increases the risk of dementia in general by 42 percent, of Alzheimer's by 80 percent, and of vascular dementia by 73 percent. Alzheimer's is the eighth leading cause of death in the United States. The researchers found no elevated risk of dementia in people who were in the healthy or overweight BMI weight ranges. Prevention or early treatment of obesity can decrease risk by 20 percent, which is important because it is expected that 50 percent of all people who reach age 85 will develop symptoms of Alzheimer's disease.

SLEEP APNEA

Many people who are obese suffer from obstructive sleep apnea (OSA)—disrupted breathing during sleep technically defined as "repetitive interruption of ventilation during sleep caused by collapse of the pharyngeal airway."[22] An estimated 15 million adults in the United States, Europe, Australia, and Asia suffer from OSA. One in five adults has mild OSA, and one in 15 has moderate to severe OSA. Most of those who have clinically significant and treatable OSA have never been diagnosed or treated. According to a large study conducted by the Wisconsin Sleep Cohort, obesity is a factor in obstructive sleep apnea.[23] Obesity raises the risk of premature death due to OSA, primarily when the degree of visceral obesity—that is, fat in the abdomen—is high. Visceral fat is associated with metabolic syndrome (discussed earlier in this chapter in the material on diabetes), and the higher the volume of visceral fat—often seen most obviously in the "beer belly" or potbelly appearance—the greater the risk of cardiovascular disease, regardless of BMI. Men in particular are at greater risk of death from OSA; men who have OSA and a beer belly but are otherwise not so fat are at increased risk of dying from heart disease. Additional factors associated with OSA include hypertension, type 2 diabetes, and cardiovascular disease. Untreated OSA is associated with an increased rate of cardiac events and cardiovascular mortality. Not only is it important to lose weight if you are obese, and especially if you have a beer belly, but it is also necessary to see your doctor to treat excessive snoring and other symptoms of OSA such as daytime sleepiness.

TIP For more information on metabolic syndrome or Syndrome X, visit **www.nhlbi.nih.gov/health/dci/Diseases/ms/ms_whatis.html** or check out **www.americanheart.org**. For more information on OSA, visit **www.medscape.com/viewarticle/568404_7**.

EXCESS MORTALITY

Despite much controversy, research evidence demonstrates that obesity—defined as a BMI equal to or greater than 30—is strongly associated with increased mortality and impaired quality of life in men and women of all racial and ethnic groups.[24] Some people argue that this conclusion does not apply to those who fall into the overweight category (based on some evidence that a few extra pounds do not pose a threat). However, an article published in 2006 in the *New England Journal of Medicine* of research that followed over 60,000 participants over 10 years stated that significant excess body weight during midlife (over age 50) is associated with an increased risk of early death.[25] In further analysis, after controlling for health status and smoking, a higher risk for death was still associated with being overweight, as well as being obese. The results suggested that men and women in mid-life (aged 50–55) who had never smoked but were overweight or obese had a 20–40 percent increased risk for premature death. Another study published in the *Journal of the American Medical Association* provided some good news: the older an overweight person is—that is, the longer he or she has already survived—the less his or her risk of premature death due to overweight.[26] If overweight and obesity don't get you by the time you are a senior, they become less of a threat to dying prematurely later in life; some people do survive excess weight.

Obesity and Mental Health

Overweight and obesity are associated with psychological problems as well as social difficulties. Studies of children's preferences have found that a child who is overweight is less acceptable to other children than a child who has a perceived physical defect such as a harelip or large ears. Normal-weight children are considered more attractive, are preferred by parents, teachers, and peers, and are rated as possessing more positive traits of every kind than are overweight children. Discrimination based on appearance is a fact of life, for both children and adults, and the obese are often the most blatantly ostracized. Social rejection contributes to low self-esteem, and even self-hatred.

BODY DISSATISFACTION

Body dissatisfaction is pervasive among those who are obese. Even those who are overweight and not obese are often extremely self-critical and obsessed about their shape and weight. Increasingly, this applies to men as well as women. Even though some people subscribe to the Health at Every Size concept of size acceptance, most obese people would prefer to be thinner. Remember, it is possible to be healthy at a higher than desired weight if you are eating a well-balanced diet, getting enough exercise, keeping calorie intake moderate, and don't have any of the health risk factors mentioned earlier.

> **TIP** For more information on body dissatisfaction, visit **www.psychcentral.com/library/id188.htm**.

Not surprisingly, overweight and obesity are likely to contribute to depression and anxiety. The diagnosis of an eating disorder is often appropriate for those who are obsessed with food, eating, shape, and weight; who binge eat; who suffer guilt, shame, or self-criticism about eating; who detest their appearance; or who use eating as a means of coping with stress and emotions.

DEPRESSION

Depression often accompanies overweight and obesity. One type of depression is characterized by an increased appetite and a need to sleep a lot, as well as low self-esteem and other symptoms. Alternatively, depression may be characterized by loss of appetite, loss of weight, and difficulty sleeping. Both types can be symptoms of a major depressive disorder. Another kind of depression is a chronic and persistent feeling that life just isn't very good. A study of 200,000 adults in 38 states found that respondents who were currently depressed or who had a previous diagnosis of depression were 60 percent more likely to be obese, and twice as likely to smoke, as those who were not depressed.[27]

Feeling depressed can cause some people to seek food as a relief. Eating is often used as a salve for painful emotions, including boredom, loneliness, sadness, and anger. It also provides entertainment and pleasure to counteract down feelings. Although exercise has been shown to help mild depression as well as antidepressant medication does, most obese people don't engage in regular exercise of intensity adequate to alleviate depression. Those who succeed in losing weight with the more invasive type of bariatric surgery—the Roux-en-Y procedure—find that their depression lifts as they begin to lose weight. For others, dieting without success can itself contribute to depression. It is not known whether depression causes obesity, or the reverse. However, eating is often a means of coping with depression—whatever its source. When symptoms of depression are evident, the help of a therapist or physician is indicated.

ANXIETY

Anxiety is a common ailment that brings people into therapy. Anxiety can interfere with sleep and makes daily life exceedingly uncomfortable. People who are overweight or obese typically use food and eating to assuage anxiety. They may even become anxious at the thought of not having enough food in the house in case they need to eat.

Many who are obese suffer from social anxiety—anxiety about being around strangers or authority figures, or having to perform at work or in public. Those with social anxiety tend to isolate and avoid social contacts whenever possible. If they isolate themselves, and thus avoid the anxiety of being around others who they fear will judge them, they are more vulnerable to eating out of boredom or loneliness. Some people also use alcohol to escape anxiety, which can lead to weight gain.

SEEKING PROFESSIONAL HELP

Depression and anxiety are best treated by seeing a professional such as a psychiatrist (M.D.), a psychologist (Ph.D., Psy.D., Ed.D.), or another type of therapist such as a Marriage and Family Counselor or a Licensed Clinical Social Worker. Only psychiatrists or other physicians can prescribe medication and some psychiatrists also provide therapy. Psychologists and other therapists provide talk therapy of various kinds. Cognitive-behavior therapy is symptom-focused, whereas psychodynamic therapy focuses on past relationships and how they are related to current behavior. Some people avoid or delay seeking help because of a perceived stigma about "being in therapy." Most people who suffer depression do not seek treatment. However, the best course is to seek professional help if you suffer from either of these problems.

 Many therapists now have websites or are on Internet referral lists. Some good sources for referral are **www.abct.org** and **www.adaa.org**.

Ask for a referral or recommendation from a doctor or a trusted friend, or check out the website of one of the organizations that provide referrals of therapists, such as **abct.org** or **adaa.org**. Once you have names of potential therapists in your area, contact them and ask how they would work with you and your issues. (It may be best to avoid therapists who provide only online therapy.) That first contact should tell you a lot about that therapist. If he or she spends some time on the phone asking about your situation and explaining how he or she works, make an appointment. If necessary, see several therapists before making a decision whom to go with. Allow yourself a few sessions with that therapist to finally decide whether he or she is right for you. You should feel that the therapist understands you, and you should feel safe talking to him or her.

Medications for Treating Obesity

Several prescription medications are available to treat obesity (BMI >30) and those who have an increased medical risk because of their obesity. However, these drugs are not cure-alls, and are most often useful in producing a rapid initial weight loss. In general, these medications are modestly effective, leading to an average weight loss of 5–22 pounds above that expected with nondrug obesity treatments. People respond differently to such medications; some lose more weight, and some lose little. Maximum weight loss usually occurs within four to six months of starting medication, after which weight tends to level off, or increase, during the remainder of treatments. Research studies conducted in people with obesity all show that people who eat less, increase physical activity, and take medication lose considerably more weight than people who use medication without lifestyle changes. Medication alone is not a substitute for exercise and cutting calories.

Most weight-loss medications are approved for only a few weeks or months of use, although some of the newer medications may be used for longer periods. The possible benefit of these drugs in the short term includes weight loss, which may lower obesity-related health problems. Whether these drugs actually improve a person's health over the long term is not known. All medications have side effects that should be discussed with a doctor.

PRESCRIPTION MEDICATIONS FOR LONGER-TERM USE

Currently, most available weight-loss medications approved by the U.S. Food and Drug Administration (FDA) are for short-term use. The only medication approved for longer-term use is Xenical® (orlisat), although the safety and effectiveness of this drug has not been established for use for longer than one year.

Meridia® is a non-amphetamine appetite suppressant that was claimed to promote weight loss by decreasing appetite or increasing the feeling of fullness. It also had some anti-depressant properties that addressed mood issues. However, it caused increases in blood pressure, and thus required regular monitoring. It could not be taken with other antidepressants, in order to avoid serotonin syndrome—a rare but serious condition. In 2010 Meridia was taken off the market by the FDA for safety concerns, and because it did not stand up to the claims made for it.

Xenical® is a fat-absorption inhibitor that works by preventing the body from breaking down and absorbing about 30 percent of dietary fat eaten with meals. The undigested fat is then eliminated in bowel movements, thus lowering calories absorbed. The undigested fat causes an increased frequency of bowel movements, which are likely to be oily in consistency. Side effects include oily spotting, gas with discharge, and urgent need to use the bathroom. Patients who take Xenical® must adhere to a reduced-calorie diet that contains no more than 30 percent fat, lest the effect on bowel movements be more pronounced. The medication will also block digestion of the fat-soluble vitamins A, D, E, and K, so supplements should be taken.

Some antidepressant medications have been studied as appetite-suppressant medications. While these medications are FDA-approved for the treatment of depression, their use in weight loss is "off-label" (i.e., not been officially approved for the purpose by the FDA). Studies of these medications generally have found that patients lost modest amounts of weight for up to six months. However, most studies have found that patients who lost weight while taking antidepressant medications tended to regain weight while still on drug treatment unless they also made concurrent lifestyle changes.

CHAPTER TWO

Getting and Staying Motivated

OLIVIA WANTED TO LOSE WEIGHT *for her daughter's upcoming wedding. One obstacle to her weight loss was that Olivia and her husband liked going out to dinner and socializing with friends. Olivia was about 15 pounds overweight, but her husband didn't mind: "I like a woman with meat on her bones." Although Olivia was already a well-dressed woman, she wished she could wear a smaller size. It was hard for Olivia to get enough motivation to undertake a serious weight loss effort. She had to carefully examine her reasons for wanting to lose weight. Perhaps she just needed to make some changes to make her lifestyle healthier. One thing she realized was that she wasn't exercising as much as she could. She found a smartphone application called **LoseIt** that helped with goal-setting for food and exercise as well as offering feedback and social support. The support she found helped her get motivated to make some important lifestyle changes.*

What Is Motivation?

Motivation can be elusive. The dictionary defines it as "that which causes a person to do something or act in a certain way." Motivation causes you to do (or not do) certain things. Both internal factors, such as thoughts, and external factors, such as friends or events, stimulate your desire to exert effort to attain a goal. Expectations about the likely consequences of a behavior also affect motivation: if you expect a pleasant reward, you are more likely to be motivated to act; on the other hand, if you think the behavior will lead to something unpleasant, you are likely to be motivated to avoid that action. If your friend invites you to walk with her several times a week, you may be more likely to do it than if you had to walk alone.

TIP The **LoseIt** program is easy to use, and free—as is its app. It allows you to track calories you take in from the foods you eat and calories you expend in exercise. The iPhone app is particularly handy because you can keep it close at hand to track your progress. The free companion website provides stats, charts, and backups of your data. Among the motivating features of **LoseIt** are goal-setting, tracking, feedback, and the ability to print reports that you can give to a therapist or support person.

Generally a normal human being seeks to experience things that feel good and avoid those things that feel bad, at least in the short run. Tasting something good motivates you to take another bite. The motivation to keep eating generally continues until you are full or satisfied—or until the food is all gone. Motivation to stop is signaled by a cue, such as a feeling of satiety or the sight of an empty plate or food container. Such motivation is governed not only by cues, but also by the rewards expected or gained from behavior.

Motivation can come from learning alone; experience is not always necessary. Getting burned by a hot stove motivates you to avoid touching stoves or other heat sources in the future, or at least to generally be more careful around them. Fortunately people don't have to be burned to avoid a hot stove; they can learn to avoid hot stoves merely by being warned not to touch sources of heat. Being told not to touch something, lest you be hurt, is usually enough to motivate you to move away from a heat source. Similarly, learning that red meat contains lots of saturated fat might motivate you to limit your red meat consumption. In this case, warnings about eating fat motivate you to choose other food options.

Motivation also comes from thoughts, beliefs, expectations, goals, and personal values, without any external cue having to be involved. You may feel motivated to take food to a grieving neighbor because you think it will help, and because you believe that neighbors should help neighbors in time of need. You do this because you have a personal value of being kind to others in need, and also because "it feels like the right thing to do." Or you might hear of a new diet that promises easy success and be motivated to try it, hoping that—this time—a new diet plan will work for you. All too often, your hopes for the diet are eventually dashed, and motivation to continue the diet disappears. What's worse, you may tend to blame yourself, not the fad diet, for your failure. Your renewed belief that you are one of those persons who can't lose weight decreases your motivation to try again.

Sometimes what starts as motivation eventually evolves into habit—behavior a person engages in without complete, conscious control, and even without the desire to do so. Habit results from doing the same thing so consistently that it becomes routine. With repetition of a behavior, the initial motivation to seek pleasure or avoid pain through a behavior dissipates and is replaced by a habit that involves little, if any, conscious thought. For example, consider walking by a coworker's desk and taking a handful of M&Ms: if you do it almost every day, it becomes a habit. At one time, this behavior was pleasurable but that pleasure may have been forgotten or diminished as now you act simply out of habit. Taking the elevator when you could take the stairs can also become a habit. This habit is one of avoiding the energy expenditure of walking the stairs. (Please refer to Chapter 3, Changing Behavior, to read more about the ABCs of behavior and what factors energize behavior.)

TIP You can obtain a free motivation kit by going to **www.motivation123.com/freekit-online.html**. That website also has helpful hints for encouraging motivation. A variety of programs and applications are available through the Internet and smartphones to help bolster motivation.

Motivation and Goal Setting

Setting appropriate goals is a valid and useful way of increasing motivation. To be motivating, goals need to meet certain criteria; they need to be specific, measurable, attainable, relevant, and time-bound to be most effective. Dr. Edwin Locke's pioneering research on goal setting and motivation showed us that clear goals with appropriate feedback are the key to improved performance.[1] Locke's research indicated that there is a relationship between how difficult and specific a goal is and people's performance of a task. Specific means the goals are defined in terms of behavior, are measureable, and have a timeframe. For example, saying, "I will take at least 6,000 steps (behavior) today (timeframe) as measured on my pedometer (measurement)," is more motivating than, "I'll try to go for a walk later."

Likewise, the *difficulty* of accomplishing a goal is important. Difficulty can range from easy to hard. A goal that is too easy will not be challenging enough, and therefore not very motivating. A goal that is so hard that it is unlikely to be achieved can also be unmotivating, especially because of the good chance of failure. Thus a goal must be reasonably attainable, yet challenging enough to be worth doing. And it must be relevant to the larger goal or value as well—as setting a specific goal of walking 6,000 steps a day is relevant to the larger goal of managing weight and living a healthy lifestyle.

Specific and sufficiently challenging goals lead to better task performance than vague or easy goals. Achievement is also motivating and important. That first time the scale shows a decrease in body weight is rewarding and stimulates more effort. More success boosts enthusiasm, as well as the drive to keep trying. Some research shows that those who lose weight early in a weight-loss effort (within the first four weeks) tend to be more successful in the long run, whereas those who do not lose weight in the first few weeks tend to drop out. Even though the scale is a poor measure of body fat, it is a common source of feedback and motivation.

FEEDBACK AND PROGRESS REPORTS

Feedback can come in a variety of forms. As mentioned, your bathroom scale is one means of assessing progress. Tracking steps or mileage on a pedometer is another. Monitoring daily calories or calories consumed over time is yet another type of feedback. Even changes in the ways clothes fit, though difficult to measure precisely, can be motivating.

In addition to setting goals, feedback about progress is also important for motivation. Feedback provides opportunities to make adjustments in your goals or program. A regular progress report allows you to measure success along the way, something that is particularly important if it is going to take you a long time to reach a major goal—such as losing a lot of weight. In such a case, it is necessary to break down the larger goal of losing weight or getting fit into smaller goals (that ultimately lead to the larger goal) and link feedback to the intermediate milestones.

This book provides a variety of means for feedback and charting progress. One is the calendar-and-stickers method, which can be individualized to any smaller type of goal. (See Chapter 3, Changing Behavior, for more about the calendar-and-stickers method.) Charting steps on a graph when using a pedometer is another. Many programs available online, as well as many smartphone applications, provide charting of progress and feedback; by using these you can keep count of calories consumed throughout the day or calories burned in daily exercise, as well as tracking weight loss and graphing exercise. Of course, keeping a food journal or tracking food eaten is also a powerful means of change. Some people prefer to use the old, reliable paper-and-pencil method of journaling and tracking. Each member of Weight Watchers keeps track of daily "points" in a small weekly journal provided by the program that can then be collected in a larger binder.

Motivation and Values

Motivation is influenced by values. Your actions are guided by that which you value, or the guiding principles in your life. For example, if you value being an honest person, you generally don't tell lies. Motivation comes when a person embraces and refers to his or her personal values. Maybe you make sure to get some exercise every day because you value being healthy and believe that participating in regular exercise is a necessary means of achieving physical well-being. Being physically fit is your value. Likewise you may choose to eat reasonably sized portions in an attempt to eat healthily. Getting exercise and making healthy food choices are in alignment with your value of striving for good health.

Values are a key concept in mindfulness- and acceptance-based therapies. Values, as defined by ACT, an acceptance and commitment therapy supported by research, are global, desired, and chosen life directions.[2] They embody intention and are exhibited in every purposive act. Usually values are deliberately chosen combinations of verbs and adverbs. For example, *relating to others lovingly* is a value. *Paying bills on time* is a value. *Making healthy choices* is another value.

> **TIP**
>
> To learn more about ACT, go to **www.contextualpsychology.org** and click on the "public" section of the website. Another helpful website on acceptance-based therapy is **www.actmindfully.com.au/acceptance_&_commitment_ therapy**. An excellent article on ACT can be found at **www.actmindfully.com. au/upimages/Dr_Russ_Harris_-_A_Non-technical_Overview_of_ACT.pdf**.

A personal value, such as *being honest*, might motivate you to give back money to the insurance company if you find the lost item that had been insured after you had mistakenly reported it as lost and been reimbursed for it. Of course, the goal of personal gain might motivate you to forget your value of honesty and keep the money, especially if you think you would not be caught. If you generally think of yourself as an honest person, your mind might try to trick you with rationalizations such as, "It's just a big insurance company and they make lots of money anyway." Any value, such as that of being honest, doesn't stop and start depending on circumstances. It is something you *do* consistently, not just now and then, or in the future, or when it is convenient. Of course, many people stray from their values occasionally, but even so they return to their values as soon as possible. But motivation is influenced by goals as well.

GOALS VERSUS VALUES

People are endowed with the capacity to conceptualize a future. For example, wanting to become a firefighter or a doctor provides inspiration and motivation to take actions to realize such long-term goals. These goals are in service to the larger value related to career direction. Goals are things you can obtain, like owning a Corvette, for example, or getting a graduate degree. They are concrete events, situations, or objects, and they can be completed, possessed, or finished—not so values. Over time, and with experience, goals may change, but the personal value system that guides your actions is not so changeable. Values help you define what your life is about. They point you in a direction, but they are not a destination. Values are about having a particular code or philosophy that you live by—like honesty, reliability, integrity, treating others respectfully, and so forth. They are like a compass that guides your life actions. Most important, values are chosen.

DEFINING YOUR VALUES

Identifying your own values and associated guiding principles is important for motivation and for choosing healthy behavior. This may seem like a daunting task. You may never have thought about your values, or about what principles you want to guide your life choices—you may even conclude that you have no values. But answering just one question can start you on the road to being aware of, and defining, your values. The question is simple: "What do I want my life to be about?"[3]

It is not uncommon for people to deny that they have any values at all. It can be painful to look at your past actions and inquire about what values they express. For example, it may be easier to profess an absence of values than to acknowledge to yourself that binge eating suggests a disregard for health, or perhaps an easy way to avoid unpleasant feelings—or that lack of exercise might suggest negligence when it comes to healthy behavior. The good news is that it is never too late to examine and redefine your values.

Most people learn values in the context of their family and the culture. If your family put great stock in doing the "right" thing, you probably do, too. If you were imbued with the idea that paying your bills on time is important, that is what you are likely to do as well, because you learned this value. If your parents were spendthrifts, you may not have learned to budget or to stay within your credit limits. All of your experiences inform your values, and your behavior expresses them. As an adult, with hindsight and the ability to discover what is working and what isn't in your life now, you have a choice about your values.

The values you choose to live by define who you are and what your life is about. It helps to think of values in terms of verbs and not as nouns. So instead of *honesty*, a value might be expressed as *being honest without hurting others*. Instead of *health*, a value might be *making life-enhancing choices*. Frame your values so that they point to actions. Table 2.1 features a list of some domains of values framed as actions (verbs and adverbs).

Living consistently with your values and guiding principles may allow you to feel good at times, but not always. Giving back a large sum of money to a faceless insurance company may be painful, at least initially. You may wonder if you really should have done that, especially if friends question your actions. Getting out and exercising five days a week may not always be what you want to do, but you do it because of the value you place on the benefits of exercise. Note the difference between this *value* of exercising for health and a *goal* of getting exercise today. Goals are changeable; values inform a higher level of meaning in your life. Goals can be discarded; values may hit bumps in the road, but still you persist in the direction they point. A person who values creating a loving family may nevertheless have to go through a divorce. To adhere to this value during a divorce would mean not allowing children to be used as weapons against an ex-spouse, and it would mean agreeing to a fair division of assets. Even when you have failed to live up to your values, you can take corrective action and bring your life back into alignment with your values.

Table 2.1
VALUES FRAMED AS ACTIONS

Value Domain	Value expressed as a chosen life direction
Health	Making healthy choices
Relationships	Treating others respectfully
Family	Creating loving relationships
Friendship	Nurturing friendships
Career	Doing my job well
Education	Pursuing personal development
Recreation/leisure	Engaging in revitalizing activities
Financial	Being financially responsible and secure
Spiritual	Feeling connected to something larger than myself
Citizenship	Contributing to society and the community

Values are the overarching guides that give direction to behavior and make life meaningful. Goals are the targets for action that help you live the life you say you want. Behavior is directed toward attaining a goal and should be consistent with personal values. Goals are also motivators of action. You need to have plans for putting your intentions or goals into action. How many times have you said, "I'll start tomorrow," but then tomorrow never seems to come? You may have an intention, but you have no way to implement it. Good intentions and lofty goals alone are not enough to get you where you want to go.

Motivation is helped when you define and stay in touch with what you want for yourself in the long run. Of course, some people have never given much thought to the direction they want their life to take. They may simply follow opportunities as they present themselves. And even those who have thought about what they value in themselves may still struggle with behavior change. A helpful way of understanding this is through the Stages of Change model, which characterizes different phases of the change process.

The Stages of Change

Behavior change is rarely a discrete, single event. Instead, the person who wants to change moves gradually from being uninterested in changing to considering a change to deciding and preparing to make a change to, finally, actually changing. The person eventually takes genuine, determined action and, over time, works to maintain the new behavior. Lapses or backsliding slips are almost inevitable, but they are not excuses to stop taking action. Rather, they are simply part of the process of working toward permanent lifestyle change.

The five stages of change describe how a person can modify a problem behavior or acquire a new and healthier behavior.[4] Pre-contemplation is the stage at which there is little or no acknowledgement of the problem and no intention to change behavior in the foreseeable future. A person in this stage may be unaware of his or her problems or be in denial. He or she probably has not thought about his or her values. In the Contemplation stage a person may be aware that a problem exists, may even acknowledge this and be in the process of seriously thinking about overcoming it, but has not yet made a commitment to take action. The person may not yet be clear about his or her values. Preparation is the stage in which a person is intending to take action in the next month or so or has unsuccessfully taken action in the past year. At this stage the person has more clearly identified and embraced personal values. Action is the stage at which a person takes steps to modify his or her behavior or environment in order to overcome personal problems. This stage requires considerable commitment of time and energy to actually change behavior patterns. Successful action is guided primarily by values. In the Maintenance stage, a person works to prevent relapse and consolidate the gains attained during the Action stage. Even when there is a slip, values guide behavior back on track.

These stages are not lockstep, and people may slide back to a previous stage or move back and forth between stages. Learning to recover from small slips so as to prevent total relapse is important. The first two stages of change—Pre-contemplation and Contemplation—are characterized primarily by thinking and emotions, whereas taking action is the focus of the latter two stages—Action and Maintenance. The third stage, Preparation, involves both taking action and cognition (thinking and feeling).

PRE-CONTEMPLATION

People may be in the Pre-contemplation stage because they are uninformed or underinformed about the consequences of their behavior, or because they simply don't want to acknowledge the negative consequences of their current behavior. They are in denial. Recall that Chapter 1, Understanding the Relationship between Weight and Health, of this book aims to inform readers of the consequences of unhealthy behavior related to eating, exercise, and weight. Some who are in the Pre-contemplation stage may have tried to change their behavior a number of times but have become demoralized about their inability to change. Both those who are uninformed and those who are discouraged may tend to avoid reading, talking, or thinking about their high-risk behaviors. They may be "resistant" or "unmotivated," but the end result is that they avoid or discount any disturbing information about their health. They just don't want to deal with a problem or issue. They may even find arguments to refute the existence of health risk from obesity.

If you are in the Pre-contemplation stage, it is important to realize that you are not ready to jump into action of any sort, except for giving thought to your personal life direction and values. There are important questions for you to answer first: What do you want your life to be about? What do you value? (That is, what principles do you want to guide your behavior?) What are your goals? Do your current behavior patterns actually serve your larger goals and values related to leading a healthy and a fulfilling life? What would have to happen for you to believe that significant overweight or obesity or lack of exercise is a problem for you? Naturally the answer to these questions and the decision to change is entirely yours. But before answering these questions, acquaint yourself with the health risks you face if you do not understand and accept the research evidence about what constitutes a healthy lifestyle. Go back and read Chapter 1, Understanding the Relationship between Weight and Health.

CONTEMPLATION

If you are reading this book, you are probably in the Contemplation stage or a later stage. In the Contemplation stage, you are thinking about change but don't yet know if you can, or will, make changes in your life. You are aware of the pros of changing but are also acutely aware of the cons. In essence, you are sitting on the fence. The balance between costs and benefits of changing or not changing can produce profound ambivalence that can keep you stuck in this stage for long periods of time. The prospect of giving up an enjoyed behavior that has helped you cope can cause you to feel an anticipated sense of loss despite the possible gain in changing.

Completing the cost–benefit analysis provided later in this chapter (Tables 2.3 and 2.4) is meant to tip the balance toward the Preparation and Action stages of change. It is intended to help you evaluate the pros and cons of behavior change. During the Contemplation stage, it is important to assess the barriers to change, such as time, expense, hassle, fear, and uncertainty, as well as the benefits of changing. At this stage of change, the potential to change exists and the threat of inertia prevails.

Important questions to answer are: "What are my reasons for changing?" "Why am I thinking about change at this time?" "What would keep me from changing at this time?" "What difficult challenges have I faced and overcome in the past?" and "What might help me overcome barriers to change?"

PREPARATION

The Preparation stage is marked by experimentation. In this stage you are testing the waters. In all likelihood, you are thinking about what specific changes you could make. You may experiment with small changes as your determination to change increases. All this is preparation for taking action in the immediate future. Perhaps you have already taken some significant action, such as talking to your physician or checking online for a weight-loss program. You may have other action items in mind, such as joining a gym, calling a therapist, or reading and completing the exercises in this book. Maybe you have already made some changes in what you eat or in your exercise habits—for example, you may have already tried eating smaller portions as a first step towards more dietary modifications.

Now is the time to identify your future plan of action and assess obstacles. Seek social support for your plan to change. Talk to friends, family, or professionals who are likely to be supportive. Contact others who are interested in managing weight, and plan to do things with them. Get them involved. Check out some websites that offer tools and blogs for social support. Start with small initial steps. Preparing and planning your approach is an important step before swinging into full action.

ACTION

In this stage you are already undertaking changes in your lifestyle. Within the past six months you have made positive changes to your eating behavior or have been working out, perhaps with a trainer or in a gym. You are restructuring your environment to better manage eating cues or are using rewards to reinforce new behaviors. You may be using the tools provided by many websites and apps to help with food and exercise. If you have been a binge eater, you are taking care to eat three adequate meals a day, plus planned snacks as necessary. You are implementing new ways of managing stress to avoid emotional eating. You have someone who listens when you need to talk. You may have enlisted a "buddy" or joined a social network to support you during your change process; perhaps you have joined a forum or blog for support.

During this stage you may have feelings of loss about your old ways of eating or using food, and you need to reiterate to yourself the long-term benefits of managing weight and living a healthy lifestyle. It is helpful to be aware of the causes, consequences, and cures for problematic lifestyle behaviors.

At this point, a vigilant response to relapse becomes critical. Relapse or backsliding is common during lifestyle changes but need not spell the end of motivation. A slip is an opportunity to learn something new about yourself and the process of changing behavior. After a slip, deconstruct what happened: What were the triggers? What was the function of the behavior? Knowing what you know now, what would you do differently? Problem solving, not self-blame or giving up, is in order. Evaluating what triggered a slip or lapse, and learning from it, is important for recovery.

You need to learn to recover from small slips before they lead to a total relapse into old habits. If you slip, reassess your motivation and reaffirm your plan to overcome the barriers to permanent change. Learning coping strategies is important. As you become more confident in your ability to sustain change, your awareness of the cons of changing—the difficulties—starts to shift to an awareness of the pros of changing—the rewards. In this stage, to be successful you have redefined who you are and what you do with regard to your life values about health.

MAINTENANCE

In the Maintenance stage, the change process is mostly complete and your new lifestyle has become part of your new self-definition. You must still prevent relapse and recover from lapses, but you are more confident about handling small slips. There is less need for external rewards, because you have internalized the rewards of a healthy lifestyle. Your beliefs about how you choose food and what you do for exercise guide your actions. You think of yourself as a person who leads a healthy lifestyle. You have a firm commitment to sustaining your new lifestyle and have incorporated the new behavior for the "long haul."

Benefits and Costs of Losing Weight

To create and maintain motivation, especially in the Contemplation and Preparation stages, you need to assess the benefits and costs of either undertaking a change effort or not doing so. The first step is to examine and strengthen your reasons for wanting to lose weight, if that is your goal. Your aim is to create clear, concrete goals that will guide your behavior in this regard and be kept in your consciousness over the long term.

Begin by completing the self-test, "Why Do You Want to Lose Weight?" in Self-Test 2.1. Rate yourself on each of the reasons for losing weight according to *how important that reason is in your decision to undertake weight reduction at this time.* (Be careful to avoid the common temptation to rate all or most of the reasons as "extremely important.") After you have rated each reason separately from 1 to 10, go back and choose the top three reasons you rated most important. Use the spaces provided to the left of each statement to rank the first most important reason that made you decide to lose weight at this time, the second most important reason, and the third most important reason. Later you will use this information to help bolster your motivation and to create a clear commitment that will increase your chances of success.

The reasons you cite for wanting to lose weight reflect either the benefits you expect to get by succeeding in losing weight or the costs you want to avoid paying if you remain overweight. Benefits include the rewards, pleasure, or satisfaction you perceive for losing weight. Benefits also accrue if you think you can avoid something unpleasant or bad—like avoiding gaining more weight or developing a chronic health condition. Of course, there are also perceived benefits for not losing weight—i.e., not changing. A benefit for not trying to lose weight might be that of not having to take responsibility for your food choices and eating anything

SELF-TEST 2.1
Why Do You Want to Lose Weight?

Rank	Extremely Important			Somewhat Important				Not at all Important		
___ 1. I want to wear nicer clothes.	1	2	3	4	5	6	7	8	9	10
___ 2. I want to feel better about myself.	1	2	3	4	5	6	7	8	9	10
___ 3. I want praise and approval from others.	1	2	3	4	5	6	7	8	9	10
___ 4. I want to move around more easily.	1	2	3	4	5	6	7	8	9	10
___ 5. The doctor said I need to lose weight.	1	2	3	4	5	6	7	8	9	10
___ 6. Someone I care about isn't happy about my weight.	1	2	3	4	5	6	7	8	9	10
___ 7. I have a health problem and losing weight could help.	1	2	3	4	5	6	7	8	9	10
___ 8. I want to avoid potential health problems from too much weight.	1	2	3	4	5	6	7	8	9	10
___ 9. I'm afraid of getting fatter, so I better start now.	1	2	3	4	5	6	7	8	9	10
___ 10. I don't like the criticism and ridicule I get from others.	1	2	3	4	5	6	7	8	9	10
___ 11. My weight gets in the way of my feeling sexy.	1	2	3	4	5	6	7	8	9	10
___ 12. I want to present a better professional image.	1	2	3	4	5	6	7	8	9	10
___ 13. If I don't lose weight I may lose my job.	1	2	3	4	5	6	7	8	9	10
___ 14. Other: _____ _____ _____	1	2	3	4	5	6	7	8	9	10

you want whenever you want it. Likewise, costs are associated with changing as well as with not changing. The costs are the punishments, pain, or discomfort you experience whether or not you change. Costs of changing include having to impose self-discipline about exercise and food choices, as well as accepting the expenditure of time, money, effort, or the loss of certain personal pleasures in order to succeed at changing. Costs of not changing are likely to involve diminishing health and vitality and increasing social problems.

When you believe that the rewards or benefits from doing a particular thing outweigh the costs involved, you tend to keep doing whatever produces benefits. Conversely, you tend to stop doing whatever produces punishment or displeasure or costs you more time and effort than the resulting benefits are worth. Since both benefits and costs are involved in every behavior pattern—whether it involves eating, exercise, or some other area of life—you make tradeoffs between the two.

For example, exercising may provide the immediate benefits of feeling good and the long-term benefits of improved cardiovascular fitness, but it also takes time that you might prefer to spend differently, and, in the beginning at least, may involve some discomfort. If you like feeling good about yourself after exercise and want to ensure long-term cardiovascular health, you decide to pay the costs involved in exercising, including making time for it and expending the effort.

People who exercise regularly usually have a long list of the benefits they get from exercising—feeling good, having more energy, being able to eat more than sedentary people, and so forth. If asked what they don't like about exercise, they are likely to minimize the costs. They exercise frequently because they perceive greater benefits than costs. (They also think of themselves as people who get regular exercise.) On the other hand, people who don't exercise or who used to exercise occasionally but don't anymore are more likely to give you a long list of the costs of exercise, and to minimize the benefits.

Exactly what constitutes a cost or a benefit depends on your point of view. What is rewarding to one person may be punishing to another. The benefits you derive or the costs you pay are what you think they are, not what someone else judges them to be. If you get enough benefits from behaving a certain way, your tendency is to ignore the costs that go along with this behavior pattern or rationalize them away. People who smoke, for example, manage to ignore smelling bad, persistent coughing, stained fingers and teeth, and long-term negative health consequences. By ignoring the costs of smoking and focusing on the pleasure or relief tobacco gives, they allow themselves to continue smoking. People are very good at distorting or denying the very real health costs of a particular behavior pattern—whether it is smoking, eating inappropriately, or not exercising—in order to keep enjoying the rewarding aspects of unhealthy behavior. Denying the costs of bad habits or rationalizing them is a common reason for procrastination and loss of motivation. It is this kind of denial that leads to putting off losing weight or to periodically starting some weight reduction effort and losing momentum before achieving success.

IMMEDIATE VERSUS DELAYED COSTS AND BENEFITS

Some of the benefits and costs associated with a behavior are immediate: When you eat a hearty meal, you feel satisfied. When you overeat, you feel uncomfortable. Other benefits and costs are delayed: You can eventually wear a smaller size when you lose weight. If you don't lose weight, your clothes may feel tight and you may some day develop diabetes or some other health problem.

The benefits and costs that have the most powerful influence on how you act are those that occur immediately, at the time you are acting. Results that come later have far less influence. When faced with the choice of whether to eat a hot fudge sundae and get pleasure now or to pass it up and lose weight so you can wear smaller clothes later, it is much easier to decide "I'll start tomorrow." When the alarm goes off a half hour earlier to remind you to get out and jog, the immediate pleasure of continuing to sleep is often more compelling than the idea of the exhilaration that will come an hour from now from exercising or having better health months or years down the road. That's why values are so important—they make long-term rewards more immediate by providing lifestyle guidance.

To be successful in losing and managing weight, you need to keep the delayed benefits you expect from losing weight, and the costs you pay for not doing so, in the forefront of your thinking at all times. At the same time, you need to minimize and discount the immediate rewards you get from staying the same and to ignore or minimize the costs of changing. Unfortunately, as you begin the work of changing your habits, choosing food differently, and increasing your exercise, you may find that your attention shifts to the more immediate benefits of not trying to change, as well as to the immediate costs of making such efforts.

It is crucial that you avoid focusing and dwelling on the pleasures you used to get before starting weight management. Otherwise, it is only a matter of time before you revert to old patterns and give up your weight management efforts once again. You need to constantly bring your focus back to what you expect to get by losing weight and to a realistic assessment of the costs you will pay for not losing weight—and your values. When you find yourself dwelling on the effort involved in losing weight, refocus your thinking to the motivating aspects of changing. Doing a cost–benefit analysis can help in that.

DOING A COST–BENEFIT ANALYSIS

Completing a cost–benefit analysis will help you assess the costs and benefits you expect to experience from undertaking behavior change. In the sample shown in Table 2.2, the change is that of losing weight, although you could specify some other behavior change, such as quitting smoking or undertaking exercise. Later on, when you feel tempted to return to old habits, review what you have written. Post the form in a place where you can see it readily and be re-

Table 2.2
SAMPLE COST–BENEFIT ANALYSIS

#1   Benefits of losing weight

What good things do you expect to get, now or later, from losing weight?

What do you avoid that would be unpleasant?

— *feel better physically*

— *able to put on panty hose without getting out of breath*

— *wear pretty clothes*

— *like myself more*

#2   Benefits of NOT losing weight

What enjoyable things do you get to do or have by not trying to lose weight?

What unpleasant things do you avoid?

— *don't have to deal with men*

— *don't risk getting hurt*

— *eat and drink what I want*

— *control is unnecessary*

— *don't have to exercise*

#3   Costs of losing weight

What do you have to do or give up that you don't want to do or give up to lose weight?

What do you have to do that you would rather not do?

— *give up junk food*

— *cut down on alcohol*

— *make time for exercise*

#4   Costs of NOT losing weight

What unpleasant or undesirable things are you likely to get now or in the future if you don't lose weight?

What are you likely to lose?

— *poor health*

— *feeling fat*

— *feeling bad about myself*

— *lack of a relationship*

— *hard to get around; tired, out of breath*

minded of your reasons for changing. If you are keeping a journal, put your cost–benefit analysis in the book. Blog with others about your analysis.

First, take a look at the sample cost–benefit analysis in Table 2.2. Then fill out the blank form in Table 2.3 or create your own form by drawing a line down the center of a paper and another line across the center, so as to form four quadrants or boxes. Label the one in the upper left-hand corner "1: Benefits of changing," the one in the upper right-hand corner "2: Benefits of not changing," the one in the lower left-hand corner "3: Costs of changing," and the one

---

Table 2.3
COST–BENEFIT ANALYSIS

#1   **Benefits of losing weight**

What good things do you expect to get, now or later, from losing weight?

What do you avoid that would be unpleasant?

_____

_____

_____

_____

#2   **Benefits of NOT losing weight**

What enjoyable things do you get to do or have by not trying to lose weight?

What unpleasant things do you avoid?

_____

_____

_____

_____

#3   **Costs of losing weight**

What do you have to do or give up that you don't want to do or give up to lose weight?

What do you have to do that you would rather not do?

_____

_____

_____

#4   **Costs of NOT losing weight**

What unpleasant or undesirable things are you likely to get now or in the future if you don't lose weight?

What are you likely to lose?

_____

_____

_____

---

in the lower right-hand corner "4: Costs of not changing." Changing, of course, can relate to losing weight, exercising more, adopting a particular healthy lifestyle behavior, or some other change-related goal.

In Box 1, note the benefits you expect to get both now and later from undertaking behavior change. (If this change is to lose weight, as shown in the sample, you can get some help on this from the "Why Do You Want to Lose Weight?" checklist in Self-Test 2.1 that you completed earlier in this chapter.) Unfortunately, the benefits expected from weight reduction are often not well thought-out. You need to develop persuasive but realistic ideas of the benefits you expect to receive from reducing your weight. Moreover, these benefits must be important to you, regardless of what others think. If the benefits you expect from losing weight are not powerful enough to compete successfully with the benefits for staying the same—that is, not changing—or if they are not powerful enough to overcome the costs involved in losing weight, you must give this question more thought. Your odds of long-term success will not be good unless you have powerful reasons for wanting to lose weight.

In completing this analysis, Olivia from the chapter-opening vignette wrote that the benefits she expected to get from reducing weight were to be able to wear a size 8 dress and get more compliments. She was asked if she presently got compliments about her appearance from her husband and people she cared about. Olivia replied that she did. She was then asked if her husband and friends particularly cared what size she wore. Olivia conceded that they probably didn't.

"Is wearing a size 8 dress going to be powerful enough to carry you through the tough times when you don't feel like exercising or do feel like making less healthy food choices?"

"I guess not," replied Olivia.

Olivia was given this good advice in response to her reply: "Then you need to rethink your reasons for wanting to lose weight. Try to develop some really powerful but realistic ideas about what being slimmer will do for you. Maybe there is something else that you seek, and losing weight seems like the most ready solution. Don't start weight reduction efforts until you examine the situation. Perhaps you should check the BMI chart and, if you are within the healthy range, reconsider whether you need to lose weight at all. If you are not in the healthy range, consider the health benefits of losing weight. Or even if you are in the healthy weight range, give some thought to losing some weight if you have signs of cardiovascular disease, such as hypertension or high cholesterol. Perhaps you can benefit from increasing your exercise and just making some small changes in the way you eat, such as reducing your intake of red meat."

In Box 2, indicate the benefits you expect to get now and later by staying the same—by not changing or not trying to lose weight. Examples might be "not having to exercise" or "continuing to eat whatever I want." These are the sorts of things you get to enjoy right now when you are not trying to lose weight, and these are the things that are most likely to come to mind when you are in the middle of a weight loss effort.

In Box 3, state the costs you expect to pay both now and later by undertaking change or losing weight. In the enthusiasm of a fresh start, you may be tempted to ignore or minimize these costs. Don't. Acknowledge them now so you can make an informed decision to pay the costs. It is important to recognize and acknowledge them in the beginning so that they will not come as a surprise later. When you find yourself thinking about the costs in the future, it will be easier to accept them if you have anticipated them. You will need to discount and minimize the costs *then* as much as possible and to turn your attention back to what you have noted in Boxes 1 and 4.

Finally, in Box 4, write the costs you now pay and may pay in the future by not losing weight—by not changing. Some of the reasons you checked earlier in Self-Test 2.1, on the "Why Do You Want to Lose Weight?" checklist, may give you a clue to your costs for staying the same. For example, one cost could be lower self-esteem. Once your change effort is underway, your natural tendency will be to deny or minimize the costs you pay for not losing weight. By listing them now, it will be harder to dismiss them later. Be honest with yourself here; it will be important later.

At the moment, as you anticipate beginning a change effort, the boxes that tend to exert the most influence on your behavior are Boxes 1 and 4—the benefits you get from losing weight and the costs of not losing weight. As a result, you feel motivated to get going. Box 1 is like the carrot, and Box 4 like the stick, for your motivation. People who focus on Boxes 2 and 3—the benefits of not changing and the costs of losing weight—find it hard to start on a change effort or to stay with one.

These "de-motivating" boxes are shaded on your sample and the blank forms as a reminder that focusing on these concerns is likely to steal your motivation. If thoughts about these do arise, just notice that they are there and remind yourself that these are just tricks your mind is playing and you don't have to act on those thoughts. They come from that part of you that doesn't like change and that wants you to take the easy way out. Simply acknowledge to yourself that these thoughts are coming from the part of you that isn't in touch with your values. Refocus your thoughts on the ideas in the unshaded "motivation" boxes—Box 1 (the benefits you expect to get from changing) and Box 4 (the costs you will pay for not changing). By reminding yourself of these ideas, and by staying in touch with your values, you can motivate yourself to undertake change and to stick with it.

Periodically you should go back and review your cost–benefit analysis. As you progress in your change endeavor, you may find new reasons to continue with your effort, or you may need to acknowledge and accept some costs you hadn't recognized previously. If your motivation starts to flag, review your analysis. Use it to keep your commitment clear and your motivation on track.

Social Support and Motivation

Finding other people to support your weight management efforts helps achieve success and sustain motivation. Some Internet programs and smartphone applications aimed at helping members lose weight provide for social support in a variety of ways. They may provide bulletin boards or chat rooms for interaction or other means of social networking with others who are trying to lose weight or get more exercise. Another way to get social support can be to choose a "buddy" or support person to help you in your change efforts. A buddy or friend is someone with whom you check in on a regular, perhaps daily, basis for praise, encouragement, and a listening ear when necessary. Perhaps your buddy can join with you in making lifestyle changes. Having a support person means being accountable to someone else for your actions. Because you report on your efforts to someone else, you are more likely to stay on track.

 A good website for finding others who are also trying to lose weight **is www. BuddySystem.com**. Its aim is for "buddies" to inspire and support each other while keeping a journal and tracking food and exercise in logs.

If you are participating in a group or formal weight-loss program, it is a good idea to choose your support person from among the group. In larger groups, the leader may suggest choosing a buddy. Alternatively, there are people who perform the services of a weight-loss coach for a fee. You may be able to find one near you by checking the Internet. If you are trying to lose weight on your own, try to find someone who is interested in losing weight with you. It is okay to have more than one support person. Working with a buddy is usually a reciprocal arrangement—in most cases you will act as a buddy in return.

Some people in a group program don't like the idea of having a buddy in their weight management efforts. They think they should be able to succeed without outside help, or they want their weight management effort to be a private affair. If forced to choose a buddy from the group, they are likely to find someone who shares these sentiments, and the two in effect collude to pretend to be buddies. In other cases, one person genuinely wants to have and be a buddy, but the other person isn't as committed to the idea. Perhaps the other person isn't as committed to losing weight as you are. For the buddy system to work, both of you need to believe that it can benefit you, and you must be willing to make the extra effort to stay in touch with your support person. For the buddy system to pay off, it has to be a mutually cooperative effort.

TIP One key to success is keeping in contact with others who are trying to lose weight. When there are others who are in tune with your weight-loss ups and downs, and who are committed to helping, you are more likely to lose weight and keep it off. To find a buddy, first join a weight-loss program online that appeals to you. **SparkPeople** or **LoseIt** are two possibilities; **Weight Watchers Online** is a commercial program that also provides online support. Register for the site of your choice; don't just cruise it for tips. Use the tools provided on the site. Blog often. And help others.

THE ROLE OF A SUPPORT PERSON

A good support person has an optimistic attitude. There is no place for pessimism or criticism in the buddy system. Support persons not only talk to each other about their progress, but also may engage in other helpful activities as well. They may exercise together, for example, or support each other in other ways. Support persons should

- Maintain a positive, accepting, success-oriented attitude

- Avoid judging or criticizing

- Make regular contact as mutually agreed upon

- Listen with the intent of hearing the other's feelings

- Share progress and positive experiences

- Offer advice or suggestions only when asked or given permission

- Avoid complaining or rejecting suggestions out-of-hand

- Avoid giving permission to backslide

- Be as committed as you are

CHOOSING A SUPPORT PERSON

Some people are shy about asking an actual person (as opposed to someone online) to be a buddy or a support person. To get it over with, they simply turn to the person nearest them if they are in a weight management group. A more productive approach is to get to know some of the other people in the group before choosing someone to ask to be a support person. Take some time to find out how a prospective support person feels about having a buddy and what his or her expectations are. (It also helps to have a second choice in mind.)

If you are not in a group program, consider asking a friend or coworker to be a support person. It is great if the prospective support person is also engaged in a similar change effort, but it is not absolutely necessary so long as he or she is understanding and accepting. However you find a support person, it is necessary to exchange information, including e-mail addresses, phone numbers, and the best times to be in contact and talk.

If you decide to find a support person who is not currently involved in a weight management effort, be sure to explain to them how they can be of help. Explain to the person you choose what you need him or her to do and not do. For example, you do not want your support person to watch over your every move or to comment negatively on what you are eating.

Often a willing spouse or significant other can be a valuable and supportive buddy. Spouses who also keep track of what they eat, who are also striving to improve eating and exercise habits, who praise partners for day-to-day progress and for attaining goals, and who exercise with them are the most helpful. If possible, spouses should attend weight-loss program meetings and learn more about weight management. Spouses who are involved together in weight management generally report increased marital satisfaction.

COMPETITIVE BUDDIES

Some people find that engaging in a competition is helpful to their change efforts and helps increase motivation. Often deciding to compete is done informally, such as when one person poses the challenge to another that "whoever loses 20 pounds first wins." The pair may wager some money or another prize to boost their motivation. Such an approach is more likely to work if it is done a little differently. First, instead of issuing a challenge for number of pounds, establish a proportion of body weight to lose such as 5 or 10 percent of your total weight. In that way, people of different sizes or genders can compete more or less equally. Likewise, set a time limit that allows for the reasonable possibility of losing that proportion of weight, and be specific about the prize. For example, the challenge might be, "The first one to lose 10 percent of his or her body weight by a set date (say, four months from now) will be owed $50 by the other." Next, involve a monitor for each competitor. The monitor is present when each competitor weighs in at the beginning and end of the competition and periodically asks about progress. The monitor also makes sure the prize is awarded.

Contests and competitions involving groups of people can also be helpful in promoting motivation and weight loss. Whole organizations sometimes compete against other organizations, or departments within one organization might wage a contest with one another. Just as when two individuals compete, it is important that a definite timeframe be established, with rules and an agreed-upon impartial person to monitor the process. When contest participants exercise together, monitor eating, and support one another's efforts, they are more likely to stay motivated and to succeed.

CHAPTER THREE

Changing Behavior

JADE WAS ALWAYS GOING ON A DIET. She could be "good" for awhile, but at some point— usually when stress got to her—she would have a cookie or two, at which point she felt she had crossed some imaginary line: "Well, now I've blown it. I may as well keep on eating." And all her resolve went out the window. She felt terrible about herself when she went off a diet, but when she heard of a new "breakthrough" diet, she would try again. She had heard that diets don't work, and that adopting a healthy lifestyle including exercise was the key, but she didn't know how to go about it. Then a friend recommended that she try an Internet program called **MyFoodDiary***, which provided her with tools for changing her lifestyle over time to achieve permanent weight loss. She got lots of support from others on the weight loss forum that was one of the tools, and it helped her change her behavior and increase her motivation.*

Behavior and Behavior Change

What makes a new behavior "stick"? Would doing something for 90 days make a new behavior pattern stick? Some research reported that success quitting smoking was more likely if the smoker refrained from smoking for 90 days. Of course, quitting smoking is about relinquishing a bad habit—changing an unhealthy behavior pattern. The solution for breaking bad habits is to watch out for potential slip-ups and say to yourself, "No, don't do that!" before you indulge. Vigilance and removing the opportunity to backslide are keys for changing unhealthy behaviors. But what about people who are trying to adopt healthier behaviors? One source claimed it takes only 21 to 28 days to form a new habit. Some research found that it takes an average of 66 days to form a new habit, depending on what you are trying to do.[1] (The study focused on relatively simple behaviors like drinking water regularly every day or doing 50 sit-ups each morning before breakfast.) While this may sound encouraging at first, the research also found a wide range of times for a behavior change to stick—anywhere from 18 days up to 254 days before the habits took hold. Some people took much longer than others to form their habits, and certain habits took much longer than others to form. Clearly more than the amount of time devoted to changing influences when a new behavior stabilizes into a habit.

In terms of weight management, as is the case with so many things, genes influence behavior, but so does environment. Genes load the gun—that is, they determine a vulnerability to some condition—but environment pulls the trigger. Environment makes a possibility into a probability. For example, obese parents may pass on a gene for higher weight, but exercise and eating right modify this vulnerability. Having parents model healthy eating and regular exercise behavior also makes it more likely that children will adopt healthy habits. Little can be done about genes, but you can do much about your environment—the conditions you allow to exist—and the choices you make.

> **TIP** Focusing on lifestyle change as well as weight management, for a fee but with a free trial, **www.MyFoodDiary.com** provides a forum for connecting with others who are trying to lose weight, in addition to an online database of over 70,000 foods. It allows you to track fat, cholesterol, protein, and carbohydrates, as well as calories. An exercise log calculates calories burned for a variety of exercises, and this program provides feedback and reports of progress for promoting motivation.

Environment sets the stage for behavior and influences the success of any change endeavor. It provides the circumstances for behavior—the setting that includes the external cues that prompt behavior and the rewards that follow. For example, being offered some cookies (cue) may be followed by eating a cookie (behavior)—and if one cookie tastes good (reward), you may take another. Behavior can be observable (eating a cookie) or mental (deciding you like the taste of the cookie). Thinking is a special type of behavior that you cannot see as it takes place in the mind, but it influences observable behavior, like taking yet another cookie. That is, the mind exerts its own effect on actions. However, the mind can also play tricks and cause undesirable behavior. So after eating the first cookie you may have the thought, "Now I've blown it." That thought could cause you to eat a lot more, and feel bad.

A new way of "thinking about thinking" is helping people deal with difficult situations or problematic thoughts. For example, just because you have a thought about having blown your intention to not eat something doesn't mean you must give up and keep eating—but more about this later in this chapter. First, a little review of the history of modern psychology will provide a context for understanding new ways of thinking.

The modern psychology of behavior and behavior change has had three waves or iterations: behaviorism, cognitive-behavior theory, and mindfulness- and acceptance-based change. Each of these contributes to understanding how to make behavior change stick.

A Brief History of Modern Psychology

In his now-famous experiments, Ivan Pavlov proved that dogs and pigeons could be made to respond to a *stimulus* or *cue* in the environment, which was typically unrelated to eating but that indicated food was coming. When a light came on or a bell sounded at the same time that food was presented, the dogs would salivate or pigeons would peck at the lever controlling the delivery of food pellets. After a time, when just the light came on or the bell sounded without food coming, the animals would still salivate or peck. The dogs and pigeons were now responding to the cues of the light or bell, even though food didn't always come in conjunction with the cue. These animals were said to have become *conditioned* to the secondary stimulus—the light or bell. The primary stimulus was the food itself. Pavlov's work led to the inquiry of how behavior is cued by stimuli and how organisms can be conditioned to respond to secondary cues. From this work came the first wave of modern psychology—behaviorism.

THE FIRST WAVE: BEHAVIORISM

In 1913, a psychologist named John B. Watson formulated an approach to psychology termed *behaviorism*. This philosophy of psychology is based on the idea that people and animals also *learn* how to behave—to perform physical actions. Along with this belief in learned behavior came the idea that research should study objective, observable behaviors rather than subjective, qualitative processes such as feelings or motives, or hypothetical constructs such as thoughts or unconscious processes. Other behaviorists such as Edward Thorndike also rejected introspective methods and sought to restrict psychology to scientifically accepted experimental methods involving observable behaviors.

Later, B. F. Skinner demonstrated that rewarding behavior was powerful in and of itself. He argued that *rewards* controlled behavior and themselves became cues signaling new rounds of behavior. Identify the rewarding consequences following an action, and you had the secret of why the behavior kept happening. Change the consequences to something unpleasant, and the action diminished, stopped, or changed. Consistently reward a new behavior with something desirable, and voilá!—a new habit in the making. And the behavior becomes even more entrenched when the reward is highly desirable but the frequency of reward is unpredictable—like gambling. Of course, predictability works too. The thing about food, especially sweet, high-calorie food, is that it can be counted on to taste good and make the person eating it feel better—virtually every time.

Eventually, researchers determined that teaching people how to manipulate cues or rewards themselves made them able to change their own behavior. In the 1970s, behavior modification became all the rage in research, and self-help books for weight management began to appear. People learned to monitor and manipulate cues and rewards on their own to bring about behavior change. For many people, focusing on cues and rewards worked—for awhile— but making behavior change stick was still a problem for most people.

Then there was a new question: what if you could anticipate a situation and just change the behavior the situation would ordinarily elicit, without having to eliminate or change the cues or having to manipulate reward? Could you plan to substitute another, healthier behavior ahead of time for an anticipated situation and have that work? Instead of eating the whole plateful of something, what if beforehand you could decide to set aside half to eat now and ask to take the other half home? What if you planned ahead of time to take a walk around the block when stressed, instead of going to the refrigerator? While eliminating or changing cues and rewards was helpful, planning new behavioral responses to existing cues and in the face of alternative rewards was also found to help people change. For this approach to work, an alternative behavior must be at the ready to use when an old cue or situation is expected to present itself. This solution—substituting healthier responses—is discussed later in this chapter.

Even today, instructing people on how to change behavior themselves by manipulating cues and rewards, as well as using behavior substitution, is the basis for effective weight management and successful behavior change. To design your own weight loss or health behavior change program, you need to learn the ABCs of behavior change.

THE ABCS OF BEHAVIOR

Eventually researchers combined stimulus control, behavior substitution, and reward management to formulate the ABC model of behavior. According to this model, an Antecedent (stimulus or cue) prompts a Behavior (an action), which is followed by a Consequence. And if the consequence is sufficiently rewarding, it keeps the behavior happening again and again or, alternatively, alters the behavior if the consequence or reward is unpleasant. Then the cycle repeats, with the reward or consequence becoming a cue for a new cycle.

Antecedent → Behavior → Consequence

(becomes)

New Antecedent → Behavior → Consequence, etc.

Of course, things are actually a little more complicated than that, but this simple model made it possible to instruct people how to begin to change behavior themselves and start new habits by intervening at one of these points.[2] Initially the model was only intended for observable actions. Later, it was expanded to include thoughts, beliefs, and feelings as internal actions—also called "private events."

Psychiatrist Aaron Beck at the University of Pennsylvania and New York psychologist Albert Ellis pioneered the work involving cognition and rational thinking. As a result of their work, the influence of thoughts and feelings became a legitimate focus of research. Internal private events that acted as mental cues, actions, and rewards became the subject of study in psychology. Private events were legitimately conceived as functioning as antecedents, behaviors, or consequences. Thus it was realized that thoughts and feelings can trigger eating, or eating can trigger self-criticism and feeling bad, for example. Or, feeling bad can trigger a thought about food, which then leads to eating, followed by more thoughts and feelings—often self-criticism and upset. The idea of examining overt behavior (observable actions) in conjunction with covert behavior (thinking and feeling) came to be known as the *cognitive-behavioral revolution*, or the second wave.

THE SECOND WAVE: COGNITIVE-BEHAVIOR THEORY

The word "cognition" refers to all forms of knowing and awareness, such as perceiving, conceiving, believing, remembering, reasoning, judging, imagining, and problem solving. In short, *thinking*. Thinking can occur silently in the privacy of one's own mind by "talking" silently to oneself (although sometimes thinking is done out loud). Thinking can also involve picturing things or places in our heads, imagining something that doesn't yet exist, recalling past memories, or considering what to do about problems. Research has shown that cognition is an important part of how and why behavior happens.

More and more research is investigating cognitive processes that operate in the background of conscious processing and also influence behavior. Such processes take place in what is called the unconscious or subconscious mind. Here a collection of mental phenomena manifest, though the person is not aware of them. These phenomena include automatic skills (like driving a car without knowing how you got to your destination), unnoticed perceptions (for example, nonverbal behaviors in others, or subtle physical sensations in one's own body), or unconscious thinking habits. One example of unconscious thinking habits that are covered in a later chapter is cognitive distortions, or common errors in thinking that many people make. An example? Thinking, "I'm either perfect or I'm a failure." This cognitive distortion is known as all-or-none thinking.

From the marriage of behaviorism and cognitive theory came cognitive-behavior therapy (CBT). In CBT, which many therapists today practice, the contribution of the mind to behavior is acknowledged and addressed along with observable actions. With regard to weight management and behavior change, excuses and rationalizations, self-criticism, and other kinds of self-talk and distorted thinking have been identified as important impediments to success. Cognition is so important for changing behavior that two entire chapters, Chapter 6, Managing Thinking, and Chapter 7, Challenging Your "Inner Voices," are devoted to the topic of how the mind can help or hinder behavior change.

The idea was—and still is—to use the ABC framework to identify both the overt and covert behaviors that are triggering or rewarding overeating, or other unhealthy behaviors. This involves deconstructing a behavior pattern into its parts: antecedents, behaviors, and reinforcers—both observable and cognitive—and trying to sort out what cues triggered the behavior of interest and what reinforcers followed.

To identify reinforcers, it helps to ask what the function of the behavior is: What does problem eating *do* for you? What thoughts or emotions does it allow you to avoid—or embrace? How is the behavior rewarding to you, at least in the short run? Then, in similar situations in the future, you can either change the cues or the rewards in order to change behavior, or substitute another, better response to an anticipated stimulus situation.

THE THIRD WAVE:
MINDFULNESS- AND ACCEPTANCE-BASED APPROACHES

The so-called third wave of psychology preserves many of the ideas and techniques from behaviorism and cognitive-behavior therapy but adds a focus on the *context*—how we see and understand thoughts and feelings so that they don't have to determine action—and on learning to hold thoughts lightly. (Holding thoughts *lightly* means accepting that thoughts and feelings are not always accurate and that they need not always be acted on.) This third wave emphasizes the broad constructs of mindfulness and the role of values in guiding behavior, whereas the first- and second-wave therapies focused mainly on immediate problems and relief of symptoms. For example, a CBT therapist might seek to identify and challenge cognitions, but a third-wave therapist might focus on noticing and accepting thoughts and feelings and understanding how they tie into a person's value system. The aim of the third wave approach is to *allow* change to happen by accepting what exists now and identifying and referring to values and life goals to guide behavior. In this new approach, thoughts and emotions are conceptualized as events of the mind that may conform to, or distract from, personal values. Change depends on recognizing that thoughts can be problematic and bringing behavior into line with values. This is the new way of "thinking about thinking."

Focusing on What Works

Managing the external environment that includes observable cues and reinforcements is still an important part of changing behavior. Also important is managing thinking and coping with feelings to bring about permanent lifestyle change. The new ingredient to successful change is mindfulness and the ability to observe thoughts without judging them and without becoming overwhelmed by the mind chatter they cause. To begin the process of behavior change, it helps to first focus on managing the external environment—cues and rewards.

CUES AND REWARDS

To change behavior, attention needs to be paid to external cues and rewards. Cues are the stimuli or conditions that elicit or prompt behavior or that suggest a reward is available. Seeing someone walking down the street with an ice cream cone, or seeing an ice cream store, might serve as cues for you to go buy an ice cream cone. Picking out a flavor of ice cream you think you will like promises a reward. Seeing your running shoes by the front door or the exercise clothes you set out on the dresser the night before are cues to remind you to exercise. Anticipating a warm shower after exercise promises a reward for your hard work.

What if healthy behavior is rewarded, say, by an employer such as Safeway? In fact, the Safeway grocery chain did initiate a program whereby employees who stopped smoking or who lost weight were rewarded. That action got some of them to adopt new behavior. Is such behavior change lasting? Maybe. But for many people who participate in similar programs, the new behavior lasts only as long as the reward is in effect. Once the environment reverts—in this example, once Safeway ends the program—old habits often come back.

Behavior is influenced by many cues happening at the same time. Likewise, there are likely to be a number of rewards available for any given behavior. Think of a time when you went out to dinner with friends. Feeling good about being in a social setting was one cue. Being in a nice restaurant was another cue—and probably part of why you were feeling good. Finding appealing dishes on the menu stimulated interest and excitement—more cues for the desire to eat. All these cues set the stage for choosing food. Anticipating what would taste good promised a reward. Once you ordered and started dining, your physical sensations were pleasant and rewarding, which made you keep eating. Feeling satisfied with your entree and wanting to keep feeling good—and being excited by some dessert choice on the menu—may have prompted you to order something sweet at the end. The rewards of the experience made you want to go out to dinner again, probably with the same people. Of course, if you didn't like the restaurant or the people you were with, you would decline the next invitation. This is how cues and rewards work. But beliefs and mindfulness also influence behavior.

BELIEFS AND MINDFULNESS

Manipulating the environment so that cues are changed and new behaviors are stimulated and rewarded is important. But behavior really only "sticks" if it is internalized as the natural outcome of guiding principles and life values. A value is a belief or philosophy that is personally meaningful. Whether you are consciously aware of it or not, every individual has a core set of personal values. Values can range from the commonplace, such as belief in hard work and punctuality, to the more psychological, such as self-reliance, concern for others, and harmony of purpose.[3] Mindfulness is having an open and nonjudgmental attitude in the present moment; mindfulness helps you stay in touch with your beliefs and values.

Those who value their health and well-being find it easier to engage in behaviors that reflect their beliefs and values. A new habit sticks if it is in alignment with values held and if mindfulness is maintained. In order to change behavior permanently, it is necessary to evaluate your personal values. There must be a basic change in the way you view yourself and the values you want to live by. Otherwise, old habits eventually return.

TIP　A good, albeit long, article on personal values, including a list of common values, can be found at **http://gurusoftware.com/Gurunet/Personal/Topics/Values.htm**. If you are having trouble deciding on your values, also check out **www.selfcounseling.com/help/personalsuccess/personalvalues.html**. For an interesting article on living your values, visit **www.stevepavlina.com/articles/living-your-values-1.htm**.

You may be one of those people who in the past has undertaken a serious effort to lose weight at least once—perhaps you even succeeded for a while. Maybe you were able to take weight off and keep it off for some period of time. If you eventually regained weight, it was probably because you gradually—or quickly—returned to old behaviors. Old habits encroached on, and eventually overtook, your success. Having returned to previous behaviors and your prior weight, you were probably left with the unsettling feeling that you might never really succeed in losing or maintaining a healthier weight. And you were also left with a question: How can I change behavior and make such changes permanent?

Changing Behavior Patterns

The first step in changing behavior is to uncover your behavior pattern by keeping a record of the circumstances of the habits or behaviors. (Notice that the behavior pattern in question could be eating, or it could be exercise—or some other behavior such as smoking, gambling, spending, skin-picking, etc.) Remember that thoughts and feelings are also behaviors, albeit mental ones. Recording the cues to behavior, what actions you took, and the consequences—including your thoughts and feelings—are the circumstances of interest.

SELF-MONITORING

Behavior doesn't just happen. It is embedded in a context that includes the events—both private thoughts and feelings and observable events—that elicit or cue behavior and that reinforce behavior. These include the time of eating, the location, related thoughts and feelings, the anticipated and real results of the action, and a variety of other influences. You need to uncover the circumstances of the behavior you want to change in order to change it. One approach to identifying behavior patterns is with *self-monitoring*. Self-monitoring involves keeping a daily record of behavior and the circumstances—i.e., cues and consequences that surround the behavior. The following information should be recorded each time you eat:

◎ **When:** What time of day or night did you eat? Keep a separate record for each day.

◎ **What:** What did you eat? Giving a brief description of the food should suffice, but some people find it helpful to track calories or nutrients.

◎ **Degree of hunger:** How hungry were you at the time? Rate your hunger from "not at all hungry" to "ready-to-eat hungry" to "overly hungry."

◎ **Location:** Where were you when you were eating (at the kitchen table, in the car, at the computer, at your desk, etc.)?

◎ **Triggers:** What triggered your eating? What were the cues for eating?

◎ **Stressors:** What stressors were involved—people, thoughts, emotions? That is, what was stressful to you that might have led you to eat?

◎ **Emotions:** How did you feel about eating or the circumstances surrounding eating? What were your feelings before, during, and after eating?

◎ **Reward:** What were you getting (besides food) from eating (e.g., relief from emotional distress, escape from boredom, pleasure from eating, satisfying hunger, following a routine, avoiding thinking, etc.)?

◎ **Binge:** If you felt out of control with the food when you were eating, you were probably in the middle of a binge; indicate this on your record. You might also want to check out Chapter 9, Stopping the Binge Cycle. If you simply ate a lot but didn't feel out of control, it probably wasn't a binge.

It is highly recommended that you keep your self-monitoring record at the ready so that this information can be recorded *at the time the behavior occurs*. Unfortunately, many people who try to self-monitor do not record as they eat. Instead, they write down the information at the end of the day—that is, they record what they can remember, which usually results in an inaccurate record. Some wait even longer to record—perhaps the next day—further diminishing the usefulness of self-monitoring as a behavior change strategy.

Keeping a simple paper record on hand is probably the best way to make sure you can record the circumstances each time you eat, but these days, a paper record is not your only option. With many Internet programs people can input their daily calorie intake and calorie expenditure information. Few of the online programs currently allow recording of thoughts and feelings except in blogs and on forums. Some people prefer to create and update their self-monitoring record on a personal computer, although this may require data entry some time after the behavior occurs. They may keep track of their food consumption and the context of eating on a spreadsheet. Smartphones have a number of applications for counting calories and nutrients by recording food eaten and also allow you to keep track of your exercise. In some cases these records can be printed out to show your therapist, dietitian, or support person.

Research has shown that about a quarter of weight-control success is attributable to consistent self-monitoring.[4] However it is done, self-monitoring remains a powerful, if underused, tool for understanding and changing behavior patterns. Self-monitoring helps determine the times of day that are most problematic (usually later in the day, after about 6:00 p.m.), whether overeating at meals or snacking is an issue, to what degree becoming overly hungry is a factor in overeating, where eating takes place (cues), who may be involved (stress factors—which are also cues), and what thoughts and feelings (internal or "private" events that may influence behavior) play a role in inappropriate eating.

Changing Cues

Some people don't think they need to use self-monitoring because they already know what triggers their eating. They are aware that they skip breakfast and perhaps lunch and then overeat at dinner because they are so hungry. By that time, hunger is a powerful stimulus to eat and is hard to deny. Or they may know that emotional eating is their problem, or that mindless snacking is the real issue. They may recognize that just the sight or smell of food can trigger the urge to eat—for example, seeing food in a movie or in an ad, walking by the window of a bakery, or smelling meat grilling. Perhaps they know that having food readily available and in view is a cue to munch without much thought or to give in to a momentary desire.

Not thinking—that is, not staying conscious of behavior—can also lead to inappropriate eating. Eating without thinking and in the absence of hunger is mindless eating. Mindless snacking that starts in late afternoon and extends into the evening is common. Using food to alleviate sadness, boredom, anxiety, loneliness, and other emotions is a big contributor to emotional overeating. Even fun social occasions are common times for overeating or making poor food choices. For some women, the time just before their menstrual period is fraught with bad eating choices. Eating can be a way to deal with the anxiety, touchiness, and hypersensitivity that can accompany monthly hormonal changes. Likewise, transition times—the time when we finish one task and before we start another—often serve as cues to get something to eat.

Cues are numerous, but there are many ways to address their presence in your life. Most important, you need to consistently refer to your values and guiding principles with regard to health and well-being. If you are not clear on your values, reexamine what gives your life meaning and purpose, and clarify these. With your values in mind, decide, "This is what I eat and what I do with regard to exercise and physical activity." Shifting your view to a new definition of yourself in relation to food and exercise will help you act in accordance with a higher level of value focused on making healthy choices.

TIME OF DAY

Using self-monitoring, watch for a particular time of day that snacking or overeating starts. For many people this is late in the afternoon or early in the evening. One woman, Vera, finished work at 4:30 in the afternoon. When she got home she got something to eat, but her eating continued on into the evening. Sometimes she even skipped supper and just snacked till bed. Vera solved this problem by bringing an appropriate and satisfying snack to work and eating it in the afternoon before she went home. Once she got home, she got herself busy with other tasks or just relaxed with a book before starting supper.

Evening snacking in front of the TV or the computer is a problem for many people. One solution, of course, is not to have snack foods available. Another approach is to plan a snack for later in the evening. Make it something substantial and that you enjoy eating, but also something that is healthy. Decide that after finishing dinner, your next eating will be at the appointed snack time, and stick to that schedule. Don't eat between times. Also tune into the function of inadvertent snacking. Is it to give your mouth and hands something to do? Or could you be using snacking at these times to actually stay awake? Think of Eva, a college student, who was able to pull all-nighters by snacking while studying.

Some people eat dinner late in the evening and find themselves overeating when they finally sit down to their meal. If your dinner is likely to be late, be sure to have a late-afternoon snack to carry you through. Also be careful about snacking in unhealthy ways before a late dinner. A couple of glasses of wine and cheese and crackers can add a lot of daily calories.

HUNGER AND FATIGUE

Being overly hungry creates a strong need to eat—and you may overeat as a result. To overcome such eating, be sure to eat three regular meals a day, including breakfast, lunch, and supper, as well as planned snacks as needed. You need to plan ahead for food, especially if you work a stressful job that demands overtime. Some bariatric surgeons advise having only three meals a day and no snacking whatsoever. For some people, eating four, five, or more small meals a day works best. All experts agree that breakfast is an essential meal that should never be skipped.

Skipping breakfast may have become a bad habit. Some people say, "I *can't* eat breakfast," meaning, "I don't have time for eating breakfast," or "I just can't face food in the morning." Such excuses mean that you probably overate late last night, didn't get enough rest, or didn't plan ahead (or all three). For some people, knowing they overate the previous night, together with the attendant guilt, can reduce the desire for breakfast in the morning. Others may use the excuse, "Once I eat, I'm hungry all the time." If this is you, you need to learn to live with food, and that means breaking the fast of the night and feeding yourself regularly throughout the day with healthy food choices. Trying to stave off overeating by not eating is a strategy that inevitably leads to mindless eating or overeating later in the day. Eventually hunger makes itself known, and it will cause you to take in excess calories.

Likewise, fatigue will make you vulnerable to overeating. Be sure to get enough rest at night—eight hours is usually recommended. Practice good sleep hygiene: Be sure your room is quiet and dark; don't eat or watch television in bed; and have set times for going to sleep and rising. Don't do anything too stimulating before bed, like vigorous exercise or watching a scary movie. Remember that too much alcohol disturbs sleep, so be careful about what you drink before bed. You might think it will help you fall asleep, but drinking a lot of alcohol is likely to make it harder to get restful sleep. If you wake in the middle of the night, have a glass of water and go back to bed. Don't even *think* about eating in the middle of the night. (If you find yourself eating in the middle of the night and barely remembering it, check with your doctor; you may have a sleep disorder or be having a reaction to medication.)

TIP To learn more about sleep and good sleep hygiene, visit **www. sleepeducation.com/Hygiene.aspx**.

LOCATION

Location can provide cues to snack inappropriately or eat mindlessly. Keeping food in your desk at work or in the car is ill advised unless it is part of a planned snack program. Planning ahead about what you eat and when and where you will eat improves chances for success. Some people have access to a refrigerator at work and can keep planned snacks such as yogurt or cottage cheese handy. Items like apples and nuts packed in portioned bags don't need refrigeration. Candy and chips, however, are not part of a healthy, planned snack program. At work, avoid the vending machines. At home, passing through the kitchen and snacking haphazardly as you go is mindless eating. Don't fool yourself: standing at the kitchen counter for a quick snack adds unwanted calories. Eat your planned snack sitting down at a place appropriate for eating.

DISTRACTIONS

Don't leave food in sight; this means no cookies set out for the kids and no candy dishes for passersby. Sit down while you eat, and avoid multitasking such as reading the paper or watching television while you eat. Eating without the television on, or without something to read at hand, promotes mindfulness of eating and is a healthy habit to get into. Take time to savor your food and eat without guilt. Eating in front of the television may make you feel like you are not alone, but it robs you of the pure experience of enjoying your food. The distraction of the television or reading while eating can lead to eating too fast and overeating—plus you miss the full enjoyment that food should bring. Don't snack while you are surfing the Internet or working on the computer; such mindless eating contributes to consuming excess calories.

For an introduction to the Zen of mindful eating, go to **http://zenhabits.net/mindful-eating/**.

INFLUENCE FROM OTHERS

But what if your spouse or a family member buys and leaves tempting food around the house? How do you cope with those triggers for eating? This presents a difficult problem, but one that has some possible solutions. First, request that food not be left out for you to see (and probably eat). Stay out of the kitchen if that is where food is on display. If food is still readily available, distract yourself by getting involved in a project.

What if you are not the one who does the shopping or the cooking? You need to speak up and ask for what you want or need. Be respectful, of course; you want to maintain the goodwill of others. If all else fails, decide to eat smaller portions and make the healthiest choices possible from what is available at the time.

Unfortunately, sometimes drastic action is needed. Erin's mother, who was overweight, always had chips, dip, cookies, ice cream, and other tempting foods in the house. For two years, Erin refused to eat any of this, or even healthy foods that her mother served. Eventually, at age

17, she became anorexic. Still, the presence of all this tempting food eventually broke through her resolve, and Erin started binge eating. Her solution was to eventually move out of the house and do her own shopping. With time, she was able to overcome her disordered eating, shop for fresh and unprocessed foods, and live a healthy lifestyle by avoiding the undue influence of her family's food preferences.

What you often need most from others in your household is that they *not* comment on your weight or your weight loss efforts. If others are sharing opinions that dishearten you, thank them for their concern and request that this topic not be brought up. Ask them not to make any comments about or allusions to your weight, your eating, or your efforts.

Your family or friends may believe that they have the right to question you about your eating and exercise, which can make you feel pressured and perhaps guilty. In that case, you need to be more assertive with them. (Assertiveness skills for weight management are addressed in Chapter 8, Addressing Stress.) People also commonly comment on weight loss they observe in others, and usually they mean this as a compliment, or mention it out of curiosity. This can bring unwanted attention to you and may be uncomfortable. You may feel that people shouldn't do this. Unfortunately, they do—so you need to be prepared with what you will say when they do. Again, call on your assertiveness skills.

STRESS AND EMOTIONS

Managing stress and coping with emotions are covered more thoroughly in subsequent chapters. For now, be on the lookout for situations or feelings that trigger overeating. Binge eating is often triggered by unpleasant emotions such as sadness, anxiety, loneliness, and boredom. Eating is a way to avoid the experience of these feelings. You know you are a binge eater if you feel you lose control over food. If you think you might be a binge eater, be sure to read about binge eating in Chapter 9, Stopping the Binge Cycle. When assessing your cues for eating, note how others may be causing you to engage in stress eating. Perhaps the stress of a boss who micromanages your work is driving you to the vending machine too often. Review the previous information given in this chapter as well as the chapter on managing stress and difficulty with relationships for more assistance.

CRAVINGS

A craving is an intense desire or longing for a particular substance. About 50 percent of obese binge eaters report having cravings for sweet and sugary foods. Both hunger and negative emotions can set off food cravings. Likewise, just imagining and thinking a lot about something that would "taste good" can trigger a craving. When your desire overpowers your determination, you cave in to a craving. The desire for sweet, rich foods results from the all-too-human drive for pleasure. A craving can be triggered by any manner of things: seeing an advertisement for a desirable food or just seeing food depicted in some way, having an attractive leftover available—like surplus birthday cake. The more you dwell on the idea of eating a particular food, the more intense the craving becomes. The leftover food seems to "call to you" from the kitchen or refrigerator. Table 3.1 provides tips for coping with cravings and urges to eat.

Table 3.1
TIPS FOR COPING WITH CRAVINGS

1. **Catch a craving early.** A craving needs to be interrupted early on, before it gets out of control. Before you start ruminating about eating something, turn your attention to something else. Think about a project you are working on or a recent vacation; don't let yourself focus more and more on eating. If you continue thinking about eating a particular food, your mouth will begin to water, and your focus of attention will narrow until you lose control.

2. **Interrupt your taste buds.** Brush your teeth and gargle with strong mouthwash. It's difficult to feel like eating afterwards. Or put a strong mint in your mouth—anything to spoil your taste buds. Alternatively, try dabbing some cologne or strong-smelling ointment under your nose. These are short-term ways to stop a craving in its tracks.

3. **Leave temptation behind.** Get out of the area of the temptation. Cross the street if you see a bakery looming in the distance. Stay away from the food table at a party. Hang out anywhere but in the kitchen.

4. **Substitute, substitute, substitute.** Drink water—lots of it. Take a walk. Take a shower. Get on the Internet. Do whatever it takes to distract yourself from wanting something to eat.

5. **Manage your environment.** Put away leftovers, and don't keep tempting food in sight. If you don't buy it, you are less likely to eat it.

6. **Manage your self-talk.** Don't get persuaded by defeating self-talk; stay in touch with your goals and values.

7. **Indulge a craving with moderation.** If all else fails, let yourself eat in moderation. Watch your portions. But if you indulge, do it without guilt.

8. **Remember that cravings pass.** Cravings peak and subside like waves in the ocean. Learn to "surf an urge," that is, ride it out. It will pass. Tell yourself to wait ten minutes and then decide whether or not to eat. In the meantime, get busy doing something else. Tell yourself something like, "It won't kill me to wait. I can handle it."

9. **Avoid becoming overly hungry.** Don't skip meals. Eat at least three meals a day, with planned snacks. Never go more than three to four hours without eating.

Another approach to coping with cravings and urges is to use the Five Ds:

◎ *Delay* at least ten minutes before eating so that the impulse can pass.

◎ *Distract* yourself in the meantime by getting involved in a project or doing something engrossing.

◎ *Distance* yourself from the food or temptation; ruin it or put it in the trash if you really don't want to eat it.

◎ *Determine* how important it is for you to eat this food. Does it fit with your values? Are you making a conscious choice? (Remember—occasional treats are okay.)

◎ *Decide* whether to go ahead and eat it; if you do, choose a moderate amount to eat. Be mindful; enjoy it slowly and without guilt if you decide to eat it.

SHOPPING FOR AND STORING FOOD

You can manage your environment in other ways to reduce your vulnerability to existing cues to acquire and eat problem food. When shopping, take a list and buy only items that are on that list. Don't go shopping when you are really hungry or tired. Plan ahead to avoid the aisles that are problematic for you—like the ice cream case or the candy aisle. Ignore the candy displays at the checkout counter. If you don't have it in the house, you are less likely to eat it. Yes, you could still go out and get it later—and certainly some people do, even in the middle of the night. But if you sanitize your pantry and your refrigerator and discard problematic food, you reduce your vulnerability to eating that food. And don't forget the freezer. You know that in a pinch you might microwave frozen food or even resort to eating it frozen!

TIP Want help with shopping lists? **Shopper** is an app that replaces hastily scribbled shopping lists with an organized, uncomplicated system for building and checking off items to buy. It even helpfully groups items by aisle or store department. You can customize the order of aisles for each store you frequent so that your grocery shopping is organized according to store layout. **Shopper** has a substantial database of products, making it quick and easy to update your lists.

Remember to remove food stored in other places—like in the family room or the den. (Some people hide snacks in unlikely places, like the dirty laundry basket. One woman even hid her full-calorie Cokes in the toilet tank; it kept them cold as well as concealed them from her family, who often criticized her food choices!) The idea of not having food in the house "just in case" frightens some people. Often these are the people who use food to deal with stress and emotions. Some people say, "I can't deprive others in my house just because I can't handle food." If this is the case for you, you can try repackaging food into portions. Put cookies in plastic zipper bags containing a few cookies (an appropriate child-sized portion) to hand out to the kids as needed. (Of course this begs the question: Why not give them fruit instead of cookies—why train them to eat foods made of white flour or sugar?) Put the kids' foods on a separate shelf or in a separate cabinet defined as "not mine," just as you would do if you were sharing living quarters with a roommate.

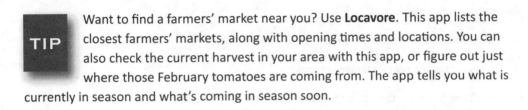

TIP Want to find a farmers' market near you? Use **Locavore**. This app lists the closest farmers' markets, along with opening times and locations. You can also check the current harvest in your area with this app, or figure out just where those February tomatoes are coming from. The app tells you what is currently in season and what's coming in season soon.

MEALTIMES

Mealtimes provide lots of cues. There are things you can do to make some cues less bothersome, though. Use smaller plates at meals so that it looks like you are getting more food. (Trick your eyes *and* your stomach!) Make eating meals an event, rather than something you rush through or wish you could avoid. Set a nice table, put on some classical music, light candles. Invite friends to share a pleasant meal. Rearrange a tight schedule so you have time for regular meals.

TIP Don't know what to fix for dinner? A good source for recipes is **www.allrecipes.com**. The associated app is **DinnerSpinnerPro**, and it offers three wheels to spin or set to find matching suggestions. Choose the type of dish, the ingredient, and the cooking time—or shake to get a random combination.

When sharing a meal with others, don't snack from their plates. Don't leave food out after a meal (especially desserts) so that people can help themselves to more, because you may be the one taking extra. And beware of the cleanup phase of meals. If possible, ask someone else to clear the table so you won't be tempted by scraps. Either throw away leftovers or save them in appropriate (non-see-through) containers for another meal. (In fact, put them in the freezer right away, if appropriate.) Don't snack on scraps or leftovers just because you don't want to waste food. Remember: *You can waste it or you can waist it.* Be aware that your mind may obsess about tempting food you have saved for later and may make you want to eat it sooner. If in doubt, trash it—and then take out the trash.

Review Table 3.2 to keep in mind the best way to manage cues in your environment.

Table 3.2
WINNING BEHAVIOR MANAGEMENT STRATEGIES

◎ Always shop from a list.

◎ Don't shop when you are overly hungry or tired.

◎ "Sanitize" your pantry; remove tempting foods.

◎ Discard leftovers, or store them in containers that are not see-through.

◎ Put away reminders of food—like the cookie jar or the partially full chip bag.

◎ Keep problem foods out of sight.

◎ Divide problem foods into portions before storing.

◎ Serve food on small plates so that it looks like more than it actually is.

◎ Choose and prepare healthy foods. Avoid frying; broil, bake, or poach instead.

◎ Slow down your eating.

◎ Let someone else clear the table and clean up.

◎ Brush your teeth before clearing the table.

Substituting Healthier Responses

Planning ahead to handle situations that can be troublesome is a good idea. Some common situations that require healthier responses include times when you are eating out in restaurants or at the homes of friends or family, or when you are entertaining guests, celebrating holidays, or taking vacations. Learning to slow down your eating and redefining your relationship to food and eating are also essential for success.

EATING OUT

Eating out in restaurants or at the homes of friends or family can be a big challenge to weight management. Business meetings over lunch or dinner can sabotage the best intentions unless you have redefined how and what you eat. Choose—or, if you must, insist on—a restaurant where you can order food that works for you, especially if you eat out a lot. Salads can be good choices, but be careful of the toppings like bacon bits and cheese, and be sure to ask for the dressing on the side. Try dipping your fork in the dressing and then take a bite of salad, or only add a little dressing at a time to the salad. Order your meat or fish broiled, grilled, roasted, or baked plain without high-calorie sauce, or ask for the sauce on the side, too. Avoid breaded and fried foods; they bring too much fat and calories. Consider choosing more meatless meals. Be sure to manage your portions.

Check the menu for the "heart-healthy" items but don't rely solely on the restaurant's recommendations. Use good judgment as well; cottage cheese and a meat patty are not necessarily a good "diet" choice. If you don't know what's in a dish, ask. Consider ordering an appetizer or two instead of a full entree. Plan to take a portion of an entree home, or ask to share an entree with your dining partner. Before you begin to eat, separate the entree into two portions on your plate before you start eating. If you get the take-home container right away, you can put the separated half to take home in it before you start eating the other half. Limit alcohol, which adds calories but no nutrition to your meal. (Besides, it weakens resolve.) Avoid or minimize your visits to fast food restaurants.

TIP **Restaurant Nutrition** is an app for the iPhone and the iPad that has a handy database of nutritional information for more than 60 national and regional fast food chains in the United States. These include Taco Bell, White Castle, In-N-Out Burger, A&W, and others. You can track what you eat as well, adding items from the database into meals that then go into your history.

EATING AT FRIENDS' OR RELATIVES' HOMES

When you will be a guest in someone's home, call ahead and let the host or hostess know any special needs or preferences you have. Don't be afraid to say you are trying to cut back on calories and would be happy with small portions. Offer to bring an appetizer, and make sure it is one you can feel comfortable eating. Forget the chips and dip; try a fresh fruit plate or vegetable *crudités*. Plan ahead and have a snack before you go out, especially if you think dinner might run late. Also decide ahead of time to manage your portions, and forgo the butter or oil if bread is served. If you plan on drinking at all, have mineral water or just plain water initially and save your glass of wine for dinner. Skip the hard liquor—and the attendant calories—entirely. Alcohol of any kind undermines inhibitions and makes it easier to give in to the temptation to overdo.

ENTERTAINING GUESTS

Entertaining at home can be easier, because you are in charge of what is served. Don't think you have to serve high-calorie food to guests. They are typically delighted just to be included in your company. Salads or light soups are generally appreciated for a first course or light supper, and it is okay to omit the bread. Choose a lean protein or fish as your entree. Keep portions appropriate. Fresh fruit is often a welcome dessert. The key to successful entertaining is in the details: nice presentation, pretty table, flowers or an interesting centerpiece for the table, or whatever shows your creativity. Don't be afraid to try out new recipes, even those lower in calories.

Epicurious.com is a good source for recipes, and it has a complimentary app, **epi**, that gives you online access to **epicurious.com**'s collection of recipes from *Bon Appétit* magazine and other sources. In addition, both the website and the app allow you to build a shopping list for selected dishes.

EATING DURING THE HOLIDAYS

Trying to lose weight during the holidays may be expecting too much (although some people manage it). Not gaining weight during the holidays may be a more achievable goal. To prepare for the holidays, think about what makes the holidays special for you. Your list might include the smell of a fresh pine tree or your family's traditional fruitcake. Maybe making cookies with the kids is your special thing. If there are foods that truly represent the holiday for you, plan to have them in moderation. Go ahead with the turkey with dressing; just exercise portion control. But go easy on the eggnog.

Holidays are often a time when some people feel sad, blue, or depressed. Perhaps some loved ones are missing; such losses can be accentuated during holidays. In addition, during the winter holidays, days are short and nights are long. Some people are especially vulnerable to a type of depression related to a reduced amount of sunlight called Seasonal Affective Disorder (SAD). Holidays are also a time when expectations are high; many people have expectations for what the holidays "should" be like, or they miss what they remember holidays used to be. Knowing this beforehand can help, as can planning ahead ways to make this particular holiday season memorable or rewarding in its own way. Having a positive attitude is important. In addition, be sure to keep up your exercise; that will help ward off feelings of depression.

TIP For tips on healthy eating during the holidays and at other times of the year, as well as for recipes, go to **www.healthcastle.com/holiday-eating-tips.shtml**.

EATING WHILE ON VACATION OR WHEN TRAVELING

Continuing to lose weight while on a vacation is a reasonable goal, especially if you plan ahead to leave your desk job behind and get plenty of exercise. Choose carefully where you will go and what you will do on vacation. Consider what food temptations you might face, and how you will cope with them. You need not deprive yourself of some special food treats that are part of the local color. Just exercise good portion control and be aware of foods with lots of sugar, fat, or salt that are likely to make you want to eat more.

These days, most hotels have exercise centers, so take your gym clothes and plan to include exercise in your day. Sightseeing often involves lots of walking, so take good walking shoes. Continue your exercise even when visiting friends. Taking a cruise can increase the risk of overeating unless you exercise good choices and portion control. Just because food is unlimited in quantity and seems "free" (avoid the common excuse "I paid for it so I'm going to eat it") doesn't mean you should eat more. Be picky about what food you choose. Even on a cruise you can still plan to get in lots of exercise by walking or working out in the gym.

When you are traveling on a tour vacation, you have less control over your schedule, and thus the times when you eat or what you eat. This can expose you to becoming overly hungry. Plan to take prepackaged snacks such as power bars or nuts that fit into your eating plan. Likewise, traveling on airplanes presents food and eating challenges. Airlines usually provide free salted nuts or pretzels (you can refuse them), but on most flights you usually must supply other food, either by purchasing it from the airline or by bringing food on board that you purchase just prior to boarding. The airline food that is offered for sale is prepackaged and often includes chips or cookies that might not fit your new eating plan. A better idea is to purchase a sandwich or salad to take on board with you.

Driving long distances by car presents other challenges. If possible, identify ahead of time the types of restaurants you would stop at for food. Take along food in a small cooler—healthy snacks such as fresh fruit or a picnic lunch to enjoy at a pleasant rest stop. When you do make rest stops, plan to go for a ten-minute walk if possible; stretching your legs will help you feel fresher and enjoy the ride more.

EATING SLOWLY

Eating slowly—not gulping food quickly—helps your brain catch up with what is going into your stomach. Putting your fork down between bites is one way to do this. Another is to take sips of water between bites. (Bariatric patients are advised not to drink anything during eating to avoid premature emptying of their smaller stomach pouch.) Take smaller bites. Chew food thoroughly. Pause during the meal. Practice mindfulness: notice the smell and texture of the food, and whether it is satisfying as you continue to eat. Stop when your stomach feels full enough or when the food no longer tastes really great. Resign from the "clean plate" club.

REDEFINING HOW YOU EAT

Developing a set of internal, guiding principles that define how you eat on a day-to-day basis is a good idea for managing weight in the long term. Consider putting foods you eat into these categories:

1. Foods I *usually* choose to eat.

2. Foods I *sometimes* choose.

3. Foods I *rarely* choose.

4. Foods I choose to *treat with care* because they have been dangerous in the past and can cause me to binge or eat too much (e.g., bread, cereal, chips, ice cream, peanut butter, trail mix, candy).

The key here is the word "choose." What you eat must be a choice, not a "have-to," for you to succeed in having a healthy weight and a healthy lifestyle. And what you choose is personal; it should be guided by your values, not by just your momentary preferences. That doesn't mean you never have ice cream, or prime rib, or one of those molten chocolate desserts. It does mean that you put these in category 2 or 3.

You want to develop *your particular menu of choices of healthy foods and your way of eating* that is different from the way you choose foods now. Avoid a dieting mentality; don't restrict foods unnecessarily. The new way of eating that you need to define for yourself is one in which you are mindful of healthy choices, you are guided by your values, and you are committed to choosing food with its legitimate purposes in mind—to sustain life and provide pleasure—not for escaping life's tribulations.

A common piece of advice is that you should never make any foods forbidden. This is because doing so makes those foods all the more tempting. Furthermore, people with an eating disorder are likely to pronounce whole categories of foods off-limits—especially any foods containing fat. While no foods should be absolutely forbidden, for overeaters or binge eaters there are often one or two foods that are "dangerous." For instance, some people say they cannot have peanut butter in the house because they will end up eating an entire jar at one sitting. If you have a danger food, you may have to put it on a special list: category 4, the foods you must treat with care. Such foods must be chosen with caution, if at all.

Using Rewards to Change Behavior

No doubt you've heard the story of someone buying a dress in a smaller size as an incentive to lose weight, only to give the dress away some time later, having never been able to fit into it. This was putting the cart before the horse. A reward must come *immediately after* the behavior is performed or the goal is reached, not before. (And as for the new dress being a cue, it is more likely that it will be a cue to feel guilty for not losing weight—and you may end up eating to forget about the guilt you feel.) There are a number of ways rewards can be used to change behavior, however. Providing incentives is one.

INCENTIVIZING CHANGE

Consider the friends who agreed to a contest with each other to see who could lose the most weight. Each wagered some money, winner take all. The idea was that winning money would be an incentive to achieve weight loss and the possibility of losing the bet would be painful enough to stimulate behavior change. This is the carrot-and-stick approach to weight loss. Maybe one of these gamblers did lose more weight than the other and collected the bounty. (Or neither of them lost much weight, and they called off the bet.) But for the one who lost the bet, in all likelihood he or she just went back to eating as usual.

Incentives for behavior can work, but punishment does not work very well. No doubt the loser of the bet just shrugged it off and got another piece of cake. In the past some misled groups for weight loss have tried punishing members for not adhering to a diet by using public humiliation. That didn't prove to be successful; those who were humiliated just quit the group. Well-meaning spouses or family members may try looking disapprovingly or making critical remarks about what they see as "bad" eating behavior to try to change another's behavior, only to have the dieter get so upset that he or she eats to spite the critics. Overeaters even punish themselves with self-criticism in an attempt to shame themselves into changing. It doesn't work.

Punishment

Punishment involves suffering, pain, loss, or an unwanted event or circumstance that usually results in feelings in the "wrongdoer" of not measuring up, being less than, feeling unworthy, or one-down. Punishment is not an effective tool for changing behavior. Reinforcement or reward is more effective in incentivizing change. Reward that influences behavior best includes getting something desirable (like a fun sticker, a desired compliment, or perhaps money) or it involves the removal or avoidance of something undesirable (like hunger or painful feelings).

MAKING CHOICES

One way to encourage desired behavior is to give yourself a choice between two alternatives. The choice would be between doing something healthy for a reward you want and that occurs soon after the behavior, or making a less than healthy choice and losing that reward. This is known as *Premack's Principle*. It involves the voluntary use of a highly desirable and frequently occurring event (such as watching a favorite television show each night or reading a book in bed before going to sleep) and making its occurrence contingent on the performance of a desired behavior. For example, you might make a bargain with yourself either to avoid using butter on your vegetables at dinner and then watch your favorite television show afterwards, or to eat with abandon and forgo your favorite television show. Giving yourself a choice between consequences can be powerful. Notice that the consequences follow very soon after the behavior. This is crucial; the reward must come very soon. Another part of making this work is to give yourself a mental pat on the back for succeeding with the desirable behavior. Not only do you get to watch your favorite program, but you also take pride in your accomplishment and feel good.

SHAPING BEHAVIOR

Rewarding behavior that approximates desirable behavior helps *shape* a positive behavior pattern in yourself and others. Don't wait for the "big" win for the reward; instead reward small approximations to the goal. For example, Jade, the woman mentioned at the beginning of this chapter, wanted to reach a goal of walking for 60 minutes five days out of seven each week. Instead of waiting until she reached this final goal to reward herself, she set up smaller, easily reachable goals, and rewarded herself for accomplishing them. Her smaller initial goal was to walk 20 minutes a day, three days a week. When she accomplished this, she gave herself a reward—and a pat on the back. When she was able to achieve her smaller goal adequately and regularly, she set a new goal of walking 30 minutes three days a week, again followed by reward. Then 30 minutes four days a week—and so on until she reached her final goal. She rewarded herself for each of the smaller subgoals as she attained them. Rewarding approximations to the desired behavior pattern is called "shaping."

USING SELF-REWARD

Almost anything that is valued can be used as a reward. There are a number of ways to use self-reward to reinforce a new behavior habit or pattern. Remember, though: you are the one who sets the rules, and no one but you can enforce them. It helps to make a game out of it. If you are going to reward yourself for desirable behavior, what you use as a reinforcer must have three characteristics:

1. You must perceive it as *valuable*, either symbolically (like a fun sticker) or in reality (for example, if it is money, it is enough money to really mean something to you).

2. The reward must be *presented as soon as possible*, if not immediately after the behavior occurs. Planning a vacation as a reward is too far in the future. Instead, putting a small amount of money in a fund towards a vacation each time a desirable behavior occurs can be an effective reward.

3. The reward must be *contingent* upon your behavior occurring. You should receive the reward if—and only if—the behavior occurs. For example, if your spouse agrees to do the dishes if you avoid snacking before dinner and then does them anyway even though you snacked, the reward (your partner doing the dishes) occurs without the behavior occurring. The reward is not contingent on your behavior. If you put money in the piggy bank for vacation even if you didn't make the healthy choice, this isn't a contingent reward.

Using rewards such as money or putting stickers on a calendar (both of these methods of reward are discussed next) is intended to be a short-term way of creating interest in and motivating behavior change. Ultimately the reward must become your own feeling of competence and effectiveness in taking charge of your health and your lifestyle. When your behavior is in line with your values, it is less of a struggle to achieve and maintain change.

Calendar-and-Stickers Method of Self-Reward

Remember when you were in grade school how pleased you were to get a star or other sticker on something you produced—some artwork or an essay or report? Well, this is still a great method to symbolically reward behavior now, even for adults. Although you may initially be put off by the idea of giving yourself a sticker for each time you engage in a new behavior, it actually can be fun and motivating. To use the calendar-and-stickers method, you need a month-at-glance calendar, preferably a large, wall calendar. Another option is to find a book-style month-at-a-glance calendar that is about five by seven inches or so, or if necessary, use a week-at-a-glance calendar. Then, you can use actual metallic stars or some other kind of small sticker (e.g., hearts, red lip kisses, happy face decals) to reward yourself for performing some desired behavior each day. Decide what each individual sticker will represent on your calendar. Each sticker would represent something related to the behavior you want to change. Maybe it is doing 30 minutes of walking a day. Or perhaps a sticker is to represent a day that you ate three regular meals. Whatever behavior the sticker signifies, apply it to the calendar for the day the behavior occurs. Post the wall calendar in a prominent place (e.g., on the refrigerator door, or somewhere in the kitchen or bathroom where you will see it) or carry the book calendar in your purse or briefcase and display it prominently when you get home. Those who are members of Weight Watchers can put rewarding stickers in their weekly booklets for each day that they meet their point budget. Not only will the stickers signal daily successes, but the absence of stickers as days go by should motivate you to get back on track once you have strayed. Each month (or each week) you get to turn over a "new leaf" and start with a clean slate. See Figure 3.1 for a calendar marked up in this manner.

Jade used the calendar-and-stickers method to motivate and reward her behavior. She bought stickers of fish and sea creatures to reward herself for each day she completed a 30-minute walk along a beach boardwalk near her home. She also bought some little stars that signified eating breakfast each day. The combination of two types of stickers, one for exercise and one for a particular eating behavior she wanted to increase, helped keep her on track with behavior change and was rewarding to her while being fun at the same time.

Money as Self-Reward

Money can be used as a way of rewarding yourself, but the difficulty is that the money you want to reward yourself with is actually your money already. So you need to use special rules to make it work as a reward. Take the example of Jade, who wanted to reward herself with money for each day she did not binge and then use the money to go to the theater in a few weeks. You already know that a reward must follow promptly upon the desired behavior, so having to wait to go to the theater several weekends from now wasn't a very powerful reward, especially when Jade was faced with a bag of chips and dip that she could easily eat now. So she created two envelopes: one was to hold her reward money to go to the theater, the other was addressed to a person or organization she did not want to support or give money to. Her bargain was for each day or time the desired behavior occurred, she put a predetermined amount of money in her theater envelope. On those times when she binged, an identical amount of money went in the stamped and addressed envelope for the disliked organization or person. Of course, it was the *idea* of supporting a cause or person she didn't want to support that hopefully would prompt her to do the right thing in the first place. This method can work because your choice is between the reward you want (in Jade's case, a visit to the theater) and giving money away.

Now you might say that having to send money to a disliked person or organization is punishing. Actually, it does not meet the criteria of causing pain, suffering, and loss of self-esteem unless you berate yourself for "failing." (There's a hint here: What you say to yourself—

July

S	M	T	W	T	F	S
	1 ☺	2 ☺	3	4	5 ☺ ★	6 ☺
7 ☺	8	9 ☺ ★	10 ★	11 ☺ ★	12 ★	13
14 ★	15	16 ★	17 ★	18 ☺	19 ★	20
21	22	23 ★	24 ☺	25 ★	26 ★	27 ☺
28	29	30 ☺	31 ★			

☺ = Eating Breakfast   ★ = Exercise Bike: 10 minutes/day

Figure 3.1
CALENDAR-AND-STICKERS METHOD

your self-talk—can be punishing or reinforcing. More about this later in the book.) Is giving money away unpleasant? Yes. That's the idea. But it isn't catastrophic to your sense of self. And you can't "lose" the money to someone you like because you could rationalize that it is okay to give them money.

Of course, the alternative is not to use money as a means of reward. Instead of losing money to a person or organization you don't prefer, you could write a short note praising them. Or you could use the calendar-and-stickers method just discussed. Using a symbolic reward like stickers may be more motivating and less anxiety-producing than losing money.

Tracking Progress

Another part of behavior management involves tracking progress. That is what the calendar-and-stickers method does in addition to symbolizing success. It is a way of tracking progress in behavior change because it shows both accomplishments and falling behind. Tracking progress may also involve tracking weight loss as well as progress toward goals.

TRACKING WEIGHT LOSS

One frequently asked question is, "How often should I weigh myself?" People want to know whether they should be keeping track of progress by weighing themselves regularly. Some research suggests that regular weekly weighing can be helpful. Other research advocates daily weighing. Daily weighing is probably not helpful for those who get upset by numbers, because fluctuations in daily weight can be misleading and demotivating. Likewise, being weighed at a doctor's office and finding a discrepancy between the doctor's scale and your own can be disheartening. (In that case, it is best to rely on the trend you see in weight loss on your own scale, and not on the numbers on the doctor's scale.) There is no hard-and-fast answer to the question of how often to weigh. You should decide what works best to motivate you.

Tracking changes in measurements such as hip and waist using a flexible tape is also an option. Some Internet fitness programs allow you to input and track your measurements as a way of judging progress. Tracking progress with exercise can be very motivating; Chapter 5, Getting Started with Exercise, will go into this in more detail.

Some people assess their progress according to the fit of their clothes. Noticing changes in the fit of your clothes can be a helpful indicator of progress, though it is not as readily apparent as tracking weight as shown on a scale or using tape measurements. Other people prefer to focus on behavior change to assess progress. This is probably a good strategy for many people.

TIP An iPhone and iPod app that tracks only weight is the **Weightbot**. It allows you to choose a goal weight and then track your weight over time. It keeps a record and provides graphs of your progress. However, you can't print out the record. You can only access it on the app.

TRACKING PROGRESS ON GOALS

To determine if you are making progress with weight loss or behavior change, it is necessary to know what your goal or aim is. In other words, what are you trying to achieve? (Remember: A goal is something that can be obtained whereas a value is a direction you are going.) What is the goal toward which your effort is directed? For the purposes of weight and behavior change, a goal is a concrete, identifiable end point that can be measured or quantified. (Refer to Chapter 2, Getting and Staying Motivated, for more information on goals.) Thus, it could be the goal of losing 10 pounds or exercising three times a week for 30 minutes each session. Generally speaking, it is better to define goals in terms of behavior to change and not in terms of pounds to lose. (You have control over behavior, but weight is subject to many factors.) However, some people need the reinforcement of seeing progress on the scale.

Short-term goals are usually those set up as a means to a larger end goal or for shaping behavior in pursuit of some long-term goal—like losing 50 pounds. Thus striving to lose a pound a week may be the short-term goal you set up in order to ultimately lose 50 pounds in a year. Exercising three times a week for 30 minutes may be an intermediate goal if your long-term goal is to participate in regular 60-minute exercise sessions four or five times a week. Focusing on short-term, achievable goals is more motivating than becoming too concerned about long-term goals that take time to acquire.

Behavior Fatigue

If you have ever been on a diet before, even one with moderate success, you know that you can reach a time when it just seems so difficult to keep going. This phenomenon is known as *behavior fatigue*. The importance of your goal to lose more weight fades in the face of competing needs and progress that may seem too slow. Boredom can set in. Interest and excitement wane. The "high" that might have been present at the beginning of the endeavor evaporates in the light of the vigilance and self-conscious monitoring of behavior that are needed for success in the long run.

People are motivated toward taking action to achieve a goal because they want to feel effective, competent, and self-determining.[5] The problem is that people are also prone to losing interest and stagnating. You may remember a time at school or work when you just couldn't bring yourself to finish a project. It was as if you had brain lockup. The task just seemed too difficult or too boring, and you couldn't seem to keep your attention on it. You had succumbed to behavior fatigue.

Motivation is vulnerable to many negative influences. Remember the time you were "watching your weight" and you went to a party that had tempting food, so you went off your diet? Or perhaps you once got caught up in the latest dietary craze that everyone was talking about and some even lost weight. Then, after awhile, interest in the craze faded, usually because people stopped doing it and talking about it, and probably because they also regained weight. And even though it worked for you for a while, you dropped it, too. If something like this has happened to you, you know what behavior fatigue is.

Behavior fatigue can also set in if you give yourself excuses and rationalizations for quitting a weight loss effort. If you think of your effort as a "diet" that you must follow—instead of a way you live your life—you are likely to become bored and eventually quit. Instead, recall why you are trying to lose weight (to improve your health, to feel better, to be able to move more easily) and what the values are that you want to guide your behavior.

Diets are inherently boring. People need and look for stimulation, and dieting does not provide that. Sooner or later, behavior fatigue sets in for almost everyone who goes on a diet. That's why success depends on more than just cutting calories and increasing exercise, although these are important, too. Success is predicated on your assessing your values and changing your attitude, self-concept, and lifestyle. You need to see behavior change as a gradual and *permanent* shift toward a new way of being.

You also need to see small changes as successes—and take credit for these successes. Perceived little "failures" can lead to ultimate failure. If you expect to lose two pounds a week and "only" lose half a pound, you are likely to be disappointed and feel less competent; enough such experiences will erode motivation. Getting yourself to the gym twice a week on a regular basis, when you have never regularly been involved in exercise before, should feel like progress and success. Feeling that you *have* to go to the gym and that you don't want to go produces resistance, annoyance, alienation, and eventually stopping. But just because you have such feelings and thoughts doesn't mean you have to act on them. If you remember that exercise is just something you do—that it is part of who you are—then you can ignore the momentary resistance.

To avoid behavior fatigue requires dedicating yourself to your goals and revising your self-concept. Defining yourself, for example, as "someone who exercises regularly" or "someone who eats mostly natural, unprocessed foods" is a different way of thinking about yourself and one that reinforces feelings of self-determination. You get to decide "what I eat" and "what I do" as part of your lifestyle, instead of following a diet. Choosing to adopt a lifestyle characterized by regular exercise and eating a variety of healthy foods in moderation provides feelings of competence and leads to persistence and success.

New Ways to Think about Food and Eating Behavior

The phrases "mindful eating," "intuitive eating," and "normal eating" are often used inter-changeably on the Internet. Mindful eating involves paying attention, on purpose, to your ac-tual eating experience, in the moment, without judgment. While mindful eating, also called conscious eating in some circles, is compatible with intuitive eating, intuitive eating is a broader philosophy. It includes mindful eating, physical activity for the sake of feeling good, using nu-trition information without judgment, and respecting your body, regardless of how you feel about its shape.

INTUITIVE EATING

The concept of intuitive eating involves using mindfulness to guide behavior. This has im-portant implications for eating and physical activity and involves the mind and the attitude you bring to your lifestyle. Two registered dietitians, Evelyn Tribole and Elyse Resch, have proposed a new way of approaching eating and the body which they describe in their book *Intuitive Eat-ing*.[6] This book was originally published in 1995 and is now in its second edition, with a new audio version published in 2009. Table 3.3 is a list of principles adapted, with permission, from the book.

MINDFUL EATING

Mindful eating is similar to intuitive eating, with its focus being primarily on the activity of eating. If you are like most people, you are usually doing something else while eating—like watching television or working on the computer. Most people multitask and do something else while eating. As a result, they aren't in touch with their bodies while eating. Ask yourself: do you pay attention to your body's signals to stop eating, or do you ignore your body's feed-back? If so, you may be eating mindlessly. Mindless eating involves not paying attention to eating, to the circumstances of eating, and to the body's signals of hunger or satiety. Mindless eating almost always leads to overeating or making poor food choices.

  Mindful eating, a concept first introduced in 1990 by Jon Kabat-Zinn,[7] is about being conscious of why, and how, you are eating. If you are eating mindfully, you are aware and attentive to all dimensions of eating, including mindfulness of the mind, body, thoughts, and feelings. Mindfulness is the moment-by-moment awareness—really paying attention—to all aspects of eating. According to Susan Albers,[8] there are four foundations of eating mindfully, as shown on page 84.

Table 3.3
PRINCIPLES OF INTUITIVE EATING

ADAPTED WITH PERMISSION FROM THE BOOK *INTUITIVE EATING*, 2ND ED.
BY EVELYN TRIBOLE, MS, RD, AND ELYSE RESCH, MS, RD, FADA

1. Reject the Diet Mentality

Find out what works for your body. Never make any foods forbidden. Forget the promise of diets and diet books; revise your relationship with food instead. Decide what it is that you choose to eat or not eat. You need to become the expert on your body.

2. Honor Your Hunger

Keep your body biologically fed with adequate energy. Avoid excessive hunger. Learn to listen to your body, and recognize biological hunger. If you don't seem to experience hunger signals over long periods of time, you might want to try eating every three to four hours. Eventually, your body will get used to being fed regularly and will begin to provide you with dependable hunger signals.

3. Make Peace with Food

Stop the food fight! Give yourself permission to eat what tastes good and what pleases you, and eat food without guilt. Observe how your body feels when eating any food and how satisfying it is to your tongue.

4. Challenge the Internal "Food Police"

Scream a loud "no" to thoughts in your head that declare you're "good" if you eat one way but "bad" if you eat another way. Stop being a policeman to your eating, following unreasonable rules of some diet. Learn to talk to yourself in helpful ways. Watch out for hindering or negative self-talk and thinking errors such as black-and-white thinking, catastrophic thinking, or pessimistic thinking. (And if others play food policeman to your eating, assertively tell them not to do so.)

5. Feel Your Fullness

Listen for the body signals that tell you that you are no longer hungry. Observe the signs that show that you're comfortably full. Pause in the middle of a meal or when eating and ask yourself how the food tastes, and what your current fullness level is. Eat slowly; put your fork down between bites.

Table 3.3
PRINCIPLES OF INTUITIVE EATING
(CONTINUED)

6. Discover the Satisfaction Factor

Pleasure and satisfaction are legitimate goals that result from eating. Pay attention to the sensations of eating like taste, texture, aroma, appearance, and so on. Think about how your body might feel when you finish eating. Eat as soon as you are gently hungry rather than waiting until you are overly or excessively hungry. Eat slowly and savor every bite. Don't settle for less than the best: if you don't love it, don't eat it, and if you love it, savor it. Become a "food snob" (like a wine snob—demand the best).

7. Cope with Your Emotions without Using Food

Ask yourself, "Am I biologically hungry?" If not, ask yourself, "What am I feeling?" Often it is anxiety, not hunger. Then ask yourself, "What do I need to do to feel better?" (Hint: *Eating* is not the answer.) Find other ways to meet your emotional needs.

8. Respect Your Body

Stop body bashing. Every time you focus on how you think your body is imperfect, it creates more self-consciousness and body worry. Replace disparaging comments about your body with kind and accepting body statements—and a rededication to taking care of it better.

9. Exercise—Feel the Difference

Forget militant exercise. Just get active and feel the difference. Shift your focus to how it feels to move your body—and to be able to move your body with greater ease. Activities of daily living count. Make movement a nonnegotiable priority in your life.

10. Honor Your Health with Gentle Nutrition

Make food choices that honor your health and taste buds while making you feel well. Remember that you don't have to eat perfectly to be healthy. The problem is not the occasional treat; it's what you eat consistently over time that matters. Progress, not perfection, is what counts. Gentle nutrition includes variety, moderation, and balance. Don't be duped by the *fat-free trap*. Fat free doesn't mean calorie free or nutrient dense. Likewise, don't fall into the *no-carbs trap*. Your brain needs carbohydrates. Notice how your body feels when you offer it vegetables, fruits, whole grains, and beans. Also notice which foods cause insulin spikes and blood sugar crashes.

◎ **Mindfulness of the *process*.** Pay attention to what you are doing. Observe the taste, texture, smell, and sound of food. Stay in touch with each bite.

◎ **Mindfulness of the *body*.** Listen to your body. Pay attention to hunger pains, a rumbling stomach, your energy level, and muscle tremors, and feel your body. Notice when your body signals that it is satisfied and stop eating. Eat when you are physically hungry and not when you are stressed or driven by physical distress.

◎ **Mindfulness of *feelings*.** Notice your feelings as you seek food, find it, and eat it. Get in touch with the emotions that might be driving the need or desire for food.

◎ **Mindfulness of *thoughts*.** Listen to your thoughts. Observe whether you have "should" or "should not" thoughts, critical thoughts, food rules, or "good" or "bad" judgments about food. Avoid using excuses or rationalizations that allow you to eat something less healthy.

Mindful eating is a relatively new concept on the weight and health management scene, although the practice of mindfulness is centuries old. It has the potential to transform your relationship with food and eating. The Center for Mindful Eating[9] sets forth the important components of mindful eating from their perspective:

◎ Learn to make choices in beginning or ending a meal based on awareness of hunger and satiety cues.

◎ Value quality over quantity of what you're eating.

◎ Appreciate the sensual, as well as nourishing, capacity of food.

◎ Feel deep gratitude that may come from appreciating and experiencing food.

Mindful eating helps focus your attention and awareness on the present moment, which in turn helps you disengage from unhealthy habits and behaviors.

TIP A good website for a system focusing on mindful eating can be found at **www.mindfuleating.org**. Their approach is called CAMP (Control, Attitudes, Mindful eating, Portions) and is based on sound mindfulness principles as well as portion control and the right attitude.

"NORMAL" EATING

Some people think that "normal" eating means not having to think about food choices. In fact, people with "normal" eating patterns do make conscious choices. They just don't obsess about them. They have internalized "the way I eat" or the food choices they typically make, and they monitor their behavior—but "lightly." Their relationship with food isn't automatic, but it is easy because it is in alignment with their values and who they believe themselves to be. This is the secret for changing behavior: to know your values and live by them. The rest will follow.

Karly Pitman is a good example of someone who has come to a new relationship with food. Karly, who has struggled with her weight and is now maintaining, describes her rules for normal eating in her website, **www.divinecaroline.com**:[10]

1. **I eat when I'm hungry; I stop when I'm full.** Being hungry or irritable from low blood sugar feels terrible. Too much food makes me feel bloated, stuffed, and sick. So I eat enough food to give me energy, health, and enjoyment. And the next time I feel hungry, I eat again.

2. **I eat three meals a day, every day, including breakfast.** When I was overeating, a huge part of my bingeing stemmed from *undereating*: I would eat as little as possible during the day (because I was on a perpetual quest to lose 10 pounds) only to be starving by dinnertime. Then I would overeat, not because I had poor willpower, but because I was hungry. Eating food at regular intervals makes me feel grounded, stable, and satisfied.

3. **I eat foods that make me feel good.** I like a steak every now and then. A pizza is a favorite treat. I love colorful salads. Risotto is my idea of heaven. These things make me feel good, so I eat them. Sugar makes me depressed and whacks me out. Fried eggs give me the willies. Too many fake foods—think lots of processing and packaging—make me feel icky. So I usually abstain.

4. **I eat what I really want.** What I want to eat today may be different tomorrow. What I want in the winter may be different than what I crave in the summer. How nice that I can choose—that I don't have to eat the same four things from a "good foods" list over and over again. Right now I'm in a raw fruit and vegetable phase, stemming from the heat wave we're currently experiencing. But as the weather cools I crave warm, cooked vegetables and hearty soups. A few weeks ago, when my baby was going through a growth spurt (I'm a nursing mother), I had a hankering for nuts and nut butter. I followed my desire, got a spoon, and dove into the almond butter, without any guilt, shame, remorse, or thoughts of calories.

5. **I enjoy my food.** I love food. I always have. And I've come to glory in that, rather than feel ashamed by it. Who started the lie, anyway, that women shouldn't have an appetite? I've always had a hearty appetite, especially when I'm exercising regularly and nursing, as I am now. I have no qualms about getting a second helping, rather than undereating to be socially acceptable.

TIP Regardless of the diet or diet program you might be on, or even if you are following your own plan, **www.fatsecret.com** can provide you access to buddies who are like-minded. You can join a buddy group that shares your interests or demographics, like teachers or nurses or twenty-somethings with 50 pounds to lose. Don't be put off by the name: **Fatsecret** offers lots of other tools and is easy to use.

CHAPTER FOUR

Eating for Health

*ABBY WAS NORMAL-WEIGHT AND MARRIED WITH ONE CHILD. Her mother and sister were very thin and worried constantly about what they ate and how much they exercised. Abby felt big next to both of them, and she was confused about what was right for her to eat. Her mother and sister told her that fat should be avoided and that carbohydrates were bad. Abby perused different books in the bookstore that gave advice on food and eating, but they just caused her more confusion. One book talked about how to choose foods to improve the immune system, and another about choosing high-density foods to lose weight. Some books gave specific advice on diets for athletes, while others focused on what everyone should eat. Advice often differed depending on whether the authors' focus was on losing weight or promoting a healthy lifestyle. Abby wasn't sure if she should try to lose weight to be more like her mother and sister, though she didn't want to obsess about food like they did. She decided to download the **BMR Calculator** app on her iPhone to help her figure out her base metabolic rate and how many calories she should eat given her body. Then she found **www.caloriecount.com**, a website that provided lots of nutrition information and ways to make healthy choices. Abby decided to define her own way of eating and not let herself be overly influenced by her mother and sister.*

Basic Nutrition and Weight Loss

Sometimes it can seem like a challenge to figure out the relationship between nutrition and weight loss. You may recall that there was a time when all carbohydrates were considered "bad." (Diet books by people like Dr. Robert Atkins provide examples of this approach.) People were advised to avoid "carbs" and eat lots of protein to lose weight or avoid gaining weight. (This actually worked for some people, although many nutrition experts at the time doubted its long-term viability and faulted it for not being healthy.) Many nutrition experts advocated eating "good" carbohydrates, like vegetables and grains, because they help lower cholesterol.

(They do.) Currently, many experts recommend eating a diet low in saturated and trans fats and high in unrefined carbohydrates.

In addition, more nuanced ways of choosing foods are also seen as helpful for weight management and health. Glycemic index and glycemic load together help assess how carbohydrates affect blood sugar levels. This is important to diabetics or those who are pre-diabetic or who are becoming insulin-insensitive—which includes many people who are obese—as well as for those who are sensitive to sugar. Then there is the Fullness Factor—a measure of which foods, including those with protein, fat, or carbohydrate, produce higher satiety when eaten.[1] Satiety refers to that pleasant feeling of fullness and the corresponding reduction of hunger you feel after you eat. An old standard for making calorie counting easier is the Food Exchange System, which was originally developed to help people with diabetes manage their food intake but which has since been adopted for more general weight loss efforts. This is still a good option to calorie counting, and is easy to learn.

TIP Discover new foods similar to old favorites. **Caloriecount.com** allows you to browse through its database, indicating what foods you like to eat and adding them to your personal food log. The site then suggests healthy items you may not have tried that may appeal to your personal taste. It also assists you with social networking by helping you identify members with similar tastes.

Macronutrients

It is necessary to know a little bit about nutrition to make healthy choices and to understand all the weight loss advice out there. In this chapter, we will attempt to cover some of the basics in a way that is clear and understandable and truly useful. We will start with the basics—the macronutrients.

Food is divided into energy sources called macronutrients: carbohydrates, fats, and proteins. Carbohydrates contribute four calories per gram, as does protein, whereas fat provides nine calories per gram. All three of these energy sources are necessary ingredients in a healthy diet; the question is one of balance. (Note that alcohol provides seven calories per gram.)

CARBOHYDRATES

Your body relies on carbohydrates as an immediate and continuous energy supply. Generally speaking, about 40–50 percent of your diet should come from healthy carbohydrates, which should be mostly unrefined carbs (such as vegetables, fruits, whole grains, and legumes). Without adequate carbohydrates, the body has to rely on less efficient sources of energy that involve converting fat and body tissue to energy. Nutritionists recommend keeping to a minimum the refined carbohydrates made up of simple sugars. (You will find more on sugar and sugar addiction later in this chapter.)

 For tips on adding healthy carbohydrates to your diet, visit **www.hsph. harvard.edu/nutritionsource/what-should-you-eat/carbohydrates/**.

PROTEIN

Protein is needed by your body to grow and repair tissues. Although you only need about 45–60 grams of protein a day (the higher amount is for men), the average person eats about 70–100 grams of protein daily. Sources of protein include meat, fish, poultry, eggs, and dairy. Vegetables and legumes (and foods made from legumes, such as soy products) also provide some protein but are incomplete sources. For most people, only 10–15 percent of total daily caloric intake should come from protein. (Bariatric surgery patients need more protein, and certain diets recommend in the neighborhood of 20 percent.) For those trying to lose weight, a higher protein intake can sometimes be appropriate.

 For more information on getting the right kind and amount of protein in your diet, check out **www.hsph.harvard.edu/nutritionsource/what-should-you-eat/protein/**.

THE ROLE OF FAT

The role of fat in the diet is a little more complicated than the role of the other macronutrients. Saturated fat, the "unhealthy" fat, is found in animal fats such as red meat and butter, and contributes to heart disease. Monounsaturated fats and certain polyunsaturated fats, the "healthy" fats, come from vegetable sources such as olives, corn, soybeans, and peanuts, and are good for your heart. A few vegetable fats, such as coconut oil and palm oil, are unhealthy and should be avoided. Trans fats are manmade, the result of adding hydrogen to monounsaturated fats, turning them into more industrially valuable shelf-stable fats—that are also unhealthy for your heart. Trans fats are so unhealthy that some states, like California and New York, have outlawed their use in restaurants.

The right kind of dietary fat is needed in the diet. Dietary fat helps transport certain vitamins needed by the body. Polyunsaturated fats vary in health benefits, depending on the amount of Omega fatty acids they contain. Omega-3 fatty acids, which are found in fatty, cold-water fish such as salmon, tuna, sardines, herring, anchovies, mackerel, and lake trout, as well as in certain plant sources such as flax and walnuts, are promoted by some experts as better than Omega-6 fatty acids. Although both are good for you, Omega-3 fatty acids are known to help lower cholesterol in the blood and so contribute to the reduction of heart disease. Some people take fish oil supplements to ensure that they are getting enough Omega fatty acids; eating real fish several times a week is generally a better alternative.

It's important to avoid the wrong kinds of fat in your diet, too—the wrong kind of fat can increase more than just your risk of coronary artery disease. A high intake of saturated or trans fats can double your risk of developing Alzheimer's-type dementia[2] (as compared to diets low in these fats). This is because harmful fats in food also increase blood cholesterol levels, which in turn causes inflammation of blood vessels around the brain. This inflammation impairs memory and can contribute to the development of Alzheimer's disease.

Depending on who or what is making it, the recommendation for percent of dietary fat can be from 10 percent of total calories (very low, and hard to achieve) to 35 percent of total calories, the level recommended by the American Heart Association (AHA). The AHA advises limiting saturated fat to less than 10 percent of total calories, avoiding trans fats altogether, and getting the majority of your fat calories from monounsaturated and the healthy polyunsaturated sources. It's recommended that you have at least two servings of fatty fish a week. It's also smart to toss a few cubes of tofu into a veggie stir fry and sprinkle some walnuts on your salad a few times a week, as some of the nutrients in vegetables are more readily absorbed by the body if they are consumed with fat.

TIP   For more about the role of fat in a healthy diet and recommendations from various organizations for levels of dietary fat, go to **www.snacksense.com/good-fats-oils**.

WHAT ABOUT PROPORTIONS OF MACRONUTRIENTS?

Don't worry so much about the proportions of carbohydrate, fat, and protein. Recent studies have found that when it comes to losing weight, it pretty much boils down to total calories.[3] The DIRECT (Dietary Intervention Randomized Control Study)[4] two-year study looked at success and adherence among 322 moderately obese subjects in one of three groups: the low-fat diet group, the Mediterranean diet (high monounsaturated fats) group, and the low-carbohydrates group. The researchers found that overall each group lost close to the same amount of weight. That said, people tended to stick to the low-fat diets more readily than the low-carb diets. The study concluded that the amount of weight loss at the six-month point, not the type of diet, best predicted long-term success. In other words, early success is a good sign for being able to keep it off, and is a better predictor of success than type of diet.

Australian researchers looked at a similar topic: whether macronutrient ratios of the diet played a role in weight maintenance after one year. For this study, people were divided into either a low-carb or a low-protein diet group. Both groups maintained an average weight loss of about 32 pounds, with no significant difference between the two groups. Once again, the type of diet mattered less in terms of weight loss and maintenance success than the total calories consumed.

In another trial of 811 overweight adults, people were assigned to one of four diets with varying percentages of total calories from fat, protein, and carbohydrates. Group and instructional sessions were offered. At six months, subjects assigned to each diet had lost an average of 13 pounds, but all began to regain weight after 12 months. The researchers concluded that reduced-calorie diets all result in weight loss regardless of the macronutrient spread. The bottom line for everyone is that to lose weight and keep it off, you must maintain a lower caloric intake. The choice, then, of a diet, depends on what works for you and what is healthier. However, recent research studies suggest that a low-carb diet—one that avoids pasta, bread, rice, and alcohol—maintained for six months or more is better for reducing cholesterol.

TIP To learn what the U.S. Dietary Guidelines say about nutrients needed for growth and health, go to **www.health.gov/dietaryguidelines/dga2005/ document/html/chapter2.htm**.

Food Addiction

In his book *Breaking the Food Seduction*, Neal D. Barnard, M.D.,[5] of the Physicians Committee for Responsible Medicine, contends that certain foods—including chocolate, cheese, red meat, and practically any food that includes both sugar and fat—can become a *behavioral* addiction—that is, the behavior is repeated because the rewarding aspects of the behavior are highly reinforcing. These foods cause the brain to release its own natural opioids and certain chemicals that stimulate the brain's pleasure center. Chocolate, for example, offers a range of compounds from mild cannabinoids (cannabinoids is the main ingredient that causes people to get high from smoking marijuana) to amphetamine-like chemicals that provide yet another kind of high. Other foods are rewarding as well. Cheese is mostly fat, and the texture of fat pleases the mouth and brain. Many people snack on foods such as cheese and salty crackers (salt is another pleasuring substance for many palettes) after a stressful day.

And what about physical addiction? Although research has found that excessive sugar does not cause the same physical addiction as drugs such as cocaine or heroin (that is, it does not meet the technical definition of *physical* addiction—it is not accompanied by increasing tolerance or withdrawal symptoms when stopped), sugary foods do activate the same pleasure centers of the brain as certain drugs. Indeed, research suggests that sugar releases natural opiates and the neurotransmitter dopamine (neurotransmitters are chemicals in the brain that help transmit nerve signals) into the body, making repeated forays into eating sugary foods take on the appearance of an addiction, as Barnard's book points out.

Some people really do seem to develop real cravings for sweet foods, particularly if they frequently eat a lot of them. You may know people who call themselves "sugaraholics." You may be one yourself. These people feel that they cannot get through the day without a sugar fix, or that once they start eating sugar, they can't stop. They feel "addicted" to sugar, and sometimes to other comfort foods as well. Additionally, some women report experiencing sugar cravings in the ten or so days just before their menstrual period.

Some research has also found that high and chronic intake of sugar resulted in resistance to leptin—the hormone that curbs appetite. Over time, a high intake of sugary foods blocks the leptin signal in the brain, so leptin can't extinguish hunger. To reinstate the function of leptin, high-sugar foods must be minimized or even avoided. In particular, sugary beverages and foods such as Coca-Cola, Pepsi, Cinnabon, Krispy Kreme, Dunkin' Donuts, Entenmann's, Hostess, Sara Lee, and the like should be curtailed.

Sucrose—the sugar you find in the sugar bowl—is the manmade version of naturally occurring sugars such as those found in fruit, but it is sweeter than those naturally occurring sugars and is thus highly rewarding to the pleasure center of the brain. When it is eaten a lot, it can cause the overeater to want more and more; it is as if the brain "learns" to want sugar. Sugar by other names comes as high-fructose corn syrup, honey, maple syrup, evaporated cane juice, brown sugar, raw sugar, confectioner's sugar, crystallized fructose, dextrin, beet sugar, cane sugar, and corn syrup—to name only a few.

Sugary foods do not produce satiety—they produce yearning for more sugary foods. Eating high quantities of sugar or sugary foods causes a spike in blood sugar, followed by a sharp rise in insulin, and then a feeling of hunger soon afterward. On a scale of 0 to 5, in which the lower the number the less filling per calorie, sugar (or sucrose) ranks at 1.3—not filling at all. Nevertheless, sweetness is compelling, and for some people, sugar binges can last for days.

There is no doubt that foods high in fat or sugar are very appealing to many people and can become a regular habit and even a behavioral addiction. Fast foods are not only fast, they have lots of fat, and fat provides a pleasant texture in the mouth. Like sugar, fat-laden foods also make the brain release dopamine—the neurotransmitter associated with reward and craving. Even if not technically considered addictive, these foods are more and more used to provide quick and cheap satisfaction—and lots of calories. The best way to beat a behavioral addiction is to eat a good breakfast, containing some protein, each day, and to eat regularly throughout the day. If you must eat sugary foods, make them part of a regular meal.

TIP A good article providing more information on overcoming sugar addiction can be found at **www.pr.com/article/1058**.

DEPRESSION AND SUGAR SENSITIVITY

Sugar may present other problems as well. Research suggests that depression does seem to be related to sugar ingestion and sensitivity to sugar for *some* people. Although the exact relationship between fatigue, depression, and simple carbohydrates (sugary foods as well as alcohol, white pasta, bread, and rice) is not entirely known, recent studies have suggested that eating a lot of these simple carbs can cause fatigue, and that persistent fatigue may contribute to the development or maintenance of symptoms of depression.

Fatigue is a common complaint of those who are depressed. And some depressed people develop a preference for food that is high in both sugar and fat, such as ice cream, candy, cookies and pastries, and other simple carbohydrates such as sugary soft drinks or juice drinks. Others report feelings of fatigue and lack of vigor *following* consumption of foods high in simple sugar. Some people refer to this as a "sugar hangover." That is, like the binge eater, the person overdoing sugar can feel mentally slowed and physically tired soon after eating a large amount of sugary foods. It often takes days to get over a sugar hangover, and only then by returning to balanced eating.

According to Kathleen DesMaisons, Ph.D., a nutrition expert and author of *Potatoes Not Prozac*,[6] many people, including those who are depressed, are "sugar-sensitive." Sugar evokes endorphins and promotes the manufacture of serotonin—a neurotransmitter associated with feeling calm. Initially, the sugar makes the person feel better. But when the good feeling wears off—and it can, fairly quickly—the aftereffect is feeling down and depressed. This usually leads to eating more sugar to feel better again.

If you think you are sugar-sensitive, you should consider the information that follows in this chapter regarding glycemic index and glycemic load. This nutritional tool could help you cope with an "addiction" to sugar or sensitivity to simple carbohydrates. Even if you don't think sugar is a problem for you, you may benefit more from the nutritional tools discussed in the section that follows.

Helpful Nutritional Tools

Having discussed the basics of nutrition and weight loss, it is now time to turn our attention to some helpful nutritional tools. These include the glycemic index and glycemic load, the fullness factor, the food exchange system, and the food pyramid. Each of these provides a different way of understanding and selecting foods so that you can determine your individual guidelines for eating. Once you have decided that having good health is an important value for you, you need to discover what works for your body and your preferences. These tools are intended to help you do that.

GLYCEMIC INDEX AND GLYCEMIC LOAD

People who are diabetic or pre-diabetic (or who might have sensitivity to sugar) should consider learning to use the glycemic index (GI) and glycemic load (GL) in choosing foods. The GI is an established numerical way of measuring how much of an increase in circulating blood sugar any given carbohydrate triggers. The higher the number, the greater the blood sugar response (which is followed by a corresponding release of insulin). A low-GI food causes a small rise, while a high-GI food triggers a more dramatic spike. A GI of 70 or more is high, and is an indication that the carbohydrate causes a surge of sugar in the bloodstream. Some examples of high-GI foods include white bread, potatoes, rice milk, rice crackers, and cornflakes. (Note that "whole wheat" bread also has a high GI if it is not made from *whole-grain wheat.* Later in this chapter there is a section about what constitutes whole-grain products.) High-GI foods should be avoided to avoid a sharp rise in blood sugar followed by increased hunger. A GI between 56 and 69 is deemed to cause a "medium" rise in blood sugar, although these cutoff points are somewhat arbitrary. Carbohydrates with GIs of 55 or less are ranked as low, because they cause a lower rise of blood sugar. Some examples of low-GI foods include most fruits, legumes, barley, boiled carrots, milk, and yogurt. But GI alone is not enough to help you decide what to eat. You need to know the glycemic load of foods as well.

Glycemic Load

The glycemic load (GL) of foods takes the glycemic index into account, but gives a more complete picture than does glycemic index alone. A GI value tells you only how rapidly a particular type of carbohydrate turns into blood sugar, but it doesn't take into account the standard serving size. The GI needs to be translated into an ordinary serving size in order for you to know how big a rise in blood sugar an ordinary serving would cause. This is where glycemic load comes in. You need to know the GL to understand a serving of a food's effect on blood sugar. The carbohydrate in watermelon, for example, has a high GI (GI = 72). But there isn't much of it in a single serving, so the glycemic load of watermelon is relatively low (GL = 8). In other words, the GL is about the quality of the carbohydrate *given a standard serving size.*

A GL of 20 or more is considered high, a GL of between 11 and 19 medium, and a GL of 10 or less low. Foods that have a low GL frequently have a low GI as well. Examples of low-GL/low-GI foods include peanuts, bean sprouts, and most fruits. Some foods with a high GL also have a high GI. So, for example, white rice has a GI of 64 (high) and a GL of 33 (also high). Another dish that is high in both is macaroni and cheese, which has a GI of 64 and a GL of 30. A baked potato has a GI of 85 and a GL of 28—all red flags for blood sugar surges. Foods with an intermediate or high GI range can have GL values that range from very low to very high. For example, white bread has a low GL of 10 (for one slice) but a high GI of 70, because this latter value is based on the larger quantity of bread that is usually eaten at one sitting. Likewise, one tablespoon of sugar or honey has an intermediate GI value of 68 (you would have to eat a whole lot of sugar to cause the surge in blood sugar like you get in most sweets) but a low GL of 8 (this is what you would get in an occasional teaspoon in your tea or coffee). Both watermelon and popcorn have high GIs of 72 but low GLs of 8 and 7, respectively.

The GIs and GLs for some common foods are listed in Table 4.1.[7] In the table, the calculation of GIs is based on the glucose index, where glucose is set to equal 100. The glycemic load or GL is determined with a formula that divides the glycemic index of each food item by 100 multiplied by its available carbohydrate content (i.e., carbohydrates minus fiber) in grams. The "Serving Size" column is the serving size in grams for calculating the glycemic load. For simplicity of presentation, the intermediate column that shows the available carbohydrates in the stated serving sizes as been left out.

 TIP For additional information and values on the glycemic index and glycemic load for other foods, visit **www.glycemicindex.com**. For still more information, check out **www.mendosa.com/gilists.htm**.

A quick set of rules for managing blood sugar using GI and GL is provided by Denise Webb, Ph.D., R.D:[8]

1. Include at least one food that has a low GI *and* a low GL (like fruit) at every meal. This will moderate the effects of consuming a high-GI and high-GL food by diluting the rise in blood sugar.

2. Instead of white bread, substitute whole-grain bread or sourdough bread (research shows that the acid content of sourdough helps reduce blood sugar response).

Table 4.1
GI AND GL FOR COMMON FOODS

Food	GI	Serving Size	Net Carbs	GL
Peanuts	14	4 oz (113g)	15	2
Bean sprouts	25	1 cup (104g)	4	1
Grapefruit	25	½ large (166g)	11	3
Pizza	30	2 slices (260g)	42	13
Low-fat yogurt	33	1 cup (245g)	47	16
Apples	38	1 medium (138g)	16	6
Spaghetti	42	1 cup (140g)	38	16
Carrots	47	1 large (72g)	5	2
Oranges	48	1 medium (131g)	12	6
Bananas	52	1 large (136g)	27	14
Potato chips	54	4 oz (114g)	55	30
Snickers bar	55	1 bar (113g)	64	35
Brown rice	55	1 cup (195g)	42	23
Honey	55	1 tbsp (21g)	17	9
Oatmeal	58	1 cup (234g)	21	12
Ice cream	61	1 cup (72g)	16	10
Macaroni and cheese	64	1 serving (166g)	47	30
Raisins	64	1 small box (43g)	32	20
White rice	64	1 cup (186g)	52	33
Sugar (sucrose)	68	1 tbsp (12g)	12	8
White bread	70	1 slice (30g)	14	10
Watermelon	72	1 cup (154g)	11	8
Popcorn	72	2 cups (16g)	10	7
Baked potato	85	1 medium (173g)	33	28
Glucose	100	(50g)	50	50

Source: **www.mendosa.com/GI_GL_Carb_data.xls**.

Note: GL of 20 or higher produces a surge in blood sugar, while a GL of 10 or less is "low" and preferred. Note that white bread has a high GI but an acceptable GL, as does ice cream—but notice the serving sizes. More than a cup of ice cream (one scoop) is problematic.

3. Switch your morning cereal from cornflakes to an oat cereal or one that is less processed and high in fiber as well as low in sugar.

4. Opt for basmati rice, quinoa, or bulgur instead of white rice.

5. Cook your pasta *al dente.* Overcooking pasta raises the GI and GL by significantly breaking down more of the starch.

6. Include legumes in your diet: chickpeas, kidney beans, lentils, and dried beans.

7. Adding acid to your meal slows down blood sugar response. Have vinaigrette with your salad or yogurt on your cereal. Try lemon juice on vegetables.

8. Choose snacks low in both GI and GL such as fresh fruit, dried fruit mixed with nuts, low-fat milk, or yogurt.

9. Eat some lean protein at every meal.

10. Exercise portion control, especially with carbohydrate-rich foods. The glycemic load you consume is higher if you overeat foods high in both GI and GL.

Despite the usefulness of the glycemic load and index scales for those who are diabetic or pre-diabetic, the *Tufts Health & Nutrition Letter*[9] points out that ultimately it is total calories that count for losing weight. Paying attention just to GI and GL is not enough, though it could help with satiety and cravings. A multicenter study found that participants achieved and maintained comparable weight loss after one year, regardless of whether they were on a low-glycemic load diet or a high one, as long as they adhered to a calorie-restricted diet.

FULLNESS FACTOR

While the GI and GL are ways of assessing carbohydrates alone, the Fullness Factor (FF) can be used to evaluate all foods. **NutritionData.com** (ND) developed this FF index after studying the results of numerous satiety studies.[10] Recall that satiety refers to the feeling of fullness you feel after you eat. Values for the FF range between 0 and 5, with the lower numbers indicating foods that are less filling per calorie consumed, and the higher numbers pointing to foods that are more filling.

The FF is calculated from the food's nutrient content, using values from those nutrients that have been shown experimentally to have the greatest impact on satiety. Of course, there are many factors that influence a food's ability to satisfy the palate. A person's preferences for taste or texture are two such influences. Quantity consumed is another factor.

Generally speaking, foods that contain large amounts of fat, sugar, or starch have a low FF and are much easier to overeat, as any overeater can attest. Foods that contain large amounts of water, dietary fiber, or protein have the highest FF. These high-FF choices, which include most vegetables, fruits, and lean meats, do a better job of satisfying hunger and are also known as "high-density" foods.

TIP   For more information about Fullness Factor foods, go to **www. nutritiondata.com**.

FF can also be calculated for liquids, including soups and drinks. These usually have an above average FF initially due to their high water content, and small quantities are satisfying in the short term. However, low-viscosity fluids such as juice or soft drinks will empty from the stomach quickly and can leave you hungry again in a relatively short time if you don't consume much of them. Of course, drinking adequate fluids and water in particular is important for hydration and good health, and drinking water throughout the day is recommended for helping you to feel full. (Bariatric surgery patients are advised to avoid fluids when eating meals to avoid "washing through" the food eaten.) Choosing high-FF foods is a good way to avoid hunger when reducing calories. Table 4.2 lists the FF for some common foods. Notice that common foods with a higher FF tend to be more filling, whereas those with a lower FF are less so.

TIP   NutritionData recommends the Better Choices Diet based on the Fullness Factor. For more information, go to: **http://nutritiondata.self.com/topics/better-choices-diet**.

FOOD EXCHANGES

A food exchange system is an easier way to calculate the approximate caloric content of foods you eat than keeping track with a calorie-counting list. Food choices are grouped together into exchange lists—for example, there is a list for fruits, another for vegetables, and yet another for meats and meat substitutes. Initially there were six exchange lists; now there are additional lists for such categories as alcohol and fast foods. You can find more information on all these lists by Googling "food exchange lists" or checking out the American Dietetics Association's website.

TIP   For more details on food exchange lists, go to **www.fitnessandfreebies.com/fitness/foodex.html**.

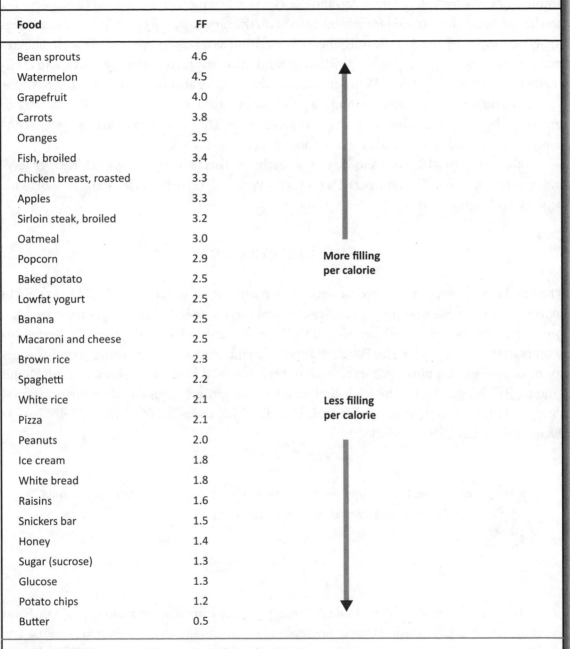

Table 4.2
FULLNESS FACTORS FOR COMMON FOODS

Food	FF
Bean sprouts	4.6
Watermelon	4.5
Grapefruit	4.0
Carrots	3.8
Oranges	3.5
Fish, broiled	3.4
Chicken breast, roasted	3.3
Apples	3.3
Sirloin steak, broiled	3.2
Oatmeal	3.0
Popcorn	2.9
Baked potato	2.5
Lowfat yogurt	2.5
Banana	2.5
Macaroni and cheese	2.5
Brown rice	2.3
Spaghetti	2.2
White rice	2.1
Pizza	2.1
Peanuts	2.0
Ice cream	1.8
White bread	1.8
Raisins	1.6
Snickers bar	1.5
Honey	1.4
Sugar (sucrose)	1.3
Glucose	1.3
Potato chips	1.2
Butter	0.5

More filling per calorie

Less filling per calorie

Source: **NutritionData.com**. Higher numbers indicate greater satiety.

Serving Sizes for Food Exchanges

For a given serving size, all choices on a particular list are approximately alike in terms of amount of carbohydrate, protein, fat, and calories per serving. Thus, one food choice on a list can be "exchanged" or traded for any other food on the same list. Lists such as these were originally developed by the American Diabetes Association as a way to help people with diabetes make better food choices. This approach was found to be helpful for weight control, and eventually was adopted by Weight Watchers early in that organization's history. It is the basis for variations on the theme, such as counting points or other ways of choosing food, that are still promoted by Weight Watchers and similar organizations. The basic food exchange system continues to be a good way to evaluate your food choices.

Table 4.3 (pages 102–103)shows six basic exchange lists (across the top), calories per serving, and serving sizes. The number of servings for various levels of caloric intake, as well as for seniors, is also provided.

THE FOOD PYRAMID

The Food Pyramid was developed by the U.S. Department of Agriculture (USDA) as a tool to help Americans make healthy food choices. Several variations of the Food Pyramid have been proposed over the years. For example, Tuft's University created a Food Pyramid adjusted for seniors over 70 years old.[11] The Food Pyramid for Seniors advocates the lower serving ranges for most food groups plus eight servings of water a day in addition to calcium, vitamin D, and vitamin B12 supplements. The Diabetes Food Pyramid groups foods based on their carbohydrate and protein content instead of their classifications based on food groups.[12,13] There is even a Vegetarian Diet Pyramid.[14]

 TIP Visit **www.MyPyramid.gov** for more information on the USDA Food Pyramid and how to use it for making healthy choices.

The Food Exchange List in Table 4.3 integrates the information from the USDA Food Pyramid as well as information for various levels of calorie intake and guidance for seniors. The Healthy Eating Pyramid proposed by Walter Willet[15] is shown in Figure 4.1, and is a good guidance option for most adults.

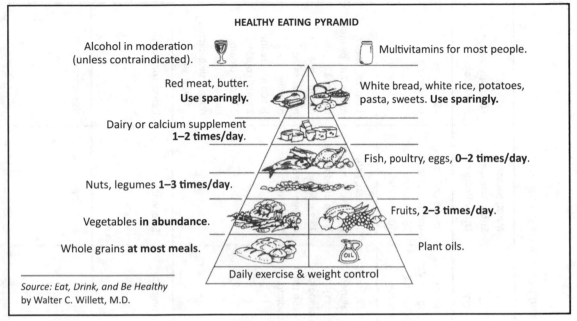

HEALTHY EATING PYRAMID

Alcohol in moderation (unless contraindicated).

Multivitamins for most people.

Red meat, butter. **Use sparingly.**

White bread, white rice, potatoes, pasta, sweets. **Use sparingly.**

Dairy or calcium supplement **1–2 times/day.**

Fish, poultry, eggs, **0–2 times/day.**

Nuts, legumes **1–3 times/day.**

Vegetables **in abundance.**

Fruits, **2–3 times/day.**

Whole grains **at most meals.**

Plant oils.

Daily exercise & weight control

Source: Eat, Drink, and Be Healthy by Walter C. Willett, M.D.

Figure 4.1
HEALTHY EATING PYRAMID

Smart Nutrition Strategies

The nutritional tools discussed in the previous section of the book can be helpful in making food choices and developing personal eating guidelines that are in alignment with your value of having good health. The following smart nutrition strategies can also serve to guide weight management behavior. Healthy snacking can help bridge the hunger gap between meals. Exercising portion control is crucial for weight management. Likewise, learning to read food labels and to plan meals are important skills for controlling your weight and making healthy choices. Minimizing fast foods is the best bet for your health as well as your weight. Finally, self-monitoring, as emphasized in previous chapters, is a proven powerful weight loss strategy.

SNACKING

Planned snacking between meals can help weight management for many overweight and obese people (although most bariatric surgeons advise against it for their patients' postsurgery). Snacking can dampen rising hunger between meals and prevent overeating at meals. If you snack, stick to smart choices such as fresh fruit or raw vegetables; low-fat dairy products like cottage cheese, yogurt, or hard-boiled eggs; snack-size low-fat popcorn; peanut butter (but

Table 4.3

FOOD EXCHANGE LISTS, CALORIES PER SERVING, AND NUMBER OF SERVINGS

Food Groups	Breads, Grains, and Other Starches	Vegetables	Fruits	Milk, Dairy	Meat, Meat Substitutes, and Other Proteins	Fats, Oils, Sweets, and Alcohol
Calories per Serving	80 calories per serving	25 calories per serving	60 calories per serving	90 calories per serving for nonfat, 120 for low-fat, 150 for whole	35–55 calories per serving for lean, 75 for medium-fat, 100 for high-fat	45 calories per serving
What is a serving?	1 slice of bread; ½ cup of rice, cooked cereal or pasta, ¾ cup dry cereal, ½ English muffin	1 cup raw leafy vegetables, ½ cup other cooked or raw, ¾ cup vegetable juice; ½ cup potato, peas, corn, or cooked beans	1 medium apple or orange, or ½ banana; ½ cup chopped, cooked, or canned fruit; ¾ cup fruit juice	1 cup milk, (note above calories differences) ½ cup evaporated milk, ¾ cup plain nonfat yogurt	1 oz meat, fish, poultry, cheese; ½ cup dried beans; 1 egg; ¼ cup cottage cheese; ½ cup tofu	1 tsp. oil, butter, margarine, peanut butter; 1 T mayonnaise, regular salad dressing; ½ cup ice cream; 2 small cookies; 2 T sour cream, half-and-half; 6 nuts; 1 slice bacon; 1 tsp. sugar
Total caloric intake of about 1,600	6 servings	3 servings	2 servings	2–3 servings	5 servings	Use sparingly
Total caloric intake of about 2,200	9 servings	4 servings	3 servings	2–3 servings	6 servings	Use sparingly

Table 4.3

FOOD EXCHANGE LISTS, CALORIES PER SERVING, AND NUMBER OF SERVINGS

(CONTINUED)

Food Groups	Breads, Grains, and Other Starches	Vegetables	Fruits	Milk, Dairy	Meat, Meat Substitutes, and Other Proteins	Fats, Oils, Sweets, and Alcohol
Total caloric intake of about 2,800	11 servings	5 servings	4 servings	2–3 servings	7 servings	Use sparingly
For seniors (70+)	6 servings	3 servings	2 servings	3 servings	2 servings	Use sparingly

Note: Women who are pregnant or breastfeeding, teenagers, and adults under 24 should have 3 servings of dairy a day.

Note: Check Table 4.4 to ascertain what a "serving" size is in a food exchange system.

COPYRIGHT © 2009 JOYCE D. NASH.

not too much); and nuts and seeds in appropriate amounts. Research has shown that people who eat a high-protein, moderate-calorie snack one hour before lunch automatically cut back their calories during subsequent meals on the same day. Remember the three-to-four rule: be sure to eat again between three and four hours after the last time you ate. Eating sooner is probably either stress-related eating or mindless eating, and waiting too long to eat invites being overly hungry—and then eating too much.

CONTROLLING PORTIONS

Portion control—keeping servings small—is crucial for weight management. But many people overestimate the amount of food in a serving. And therefore they underestimate how many servings of foods they are consuming. It is important to have a mental image of serving sizes in order to succeed with portion control. One 3-ounce serving of meat or fish is about the size and thickness of the palm of your outstretched hand, an audiotape cassette, or a deck of cards. A single serving of hard cheese is the size of a pair of dice. A portion of pasta, rice, or mashed potatoes is about half the size of your fist. A portion of salad is the size of a baseball. A single portion of French fries, potato chips, nuts, or M&Ms is one small handful—filling up the center of a slightly cupped palm of the hand. Table 4.4 lists some typical serving sizes and how they relate to the food exchange system.

Note that an ordinary portion may not be the same as a serving in a food exchange system. The definition of a single serving size according to a food exchange list varies according to the food item. For example, the food exchange system refers to protein servings in single ounces, but most dietitians refer to a serving or portion of protein in terms of a 3-ounce serving. A 3-ounce portion size of protein is actually three exchanges. A 12-ounce steak, therefore, is actually four portions, or twelve exchanges! Few people realize that a typical deli sandwich has 5–8 ounces of meat (five to eight exchanges) plus two servings of bread (two exchanges) and one teaspoon of mayonnaise (one exchange). This can easily add up to around 800–1,000 calories. A single baked potato can equal two to three vegetable servings or exchanges—plus it has a high GI and GL load and low satiety value!

READING FOOD LABELS

Food labels can help you make wise food choices. It is a good idea to learn how to read them. Most packaged foods in the grocery store list nutrition information on the package in a section called the Nutrition Facts. The Nutrition Facts label lists the serving size; the number of servings per container; total calories and calories from fat; total fat broken down by saturated fat and sometimes trans fat; cholesterol; sodium; total carbohydrate including dietary fiber (sometimes soluble and insoluble fiber), sugars, and other carbohydrate; and protein. After

	Table 4.4 TYPICAL SERVING SIZES FOR MAIN EXCHANGE LISTS		
Exchange List	Contents	Calories per Exchange	Typical Serving Sizes
Starch	Cereals, grains, pasta, breads, crackers, snacks, starchy vegetables, and cooked dried beans,* peas*, and lentils*	80	• ½ cup cereal, grain, pasta, or starchy vegetable • 1 ounce of a bread product, such as 1 slice of bread • ¾ to 1 ounce of most snack foods (some snack foods may also have added fat)
Fruit	Fresh, frozen, canned, and dried fruits and fruit juices	60	• 1 small to medium fresh fruit • ½ cup canned or fresh fruit • ¼ cup dried fruit • ¾ cup fruit juice
Milk	Milk and milk products, including skim (or very low-fat), 2%, and whole milk	90–150	• 1 cup skim, 2%, or whole milk, goat's milk, sweet acidophilus milk, or kefir • ½ cup evaporated skim or whole milk • ¾ cup plain nonfat or low-fat yogurt
Vegetable	Vegetables and vegetable juices	25	• ½ cup cooked vegetables or vegetable juice • 1 cup leafy raw vegetables
Meat and Meat Substitutes	Red meat, poultry, fish, shellfish, game, cheese, processed meats, eggs, tofu, tempeh, soy milk, peanut butter, and dried beans,*, peas,* and lentils*	35–100	• 1 ounce meat, fish, poultry, or cheese • ½ cup dried beans
Fat	Oil, butter, margarine, shortening, lard, cream, mayonnaise, salad dressing, nuts, seeds, nut butters, avocado, coconut, olives, and bacon	45	• 1 tsp. regular margarine or vegetable oil • 1 Tbs. regular salad dressing

* Can be counted as either a Starch or a Meat Substitute.

that comes a list of vitamins and minerals as a percent of two levels of reference diets (2,000 and 2,500 calories), followed by a list of ingredients. The list of ingredients shows the ingredients in descending order by weight, meaning that the first ingredient makes up the largest proportion of the food. Check the ingredient list to spot things you'd like to avoid, such as white flour, coconut or palm oil (both high in saturated fat), or hydrogenated oils (which are actually trans fats).

Note that if you eat more than the serving size listed on the Nutrition Facts label, you need to adjust the numbers from the Nutrition Facts section accordingly. For example, if you eat 2 cups and the serving size is 1 cup at 230 calories per cup, you are actually consuming 460 calories. Figure 4.2 offers more suggestions for reading a nutrition label.

How to Avoid Being Misled by Food Labels

A 2006 study published in the *American Journal of Preventive Medicine* found that only 32 percent of people studied could correctly calculate the amount of carbohydrates in a 20-ounce bottle of soda with multiple servings. Many were also confused by the nutrition label's complexity, or incorrectly interpreted information listed in the percent daily value column (the 2,000-calorie recommended daily allowance list). Not only is it hard to understand the nutrition information given—but that information is also sometimes misleading or just plain wrong.

The Center of Science in the Public Interest (CSPI), a nonprofit nutrition watchdog group, has thrown light on some of the misleading claims that manufacturers make to give their products a better image. One product, for example, claimed to be "whole grain" but only had 30 percent whole grain, and was forced by the CSPI to change its labeling. In another case, Kraft, which claimed that such products as Crystal Light Immunity Berry Pomegranate help maintain a "healthy immune system," was challenged by the CSPI. (It should be noted that some sources take CSPI to task for changing its stance on trans fats and argue with some of its findings. However, the weight of the research evidence argues that CSPI generally does a good job as an industry watchdog.) In addition, disease prevention claims on food labels require Food and Drug Administration approval before a product can hit the shelves.

Still, labels can continue to mislead consumers about such things as fiber content, or can label products "low-fat" even if that is a questionable claim. While fiber is known to be a heart-healthy nutrient that lowers cholesterol, a product may not necessarily provide those benefits if its fiber is derived from a source other than a whole grain, such as chicory root. Likewise, a low-fat food may sound healthy and even be a wise choice, but research shows that average people concerned about their weight tend to consume up to 50 percent more calories when they eat foods labeled low-fat than when they eat the original "full-fat" version of the food. This is because they think they can eat all they want of a food as long as it is labeled low-fat. But many foods labeled as low-fat have only 30 percent fewer calories than the original.

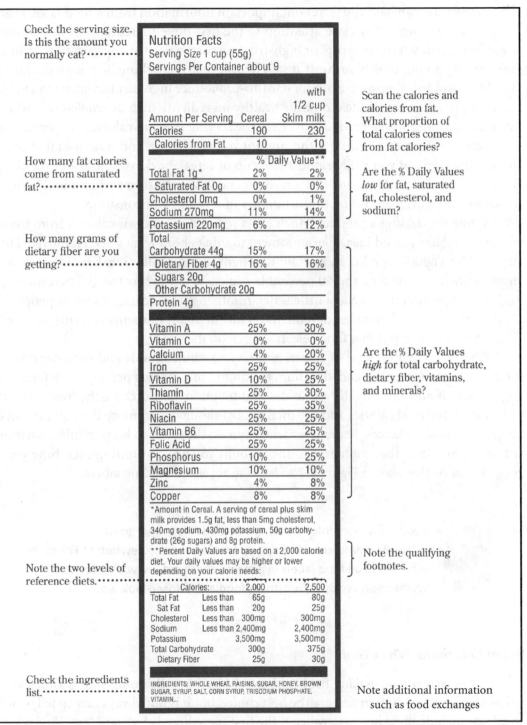

Check the serving size. Is this the amount you normally eat? ·········

How many fat calories come from saturated fat? ·········

How many grams of dietary fiber are you getting? ·········

Note the two levels of reference diets. ·········

Check the ingredients list. ·········

Scan the calories and calories from fat. What proportion of total calories comes from fat calories?

Are the % Daily Values *low* for fat, saturated fat, cholesterol, and sodium?

Are the % Daily Values *high* for total carbohydrate, dietary fiber, vitamins, and minerals?

Note the qualifying footnotes.

Note additional information such as food exchanges

Nutrition Facts
Serving Size 1 cup (55g)
Servings Per Container about 9

Amount Per Serving	Cereal	with 1/2 cup Skim milk
Calories	190	230
Calories from Fat	10	10
	% Daily Value**	
Total Fat 1g*	2%	2%
Saturated Fat 0g	0%	0%
Cholesterol 0mg	0%	1%
Sodium 270mg	11%	14%
Potassium 220mg	6%	12%
Total Carbohydrate 44g	15%	17%
Dietary Fiber 4g	16%	16%
Sugars 20g		
Other Carbohydrate 20g		
Protein 4g		
Vitamin A	25%	30%
Vitamin C	0%	0%
Calcium	4%	20%
Iron	25%	25%
Vitamin D	10%	25%
Thiamin	25%	30%
Riboflavin	25%	35%
Niacin	25%	25%
Vitamin B6	25%	25%
Folic Acid	25%	25%
Phosphorus	10%	25%
Magnesium	10%	10%
Zinc	4%	8%
Copper	8%	8%

*Amount in Cereal. A serving of cereal plus skim milk provides 1.5g fat, less than 5mg cholesterol, 340mg sodium, 430mg potassium, 50g carbohydrate (26g sugars) and 8g protein.
**Percent Daily Values are based on a 2,000 calorie diet. Your daily values may be higher or lower depending on your calorie needs:

	Calories:	2,000	2,500
Total Fat	Less than	65g	80g
Sat Fat	Less than	20g	25g
Cholesterol	Less than	300mg	300mg
Sodium	Less than	2,400mg	2,400mg
Potassium		3,500mg	3,500mg
Total Carbohydrate		300g	375g
Dietary Fiber		25g	30g

INGREDIENTS: WHOLE WHEAT, RAISINS, SUGAR, HONEY, BROWN SUGAR, SYRUP, SALT, CORN SYRUP, TRISODIUM PHOSPHATE, VITAMIN...

Figure 4.2
HOW TO READ A NUTRITION LABEL

A few rules can help you ferret out important information from a food label. First, check the list of ingredients. Pay close attention to the first three ingredients. If one of the first is sugar, honey, brown sugar, syrup, or high-fructose corn syrup (or any variation on that term), you are consuming mostly sugar. If it says hydrogenated anything, it is high in trans fat and should be avoided. Keep an eye out for hard-to-pronounce ingredients, which tend to be chemicals for preserving shelf life. Look for healthy ingredients such as *whole-grain* wheat, oats, bran, or any other whole grain. Then check the serving size and calories per serving. Be honest when you ask yourself: what is the amount you usually eat, and how does that compare to the serving size? Do you really eat just one cup of cereal, or do you pour out the cereal until the whole bowl is full? Measure out a recommended serving to see what it looks like. Be sure to adjust the calories according to the number of servings you consume.

While purchasing a product which has a reduced number of calories from the original might sound like a good idea, take a moment to think about what's been removed. For example, Welch's Light Grape Juice Cocktail: the "light" on the label translates into less sugar but more artificial sweeteners, and 60 percent less juice. Better to buy the 100 percent grape juice and cut the portion size or add a little water. Another guideline used by some people is to buy foods with no more than three ingredients on the list. If any of them are terms you don't know or can't pronounce, put that food selection back on the shelf.

Check the sodium level of frozen entrees and canned foods and consider how much it contributes to the recommended sodium maximum of 2,000 mg per day. Such foods are often high in salt; if possible, buy the reduced-sodium option. Or purchase the fresh version.

Check the total calories and the total fat. Fat should be no more than 30 percent of total calories in most instances. Remember when you do the math to keep in mind what the serving size is and how that compares to the amount you are consuming each time you eat the food. Examine the label in Figure 4.2 to learn more about reading labels.

TIP If you want more information on deceptive labeling, go to **www.eBrandAid.com** and sign up for their weekly newsletter. For more information on food labels in general, check out **www.diabetes.org/ nutrition-and-recipes/nutrition/foodlabel/closer-look.jsp**.

What Constitutes Whole Grain?

You may or may not be making the healthiest choice when choosing your bread. Most people know by now that whole grains are the best choice, but it is not always easy to tell which bread products include these healthy grains. If the first ingredient is "wheat," "enriched wheat," "enriched wheat bread," "unbleached wheat flour," or even "unbromated, unbleached wheat," the bread is mostly refined white flour. To be a whole-grain bread, the first ingredient listed must be a whole grain. Words to watch for include "whole" in front of wheat, rye, or oats. A whole grain must be listed as the first ingredient. The term "multi-grain" or "made with whole grain" on the label does not guarantee whole grain unless it is listed first in the ingredient list. Likewise, "high fiber" is not synonymous with whole grain. And you can't tell by color or texture. One good clue is to look for the "100% Whole Grain" stamp. Only products with at least 16 grams of whole grains per serving can display this stamp.

MEAL PLANNING

Like smart snacking and good portion control, planning ahead for meals is another helpful strategy for managing weight. Many who struggle with weight issues don't plan ahead. They wait until they go to the grocery store after work to figure out what they feel like eating, often having skipped breakfast or lunch and feeling tired and famished. Or they go to work without thinking ahead for lunch, only to be persuaded by colleagues to go to some restaurant where choices are problematic. Many people do not shop ahead for meals, and as a result eat what is handy regardless of its nutritional value, or end up opting for fast food.

Meal planning can be as simple as making a note the day before of what type of food you will choose for each meal the next day. This is especially important for dinner. For many people, breakfast is simply cereal or something routine—that is, if they don't skip it altogether. Lunch can be more problematic: will it be leftovers, a sandwich, a salad, or what? And dinnertime is too often governed by expediency and hunger—what can I eat as soon as possible, and what do I feel like having right this minute? This kind of approach to meals can result in poor choices.

TIP To help you with meal planning and weight management, you might want to use an online program such as **www.mealsmatter.org** to help yourself get organized. If you have a smartphone, you can use the **Notes** application or a similar app to remind you of what you plan for dinner, or purchase a specialty app to help you plan meals.

One option is to use a week-at-a-glance type of paper calendar and note the main dish for each day—for example, chicken on Monday, fish on Tuesday, a meatless entree on Wednesday, and so forth. Whether you go low-tech—and simply write a note about the next day's meal each night before bed—or high-tech and enlist your smartphone or a website, planning ahead is a proven key to successful weight management.

LIMITING FAST FOOD

In a fast-paced society, fast foods and takeout are a convenience, but they are also unfortunately a source of high levels of calories and bad fats. The healthiest choice, of course, is to avoid fast foods altogether. Fast foods have many nutritional shortcomings, but they are part of the American scene. If you can avoid them, do so, or at least minimize your visits and make the best choices you can if you go. But if you must occasionally rely on fast foods, learn how to make healthier choices in these restaurants.

Most fast food restaurants offer salads, and this is a good choice, provided you go easy on the dressing to lose weight; use half (or less) the amount in the container the restaurants provide. Avoid breaded choices in favor of grilled. For example, get the grilled chicken sandwich, not the breaded and fried version. Choose a plain hamburger instead of a cheeseburger or the burger with all the fixings. Forget the fried mushrooms, onions, and bacon that can be added to hamburgers. Try ordering the "junior" size instead of the larger size. Avoid the French fries, or—if you must—order the smallest size (or share an order with someone) and don't add extra salt. A final tip: don't eat the whole thing; leave the last two or three bites on the plate.

When ordering Mexican food, avoid the sour cream and guacamole; substitute salsa made from fresh tomatoes. Choose burritos, soft tacos, enchiladas, and tamales over cheese-stuffed chile rellenos and quesadillas, but be careful of added cheese or sour cream on any menu item. Cut your burrito in half and take the rest home. Be careful with the tortilla chips, too; they contain a lot of fat, and it is hard to control your portions when they are served in a constantly refilled community basket. (Try putting chips on a paper napkin for a few minutes and watch what happens to the napkin.)

When ordering pizza, order the thinnest-crust version available and top it with fresh vegetables. Skip the sausage, pepperoni, Canadian bacon, salami, and "double cheese." At a salad bar, choose fresh vegetables and limit bacon bits and croutons, fried Chinese noodles, marinated vegetables, and cheeses. Order dressing on the side and try dipping your fork into it and spearing some salad, rather than pouring the dressing over the salad. Get the diet drink or choose just plain water.

SELF-MONITORING OF CALORIC INTAKE

An important strategy that some people choose for losing weight is keeping track of calories. This may not be a good idea for those who tend to become obsessed with such activities, but for other people, self-monitoring of caloric intake is a helpful strategy. Self-monitoring can keep you conscious of what and how much you are eating. There are a number of online programs as well as smartphone apps for tracking caloric intake, or you can do it the low-tech way by keeping a simple diary of what you eat and its calorie content.

The food exchange lists mentioned earlier in the chapter can be helpful when it comes to recording your food intake. Instead of pouring over calorie lists of individual foods, you may prefer the simplicity of using the simple food categories and exchanges listed in Table 4.3. In the food exchange system, for example, all fruits, depending on serving size, count for 60 calories per serving. Likewise, all vegetables count for 25 calories per serving. Starches, which include breads, cereals and grains, and starchy vegetables such as corn or potatoes, dried beans, peas, and lentils, count about 80 calories per serving. Protein options, which include meat and meat substitutes, vary depending on fat content from 35 calories (very lean meat such as skinless chicken breasts) *per 1-ounce serving* to 100 calories per ounce for high-fat meat and meat substitutes, such as pork spareribs, cheese, hot dogs, and sausage. So a 3-ounce serving of lean meat is a little more than 100 calories, while the same size serving of high-fat meat is more like 300 calories per serving. Consult Table 4.4 for more information on food exchange lists and serving size.

What Constitutes a Healthy Diet?

So in the final analysis, what constitutes a healthy diet? For weight loss, your diet should focus on reducing calories and including protein, unsaturated fats, and carbohydrates in the form of fruits, vegetables, and small amounts of whole grains. In general, for a healthy diet, at least once or twice a week, choose a meatless main course. Keep saturated fat from red meats to a minimum. Don't overdo bread, pasta, or rice. If you do choose these foods, choose the whole-grain varieties and practice portion control. Minimize sugary foods and foods with added sugar (e.g., certain salad dressings, marinades, some cereals). Watch your sodium. Consume no more than 2,000 grams of sodium—preferably, less. Read the labels on frozen, canned, and packaged foods to ascertain the sodium content, which is often high. Include beans and nuts in your diet. Eat more "real"— fresh and unprocessed—foods. Choose foods that are dense in water and fiber (e.g., apples). Be careful with liquids that contain lots of calories (e.g., sugary sodas, fruit drinks, smoothies). Remember: All foods in moderation.

CHAPTER FIVE

Getting Started with Exercise

*Jacob wanted to lose weight, even though his wife, who was also overweight, was not concerned about either his or her weight. Jacob worked out in the gym three days a week for an hour each time. He lifted weights and trained with machines. Jacob's workout routine was skewed toward building muscle mass and was light on aerobic exercise and stretching. At home, his wife continued to buy tempting foods for herself and the kids, and Jacob struggled to stay in control of his eating. He started using a smartphone application that helped him adjust his exercise routine to better achieve his weight loss objectives in addition to his muscle-strengthening goals, and to get social support to motivate him to make healthy choices in the face of temptations at home. Jacob added the **C25K** (i.e., "Couch to 5K") app to his iPhone to help him incorporate running as part of his workout program. His wanted to work up to doing a 5K race. The added exercise helped him to feel better about himself and to live a healthier lifestyle.*

The Role of Exercise in a Healthy Lifestyle

Physical activity and exercise are non-negotiable components of a healthy lifestyle and successful weight management. Physical activity is any body movement that works your muscles and requires that your body use more energy than when you are resting. Exercise is a subset of physical activity that is planned, structured, and repetitive for the purpose of conditioning any part of the body. Among other examples, an exercise program can include walking, running, swimming, bicycling, working out in a gym or fitness center, doing floor exercises, or working with a personal trainer or physical therapist. Exercise improves health, maintains fitness, and helps you recover from physical disabilities. Activities of daily living are also a form of physical activity that includes pursuits such as gardening, climbing stairs, cleaning, or parking further away from and walking to your destination.

A program of regular exercise most days of the week—six or seven—together with increased activities of daily living are the goals to strive for in order to achieve optimal fitness. Many obese people are sedentary; they are often inconsistent exercisers, and they may or may not do much in the way of burning extra calories through activities of daily living. A beginning exercise plan for them may simply involve walking regularly for whatever length of time they can endure and gradually increasing the time and distance they walk as they become more fit. Eventually they may set a goal to walk a certain number of steps a day or may take up hiking for both calorie burn and enjoyment. For both adults of normal weight and those who are overweight, instituting a program of regular exercise that is of sufficient duration and intensity (i.e., raises target heart rate) is essential for reducing health risk and managing weight. Optimal fitness is the goal for preventing premature loss of vital capacities.

A number of Internet programs and smartphone apps are available to help a person get started with walking or an exercise program. Many of these programs also allow the user to monitor food consumption, calories, and weight, as well as exercise. There are also programs for those who already engage in exercise and want to challenge themselves at a higher level, perhaps by competing in fun runs or marathons or just by sharing their fitness feats with others.

TIP The **Health Cubby** app for the iPhone lets you set weekly diet and exercise goals and share your progress toward these goals with up to seven other Cubby-using buddies to get moral support or to engage in friendly competition. This app encourages you to focus on big-picture goals rather than nitty-gritty details of weight reps, mileage, or calories. **Health Cubby** syncs your data online, sharing it with the friends you've approved.

Despite the well-established role of physical activity and exercise as a crucial component of success, many confirmed dieters go from diet to diet searching for the magic answer—the diet that will finally let them lose weight easily and keep it off without having to exercise. Of course, no such magic exists. Even if there were a diet that could make losing weight easy, the key to keeping weight off is engaging in regular physical activity and eating a diet that is low to moderate in calories and that consists primarily of vegetables and lean protein. Similarly, exercise alone, without reducing calories in, does not necessarily result in significant weight loss. An abundance of research has established that long-term success in managing weight involves exercising regularly and eating moderately.

Defining Fitness

Physical fitness is to the human body what fine-tuning is to an engine. It enables you to perform up to your potential. Fitness is a condition that helps you look, feel, and do your best. There are a number of definitions of physical fitness. One of them is: "The ability to perform daily tasks vigorously and alertly, with energy left over for enjoying leisure-time activities and meeting emergency demands. It is the ability to endure, to bear up, to withstand stress, to carry on in circumstances where an unfit person could not continue, and is a major basis for good health and well-being."[1]

Another definition of physical fitness is that it is a state of being able to function efficiently and effectively without injury, to enjoy leisure, to be healthy, to resist disease, and to cope with demanding situations.[2] Physical fitness is the capacity to carry out the day's activities, pursue recreational activities, and have the physical capacity to handle emergency situations.

Despite the evidence that physical fitness is essential for good health and that expending calories and maintaining muscle mass through exercise is essential for weight management, millions of adults—and more and more children—are essentially sedentary. According to one survey of physical activity trends among residents of 26 states,[3] roughly 6 in 10 adults either were not active at all or were engaged in physical activity only on an irregular basis. Of the 4 in 10 adults who did engage in regular physical activity, only 1 out of 10 got enough exercise to promote or maintain fitness.

People who exercise more or less regularly and still don't lose weight usually have a higher calorie intake than they realize—the calories they consume are about equal to, or more than, the calories they burn. Or they may engage in less exercise than is actually necessary to lose weight, or they simply do the wrong kind of exercise. (For example, Pilates is good for building muscle, but aerobic exercise is better for burning calories.) Another problem may be that they are not achieving sufficient intensity during their workouts to make a difference, or that they simply aren't working out long enough or often enough. It takes months, if not years, of working out with a variety of exercises with sufficient intensity, duration, and frequency to obtain optimum fitness. Plus, exercise routines need to be changed regularly as muscles adapt. Working out with a qualified personal trainer can increase your chances of doing what it takes to achieve optimal fitness. Finding an Internet program or a smartphone application that helps motivate you for greater fitness is a good idea, too.

TIP

The **C25K** (i.e., Couch to 5K) app that Jacob—whose story introduced this chapter—chose is like having a personal trainer, and aims to help the "couch potato" train for running a 5K race. (Five kilometers is just over three miles.) It is a good program for those who want to challenge themselves. The program shepherds nonrunners through easy walking/jogging workouts, gradually building to a 5K race distance. It provides an effective way to ease into running without discomfort and helps smooth the transition from not running at all to actually being able to do a fun run. The routine requires a mix of timed walking and jogging, and the app handles the details for you, giving you audio prompts for when to walk or run while you listen to music of your choice.[4]

Aside from the elderly and infirm, those least likely to engage in exercise are the obese. One study found that of 1,172 American men and women, overweight females were most likely to find it hard to start or continue exercise. At the time of that study, two-thirds of subjects were not exercising regularly, and nearly one-quarter indicated they did not intend to start exercising in the next six months. Of those who tried to exercise, only 20 percent were able to maintain regular exercise for six months or longer. Clearly, many people encounter barriers to exercise despite its well-known benefits.

Benefits of Exercise

Most people think that if they exercise they must cut back on calories and lose weight to get any benefit. While this is certainly the best approach for losing weight, there are benefits to exercise even if you don't lose much weight. One study that illustrated this point included 24 middle-aged men who weren't in the habit of exercising. Eight were lean, eight were obese, and eight had type 2 diabetes. For three months, the subjects followed a fairly rigorous exercise program that consisted of an hour of aerobic exercise five times a week. The twist was they were told to eat enough to compensate for the extra calories burned while exercising so that they would *not* lose weight. Two results stood out: In all three groups, the waist size of the men shrank by about an inch, and the levels of interleukin-6 (an inflammatory chemical produced by fat and certain other tissues) declined. Most important, exercise produced a measurable reduction in health risk despite their not losing weight.

An important reason that being overweight is unhealthy is that fat tissues are metabolically active, producing hormones and chemicals that harm the cardiovascular system, the liver, and other systems. Getting and staying active with exercise helps cut down this risk. Of course, if you are overweight, exercise that brings about some weight loss is even better than exercise that does not. Both cutting calories and exercising are necessary to lose weight. But even if you don't lose weight, staying fit and active promotes better health.

Not only does regular exercise offer improved health and increased protection from heart problems as you age, but exercise can also boost your brain size and reduce the risk of developing dementia as well as other less serious memory loss.[5] Research suggests that doing aerobic exercise—mostly brisk walking—three days a week for 45 minutes a day increased the size of participants' brains. It makes sense that strength training would help, too, but the research on this isn't in yet. Your best approach is to embark on an exercise program that involves aerobic exercise, strength training, and stretching and that leads to optimal fitness.

Overcoming Barriers to Exercise

Unfortunately, many people encounter barriers to exercising. These can include attitude, schedules, fears, and worries, as well as any number of other "reasons" for not exercising. These barriers must be overcome to achieve physical fitness. Good intentions and an awareness of the benefits of exercise, though important, may not be enough to get started on, or stick to, an exercise program. Starting and maintaining an exercise program can be a daunting task, especially if you embrace perceived barriers to exercise. See Table 5.1 for common barriers cited by people who do not exercise. It is crucial to think of ways to overcome barriers such as these once you have identified them. You probably need to challenge some of your beliefs. You may also have to reevaluate your schedule to "find the time" to exercise. Be aware that you may be giving yourself excuses for not exercising that just aren't valid. For example, one man who initially claimed that he didn't have time to get out and walk admitted that he could spend less time with his ham radio activities in order to increase his physical activity.

Having the confidence that you can be more physically active, and that becoming so will help you achieve your health and weight goals, is important. With confidence, you are more likely to make every effort to overcome barriers to exercising. Part of this involves deciding that leading a healthy lifestyle, which includes regular exercise, is an important personal value for you. You must become committed to making regular exercise a part of your lifestyle. It has to be "just what I do." Undertaking exercise or intensifying your current exercise means starting from wherever you are now and setting small but challenging goals to get you to where you want to be.

WHEN TO SEE A DOCTOR FIRST

Most people find that regular exercise is invigorating and gives them more energy for other things. Worries about suffering injury or a debilitating heart event as the result of exercise are usually not warranted, but it is a good idea to see your doctor first before undertaking vigorous exercise if you are concerned. Not doing too much too soon makes health problems from exercising less likely. A common prescription for those who have had a heart attack is to get regular exercise to improve the strength of the heart as well as to improve overall fitness.

Table 5.1
BARRIERS TO EXERCISE

Attitude:	"It's boring." "I just don't feel like it."
Excuses and rationalizations:	"I don't have anyone to exercise with." "I'm too old to start now." "I can't stick with it, so there's no point in trying." "Exercise makes me hungrier."
Lack of time:	"Taking care of kids all day, I don't have any time for myself."
Fatigue:	"I'm tired and want to relax after working all day."
Worry/fear:	"What if I have a heart attack?"
Lack of knowledge:	"I don't know how to get started."
Lack of success:	"I have tried exercising before and it didn't help."
Self-consciousness:	"I don't want others to see me in exercise clothes."
Environmental barriers:	"Where I live, I can't exercise."

If you are over 35 years of age, especially if you have been sedentary and are obese, it is a good idea to check with your doctor before undertaking a relatively vigorous conditioning program. If you are 35 or younger, have not been completely sedentary for years, have no previous history of cardiovascular disease and no known risk factors, and have had a medical evaluation within the past two years, you can probably begin an aerobic exercise program without special medical clearance. If you have any risk factors for cardiovascular disease—that is, if you smoke, are obese or sedentary, have high blood pressure or high cholesterol, or have a family history of heart disease—a supervised exercise stress test may be appropriate before you undertake a vigorous exercise program. Table 5.2 lists the factors that indicate a need for medical clearance prior to undertaking vigorous exercise.

Components of an Optimal Fitness Program

Optimal fitness means being the best that you can be physically, given your age, gender, and body. This should be the ultimate goal of your exercise program, although it will probably take you time to attain optimal fitness. The components of optimal fitness include *cardiovascular* (also called cardiorespiratory or aerobic) fitness, which is achieved with endurance training; *muscle strength and endurance*, which includes core strength and is achieved

---

Table 5.2

WHEN TO SEE A DOCTOR BEFORE UNDERTAKING VIGOROUS EXERCISE

Consult your doctor before beginning an exercise program if you

- are over thirty-five years of age.

- have not had a medical checkup in more than two years.

- smoke.

- are more than 30 percent above recommended weight.

- have any close male relatives (father, brother) who have had a heart attack or stroke before the age of fifty-five or any close female relatives (mother, sister) who have had a heart attack or stroke before the age of sixty-five.

- have heart trouble or a heart murmur or have had a heart attack yourself.

- have irregular heartbeats or uneven heart action.

- have uncontrolled high blood pressure or are on medication for hypertension.

- have kidney disease.

- have insulin-dependent diabetes.

- have elevated cholesterol.

- have bone, joint, muscle, or vein problems, such as arthritis, rheumatism, bad back, or bad leg veins.

- have a resting heart rate (RHR) of more than 80 beats per minute.

- easily become short of breath doing ordinary activities.

- often feel faint or have dizzy spells.

- often experience pain or pressure in the left shoulder or arm, midchest area, or left side of your neck during or right after exercise.

- have any doubts about your health status.

---

through resistance training; and *joint flexibility*, which involves stretching and movement exercise. Two other important types of exercise that accelerate fat loss include interval training and circuit training.

To achieve optimal fitness, you need to participate regularly in a variety of exercises that address all of these components. Because exercise that develops one aspect of fitness generally contributes little to the other fitness components, different exercises should be chosen to meet individual needs and capacities.

CARDIOVASCULAR FITNESS

Cardiovascular fitness is the cornerstone of good health. Aerobic or endurance exercises that promote cardiovascular fitness are a crucial part of a well-rounded exercise program. The term "cardiovascular fitness" refers to the heart's ability to pump oxygen-rich blood to the muscles. (The term "aerobic" means "in the presence of oxygen.") Any activity that employs the large muscles of the body, especially the leg muscles, for a relatively continuous time, that is rhythmic in nature, with sufficient intensity to elevate the heart rate, and that promotes the body's ability to utilize oxygen efficiently is classified as aerobic or endurance exercise. Examples include brisk walking, jogging or running, swimming laps, bicycling hard, singles tennis, hiking hills, spinning, interval training, and circuit training.

Anaerobic exercise is brief, intense exercise such as heavy weight-lifting, sprinting, or any exercise requiring high intensity and a high rate of work for a short period of time. The term anaerobic means "without air" or "without oxygen," but it is still a component of cardiovascular and optimal fitness. Overall, anaerobic exercise burns fewer calories than does aerobic exercise and is somewhat less beneficial for cardiovascular fitness. However, it is better at building strength and muscle mass and still benefits the heart and lungs. In the long run, increased muscle mass helps a person become leaner and manage weight, because muscle burns large amounts of calories.

To achieve cardiovascular fitness you need to start wherever you are on the fitness continuum and work toward optimal fitness. Your first goal should be to get enough aerobic exercise. Walking is a good activity to begin with; later in this chapter you will learn more about walking for exercise and good health. An advantage of walking is that it is free and can be done whenever you can fit it in. If you have been sedentary, you should start at a comfortable level and gradually increase your walking until you can do more and more each day.

> **TIP**
>
> **Cychosis** is a great app for cycling that costs a small fee.[6] It provides a clean and efficient training log for cyclists letting you record nitty-gritty details about daily rides as well as big-picture goals for the year. It summarizes your rides for the week, month, year, or all time, and allows you to review the data in graphs that chart distances, average speed, and times for your rides. You can also add any number of distance goals and track your progress toward them on the Goals screen.

MUSCLE STRENGTH AND ENDURANCE

Muscle strength is the ability to exert force. Muscle endurance is the ability to sustain an activity over a period of time. With adequate muscle strength and endurance, you are able to perform all activities, including those of daily living, with less stress. Adequate muscle strength and endurance allow you to walk, stand, or sit without becoming overly fatigued or experiencing back pain. In the absence of this type of fitness you tire easily, your efficiency suffers, and your productivity declines.

Muscle fitness and endurance are achieved through resistance, strength-building, and weight-bearing activities. These include lifting weights and can involve using exercise resistance bands or tubes as well as dumbbells; working out with machines that isolate particular muscle groups; and doing a range of exercises, including floor exercises that use various body parts to provide the resistance. (Exercise resistance bands can be obtained from Internet stores like Amazon and also from stores such as Target.) Floor exercises are done on the floor and work various muscles or muscle groups; an example of a floor exercise is doing sit-ups. The current trend in fitness is to use multiple groups of muscles at a time, rather than isolating a particular muscle group. Core fitness is the first order of business in strength and endurance training.

Core fitness is the basis for being able to move without incurring injury and is required before seriously training all muscle groups. It focuses on developing strong abdominal muscles, and these exercises should be done daily. Examples of core exercises include sit-ups, reverse crunches, "bridging" (which involves pushing the mid body up from the floor using the legs and shoulders), and various other exercises focusing on the abdominal muscles. Learning to tighten the midsection of the body—known as "pulling the belly button to the spine"—is an important skill. Having a strong core reduces the likelihood of experiencing back pain.

Another advantage of striving for good, overall muscle strength is that over time it can build muscle mass. Men can do this more easily than women because they have more of the hormone testosterone. (They also start off with more muscle mass than women.) Muscles that are not exercised regularly atrophy; that is, they shrink in size over time—thus the maxim "use it or lose it." (It's not true that muscle turns into fat, but it is true that muscles shrink, and over time fat is gained.) As men and women age, they tend to exercise less and be less active in general; as a result muscle mass decreases, along with muscle strength and endurance. In addition, metabolism decreases along with muscle mass, leading to weight gain unless there is a corresponding decrease in caloric intake. The chronically sedentary person inevitably loses muscle mass without exercise and gains weight as the metabolism slows down.

To attain muscle strength and endurance in particular muscle groups, you need at least two or three sessions of resistance exercise per week to yield improvement. A range of exercises that work the muscle groups should be selected depending on your goal. Building strength requires gradually increasing weight and stressing the muscles. Endurance involves doing multiple repetitions at low weight. That is, high weight with few repetitions builds muscle, while low weight with high repetition encourages endurance.

The number of sets (a "set" is a specific number of repetitions—a set may include 10 or 20 repetitions, for example) you do depends on your goal. Start doing two to three sets of each exercise and gradually increase the number of sets or the number of repetitions per set. Proper form is key. Posture is important. You also need to move the resistance (e.g., the dumbbells) in a slow, controlled manner and avoid going too fast or jerking the weights. Maintain normal breathing and don't hold your breath. Exhale during exertion. Resistance training should be rhythmic, performed at a moderate to slow pace, and involve a full range of motion. Working with a personal trainer who is observing you and making corrections as necessary ensures that you will get the most out of your workout. Some gyms provide an initial workout and introduction to the weights and machines with a trainer at no additional cost. If you want to keep working with a trainer, there is usually a fee.

Weight training involving the large muscle groups should not be done on consecutive days, whereas exercises utilizing the smaller muscle groups can be. A day of rest between sessions involving large muscle groups allows the muscles to recuperate. Without recuperation time, the risk of injury increases. Some people do weight training five or six days a week, but they alternate muscle groups from day to day so that a specific muscle group is trained only two or three days a week. This is called a "split routine." Those who want to do a full body workout, which involves working all the major muscle groups in one session, should do this only two or three times a week on nonconsecutive days.

TIP If you want help in getting starting with an exercise program focused on muscle strength and endurance, you don't have to hire a trainer. The **iFitness** app, for a small fee, acts as your personal trainer.[7] It presents over 200 exercises, all with clear photos and instructions for how to do each exercise safely and correctly. You can browse by category or muscle group and follow a workout checklist with a suggested routine or create your own custom set of exercises. **iFitness** lets you log and chart your progress in a journal with entry screens tailored for each exercise.

JOINT FLEXIBILITY

Flexibility refers to how fully your joints or limbs are able to move. Being flexible allows for easier movements and reduced pain in joints, making it easier to perform daily activities. Flexibility is a fitness goal overlooked by many people. Adequate flexibility helps you avoid muscle pulls and strains, while lack of flexibility usually contributes to sports injuries, lower back pain, and those annoying pains and injuries that often seem to occur out of nowhere when you reach for something or bend to pick it up. Any sudden stretching that forcibly extends a muscle beyond its limits can produce injury and pain. Regular stretching exercises, in addition to helping to improve appearance by promoting good posture, protect against possible injury.

Static stretching, also known as passive stretching, is the most commonly recommended stretching exercise. It involves slowly stretching a muscle to the point of mild tension and then holding that position for a period of time—usually 10–30 seconds, or longer, until you feel the tension release or you no longer feel much tension. Static stretching has a low risk of injury, requires little time or assistance, and is quite effective. Ballistic stretching, also known as dynamic stretching, which uses the momentum created by repetitive bouncing movements to stretch muscles, should be avoided by those who are not high-performance athletes as it can result in injury if not done properly.

Yoga and Tai Chi are two forms of exercise that involve gentle movement stretching. Check local listings on the Web for classes. Another way to engage in these activities without having to join a class is to join Netflix; they have a catalog of DVDs from beginning to advanced yoga that you can rent, as well as Tai Chi videos.

TIP If you want to do yoga at your convenience and avoid traveling to classes, try the **Yoga STRETCH** app, which is available for a small fee.[8] This app is like having your own personal yoga instructor in your pocket. She won't be able to teach you poses you don't already know, but if you are familiar with basic yoga positions, you can program your own sessions with your own music (or use the default music included). **Yoga STRETCH** tells you which stretch to do and when to change. Each pose includes a silhouette of a woman doing the pose against beautiful backgrounds. You can pause your workout, skip poses, or go back to a previous pose as needed.

INTERVAL TRAINING

In terms of losing weight, *interval training* produces more weight loss than steady, moderate-intensity aerobic exercise such as walking or jogging, and is a type of exercise that should be part of any serious weight loss effort. Interval training involves bursts of high-intensity exercise alternating with periods of rest or low-intensity activity—the "intervals" in interval training. The term refers to any cardiovascular exercise—such as spinning or using an elliptical machine—that can be done in brief, intense bouts (from 30 seconds to 2 minutes) of exercise done at near-maximum exertion (measured by heart rate) interspersed with periods of lower-intensity activity. A bout of high-intensity exercise followed by a low-intensity exercise cycle is called a "set." Repeated sets done for about 20 minutes three times a week can produce significant fat loss. Part of the reason for this is that interval training drains the muscles of inbuilt energy sources and replenishment takes up to 48 hours to occur—resulting in prolonged fat burn, referred to as "afterburn."

A good source of information on interval training as well as programs for beginners through advanced can be found at **www.intervaltraining.net**.

A popular type of exercise mentioned earlier that lends itself well to interval training is spinning. Usually done in classes, spinning involves riding a stationary bike that allows for adjustments of tension. Spinning rates depend on heart rate (see the content later in this chapter about target heart rate), and the exercise is done in intervals. Kickboxing can also be adapted for interval training.

CIRCUIT TRAINING

Circuit training is a combination of high-intensity aerobics and resistance training exercises designed for muscle building and heart–lung fitness. It also helps with fat burning. An exercise "circuit" is one completion of all prescribed exercises in the program, of which there can be six or more. When one circuit is complete, the exercises are repeated for another circuit. The duration of individual circuit training stations can be in the region of 45–60 seconds and in some cases as long as two minutes, depending on the number of repetitions performed at each station. Higher repetitions put the exercise further toward the endurance end of the intensity continuum. Fewer repetitions and increased weight optimize muscle strength and bulk. Typically, circuit training boosts heart rate.

It can be difficult to do circuit training without a buddy or coach to time your circuits. The **Circuit Training Timer** for the iPhone, the iPod, the iPad, and the Android solves the problem. This app plays the role of a trainer, assisting you in composing your workout as well as timing your circuits. It provides you with audible cues to move to the next exercise as you do your circuit, so you can focus on exercise, not on the timing of sets. Listen to your favorites from your music library for inspiration as you work out.

COMBINING EXERCISES

To achieve optimal fitness, you will want to combine exercises focused on cardiovascular fitness (aerobic and anaerobic exercise), muscle strength and endurance, and stretching exercise. Doing interval training or circuit training accelerates weight loss and fitness. It is helpful if you can combine exercises that are varied and that you enjoy. One woman who was committed to improving her fitness and losing weight did a spinning class on Tuesdays and a kick-boxing class on Thursdays. On weekends she usually did a five-mile hike. Two of the other days she worked out with a trainer. That may seem like a lot of exercise if you are just starting out, but this routine is one that can lead to good physical fitness and weight loss.

Beginning Your Exercise Program

Having decided to undertake an exercise program that leads toward optimum fitness, you are now in a position to determine what you need to do to reach this goal. Warming up and cooling down are important parts of any exercise workout. This should be done each time you exercise. Learning to assess your target heart rate is a skill you need so you can know if you are exerting yourself enough while you exercise.

WARMING UP AND COOLING DOWN

You should begin every exercise workout session by warming up. The purpose of warming up is to increase the core temperature of the body and muscles to get them ready for more strenuous activity. By getting your muscles warmed up, you are helping them to become loose, supple, and pliable, which reduces the risk of injury. An effective warmup increases both your heart rate and your respiration, which helps to deliver nutrients, remove waste products, and supply oxygen to muscles. Warming up also helps get you psychologically ready for your exercise workout.

A warmup has certain key elements. The general warmup consists of light physical activity, which allows the muscles to be stretched effectively afterwards. It lasts about 10–15 minutes and usually results in a light sweat. An example would be walking at a moderate pace on the treadmill before stretching. Gentle, static stretching should be done for all the major muscle groups after the general warmup and lasts for about 10–15 minutes. After the general warmup and static stretching, the body needs to be prepared for more demands if a specific sport is to be undertaken. This involves more vigorous warming up. Activity at this time should reflect the movements and actions that will be required during the sport. For example, in anticipation of a bicycle race or long bicycle ride, some short "joy-riding" or light pedaling is a good idea. For a footrace, easy jogging for a short distance would be good preparation.

TIP   For more information on warming up and a short video on stretching, go to **www.thestretchinghandbook.com/archives/warm-up.php**.

When you have finished your exercise or activity, you need to cool down and stretch again. Cooling down is an essential part of your routine. Cooling down helps the heart rate and breathing return to normal and the muscles return to rest. The three elements of cooling down are gentle exercise (slowing down and gradually decreasing intensity), stretching, and refueling. If you have been jogging, you should drop back to a fast walk and then progressively slow down. If walking briskly is your chosen exercise, simply slow down gradually. Stretch the muscle groups you have been working. Finally, drink water, and eat a small and healthy snack after exercising.

Muscle fibers, tendons, and ligaments undergo a lot of strain during intense exercise. This produces lactic acid, a waste product that can cause muscle stiffness and soreness. A proper cooldown helps the body chemistry readjust and is vital for the removal of lactic acid from the muscles. Cooling down helps prevent delayed-onset muscle soreness (DOMS). This soreness is generally felt a day or two after a strenuous workout. Cooling down for about 10 minutes can prevent or reduce the risk of DOMS.

TIP A good source for more information on warming up and cooling down is **www.mydr.com.au/sports-fitness/ warming-up-and-cooling-down-for-exercise**.

TARGET HEART RATE

Intensity of aerobic exercise can be measured by assessing target heart rate. The target heart rate zone is the percentage of maximum exercise heart rate (MEHR) at which you will benefit most from exercise. The American College of Sports Medicine provides guidelines that indicate the percent of MEHR that will allow you to reach your fitness goals. You should choose your limits based on your present level of fitness and your exercise goals.

Sedentary persons should strive to do exercise that reaches 50 percent of MEHR. Initially, the upper limit should be no more than 60–75 percent. These limits are also recommended for older or overweight people until their fitness level improves. Those who have been exercising and who have optimal fitness as a goal need to exercise at a level of intensity that produces a heart rate between 60 and 90 percent of maximum. However, benefits start to tail off with intensity greater than 85 percent. Unless you expect to compete in a sport that requires a very high level of fitness, you probably should not exceed 75–80 percent of maximum.

Calculating Your Target Heart Rate Zone

There are several ways to determine your target heart rate zone. One is to use the following equations, which allow you to calculate the lower and upper limits of your choice for your age:

Lower limit = (220 – Your age) × 0.50 = Beats per minute

Upper limit = (220 – Your age) × 0.75 = Beats per minute

Note that 0.50 and 0.75 are arbitrary lower and upper limits; you can choose any percentage you like for these numbers. Once you get these numbers, you can divide by 6 to get your beats for every 10-minute interval. Alternatively, look up your target heart rate limit in Table 5.3.

TIP There are a number of iPhone apps for monitoring heart rate. To get a summary and overview of 25 top heart rate monitors, visit **www.iphoneness. com/iphone-apps/best-heart-rate-monitors-for-iphone/**. For example, **iHeart** is a pulse reader that lets you figure out your pulse by holding your iPhone in your hands; it can't get easier than that! Similarly, **iHeartRateMonitor** makes it easy to track your heart rate just by tapping your iPhone. It also lets you know what heart rate zone you are in. It comes with a complete guide with videos to take your

Table 5.3
LIMITS FOR TARGET HEART RATE ZONE

Age	50%		60%		75%		85%		90%	
	Beats/ Min.	10-Sec. Count	Beats/ Min.	10-Sec. Count	Beats/ Min.	10-Sec. Count	Beats/ Min.	10-Sec. Count	Beats/ Min.	10-Sec. Count
20	100	17	120	20	150	25	170	28	180	30
25	98	16	117	20	146	24	166	28	176	29
30	95	16	114	19	143	24	162	27	171	29
35	93	15	111	19	139	23	157	26	167	28
40	90	15	108	18	135	23	153	26	162	27
45	88	15	105	18	131	22	149	25	158	26
50	85	14	102	17	128	21	145	24	153	26
55	83	14	99	17	124	21	140	23	149	25
60	80	13	96	16	120	20	136	23	144	24
65	78	13	93	16	116	19	132	22	140	23

workout to the next level, and it tracks both heart rate and calories burned. **Fitview** tracks heart rate, blood sugar, and other vitals. For the more advanced, **iRunXtreme** is a highly sophisticated app that lets you monitor your heart rate using your iPhone microphone.

Staying in the Zone

Before you begin your aerobic exercise or interval training, you should determine your target heart rate zone based on your age and the upper and lower limits you have chosen. As a beginning exerciser, you need to take your pulse (Figure 5.1) three or four times or more during an exercise session, or about every 5–10 minutes, until you learn what your body feels like in the zone. Take it first after you have finished warming up. After your warmup, when you are ready to begin your exercise session, your heart rate should be approaching the lower limit of your target heart rate zone, although it would not yet be in the zone.

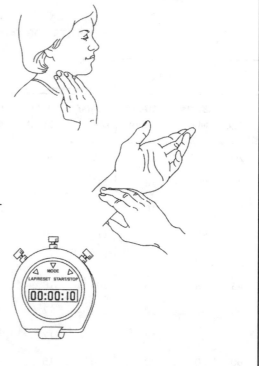

1. Locate your carotid artery with the tips of your third and fourth fingers. (The carotid artery is in the front strip of muscle that runs vertically down your neck.) Press your fingers on one side only of the neck. Press lightly with your fingers until you feel the blood pulsing beneath your fingers.

or

Find your radial artery by pressing your fingers on the inside of your wrist just below your wrist bone.

2. Using a watch with a sweep hand or with a digital read-out of seconds, count the number of times your heart beats in ten seconds.

3. Multiply the number of beats you feel for 10 seconds by six to get your heart rate (pulse) per minute. Compare this to your target heart rate zone. Adjust your exercise intensity up or down so you are in your target heart rate zone.

Figure 5.1
HOW TO TAKE YOUR PULSE

Next take your pulse about 5 minutes into the aerobic part of your exercise session. By then you should be in your target heart rate zone. If you are below the lower limit, increase your level of effort (e.g., increase your speed or intensity). If you are above the upper limit, slow down or reduce the intensity so that your heart rate recedes into the zone. Continue to take your heart rate periodically throughout your exercise session, and adjust your level of effort up or down so that you stay in your target zone.

Check your heart rate again immediately after stopping the aerobic part of your exercise session. As you become more physically fit, your heart rate will be lower for the same amount and intensity of exercise. Eventually you will need to adjust the intensity of the exercise upward to get your heart rate back up in the zone. Finally, check your heart rate near the end of your cool-down phase (when you are walking slowly or exercising with less intensity). Over time, as you reach your goal of optimum fitness, your heart rate will return to your baseline—where your heart rate usually is—more quickly. (In fact, "recovery heart rate" is one measure of fitness.)

Perceived Exertion Method

Unfortunately, not everyone can use target heart rate zone to assess intensity. Some people have a naturally high or naturally low heart rate. Certain medications, such as those containing beta blockers (e.g., some high blood pressure medications) can also increase or decrease heart rate. Pulse monitoring may not be appropriate for cardiac patients, diabetics, or pregnant women.

Such people may need to use a *perceived exertion* method.[9] Perceived exertion is how hard you feel like your body is working. It is based on the physical sensations you experience during physical activity, including increased heart rate, increased respiration or breathing rate, increased sweating, flushing of the face, and muscle fatigue. Using perceived exertion to assess intensity of exercise involves paying attention to your physical sensations. Even though this is a subjective measure, research suggests that there is a high correlation between a person's perceived exertion rating and actual heart rate during activity.

To learn more about the perceived exertion method, visit:
http://sportsmedicine.about.com/cs/strengthening/a/030904.htm.

When, How Much, and How to Exercise

If you are undertaking an exercise program for the first time, you probably have a number of questions: When is the best time to exercise? How much exercise do I need to do? How do I cope with challenging weather conditions?

TIP   A good app for beginning a program of exercise is **iExercise**, which currently costs a small fee to download. This app, which is designed specifically for the iPhone, helps you set goals for various kinds of exercise and lets you monitor how many calories you burn from exercising. There's a fairly comprehensive list of exercise activities, everything from a treadmill run to playing soccer to mowing the lawn. Just choose your activity and then enter the number of minutes you participated. You can also enter the desired amount of calories you want to burn. **iExercise** does the calculations for you. It even rewards you with Achievement Awards for reaching certain goals. It is easy to use and has a great interface. To check it out further on the Web, go to: **http://www.iexercise.info/iExercise/Introducing.html**.[10]

WHEN TO EXERCISE

There is no "best" time to exercise. Some people prefer to start off the day with exercising in the morning. Others claim that their body isn't ready to move until later in the day. Some people work out during their lunch hours, while others go to the gym after work. The hour just before the evening meal is a popular time for exercise. Some people even work out late at night at 24-hour fitness facilities. When you work out is up to you, although studies have shown that, from a motivational point of view, most people find it is better to do exercise sooner rather than later in the day. Waiting until later means that other demands can preempt exercise and take it off your calendar. Likewise, having an appointment for exercise makes it more likely you will actually do it, whether that appointment is for a session with a personal trainer or just for a walk with a friend. It is generally advisable to wait an hour or so after eating a big meal before exercising, but having a light snack beforehand is a good idea. If you exercise in the morning, you should have something light to eat first, such as yogurt. Be aware that doing stimulating exercise just before bedtime may make it harder to fall asleep. To decide the best time for you, consider the demands of your particular schedule and listen to your body.

HOW MUCH TO EXERCISE

According to the *2008 Physical Activity Guidelines for Americans* published by the Centers for Disease Control and Prevention, you need to do two types of physical activity every week to improve your health: aerobic exercise and muscle-strengthening activities. Stretching can be done every day. Different guidelines exist for how much exercise is recommended for adults, children, and seniors, depending on several factors.

For health benefits, adults who are *not* overweight should engage in at least 2½ hours (150 minutes) each week of moderate-intense aerobic activity (i.e., brisk walking or jogging) plus, on two or more days a week, muscle-strengthening activities that work all major muscle groups (legs, hips, back, abdomen, chest, shoulders, and arms). Alternatively, they should participate in 1¼ hours (75 minutes) per week of vigorous-intensity activity (i.e., running) plus, on two or more days a week, muscle-strengthening activities that work all major muscle groups, or an equivalent mix of moderate- and vigorous-intensity aerobic activity and muscle-strengthening activities on two or more days a week that work all major muscle groups.

For even greater health benefits including *weight loss*, adults should increase their activity to 5 hours (300 minutes) each week of moderate-intensity aerobic activity and muscle-strengthening activities on two or more days a week working all major muscle groups. Alternatively, adults need 2½ hours (150 minutes) each week of vigorous-intensity activity and two or more days of muscle-strengthening activities working all major muscle groups, or an equivalent mix of moderate- and vigorous-intensity aerobic activity and muscle-strengthening activities two or more days a week.

A 2010 study in the *Journal of the American Medical Association* assessed the amount of physical activity needed for older women (their average age was 54 years) consuming a usual diet of moderate calories to prevent weight gain.[11] The researchers concluded that the women in the study who were successful in maintaining normal weight and gaining fewer than 5 pounds over 13 years averaged approximately 60 minutes a day of moderate-intensity activity throughout the study.

How do you know if you are doing light-, moderate-, or vigorous-intensity aerobic activity? You need to get your heart rate up into the target heart rate zone. (Heart rate was discussed in a previous section of the book in more detail.) Moderate-intensity aerobic activity means you're working hard enough to raise your heart rate and break a sweat. Examples of moderate-intensity aerobic activity include walking fast, water aerobics, biking on level ground or with a few hills, or doubles tennis. Vigorous-intensity aerobic activity means you are breathing hard and fast and your heart rate has gone up quite a bit. Some examples include running, swimming laps, riding a bike fast or on hills, playing singles tennis, or playing basketball. If doing a mix of moderate- and vigorous-intensity activity, the rule of thumb is that one minute of vigorous activity is about the same as two minutes of moderate-intensity activity.

Remember that for fast and efficient weight loss, adding interval training (discussed earlier in this chapter) is best. Research shows that the short bursts of high-intensity exercise lasting from seconds to minutes followed by periods of rest or low-intensity exercise is more effective at inducing fat loss than simply training consistently at a moderate-intensity level.

TIP To find guidelines for physical activity for children, visit **www.cdc.gov/ physicalactivity/everyone/guidelines/children.html**. For guidelines for seniors, those 65 and older, go to: **www.cdc.gov/physicalactivity/everyone/ guidelines/olderadults.html**. Additional guidelines are provided at the CDC website for pregnant and postpartum women.

F.I.T.T. AND THE OVERLOAD PRINCIPLE

The overload principle is based on the idea that when muscles are exercised at a level above that at which they normally operate, they adapt so that they function more efficiently. Overload can be accomplished in several ways: by increasing the *frequency* of your exercise (how often you exercise), by increasing the *intensity* of your exercise (how hard you exercise), or by increasing the duration of your exercise (the length of time you exercise). Optimal levels of frequency, intensity, and duration (time) depend on the *type* of exercise involved—whether it is cardiorespiratory exercise, or resistance exercise. This principle is referred to as the F.I.T.T. (frequency, intensity, time, and type) prescription.[12]

Your individual F.I.T.T. prescription depends on your goal. For example, if your goal is to run a 5K race, your F.I.T.T prescription must focus primarily on your aerobic capacity, which involves cardiorespiratory activity. If, on the other hand, you want to be a better golfer, you will adjust your F.I.T.T. prescription for muscle strength and endurance exercises that attack those muscles you most need in playing golf—resistance exercises that focus on the core, the back, and the arms. Snow skiing requires doing exercises that puts the main focus on leg muscles. Of course, the core and other muscle groups should not be neglected.

EXERCISING IN EVERY TYPE OF WEATHER

Cold weather, precipitation, very hot and humid weather, and darkness can pose special problems for exercising safely outdoors. Rather than giving up, you can take the following precautions to promote safe exercise under adverse conditions. And always be sure to tell someone where you are going.

On cold days:

◎   Wear several layers of clothing rather than one heavy layer. The inner layer should be a material that wicks away moisture, such as polypropylene or wool. Do not wear cotton next to your skin, because it loses its ability to insulate when you perspire and it gets wet.

◎   Avoid using cotton socks for the same reason given above; choose wool socks or socks that help moisture evaporate.

◎   Use mittens, gloves, or socks to protect your hands.

◎   Wear a hat and scarf; up to 40 percent of your body's heat is lost through your neck and head.

On rainy, icy, or snowy days:

◎ Be aware of reduced visibility for both yourself and drivers. Be careful around cars and traffic. Wear bright clothing, or apply reflective tape to your workout clothes. Consider wearing ski glasses or goggles that enhance your ability to see contrasts, especially in snow.

◎ Be aware of reduced traction on sidewalks and roads. You could slip and fall, or a car might not be able to stop quickly.

◎ Consider investing in exercise clothing made of special material that repels water but that allows moisture produced by the body to escape (see the *On cold days* list above for more information on wicking fabrics). Some of this clothing absorbs body odors readily and should be washed frequently.

On hot, humid days:

◎ Exercise during the cooler hours of the day, such as early morning or early evening after the sun has gone down.

◎ Drink lots of cold water. Hydrate with water before you start to exercise. Avoid using electrolyte-replacement drinks (they slow down the absorption of fluids from the stomach) unless you drink lots of water, too.

◎ Wear minimal light, loose-fitting clothing so that your body sweat can evaporate easily.

◎ Wear sunblock and a hat to prevent overexposure to the sun. Remember that even on cloudy days the sun can damage your skin.

◎ Avoid clothing that makes you sweat, such as sweatpants.

◎ Watch out for signs of heat stroke—dizziness, weakness, lightheadedness, or excessive fatigue.

At night or on dark days:

◎ Wear bright, reflective clothing, preferably with special reflective tape or markings.

◎ Carry a flashlight or wear a headlamp.

◎ Put reflective tape on your shoes.

◎ Attach a blinking red light to the back of your clothing or bicycle.

COPING WITH DISCOMFORT

Some discomfort is a natural consequence when you first begin to exercise, but the old maxim "no pain, no gain" is outdated. The overload principle of fitness states that a greater than normal stress or load on the body is required for training adaptation to take place. What this means is that in order to improve fitness, strength, or endurance, you need to increase the workload accordingly. However, this does not mean pushing muscles to the point of experiencing pain. Pain is the body's signal to stop, and it should always be heeded.

When you first start a regular exercise program, you may find that you become easily fatigued and sometimes after the session you may feel muscle stiffness and soreness (although adequate warmup, cooldown, and stretching should reduce the risk, and intensity, of this). By starting exercise moderately and gradually increasing frequency, intensity, and duration of exercise, discomfort can be minimized, especially if you take time to stretch before and afterward. Using the principle of overload will naturally create some fatigue.

At the beginning of an exercise session, you may sometimes find that at first your body feels uncomfortable and leaden; you have to push through this feeling, which should last no more than five or ten minutes. Usually an adequate warmup will help you overcome this initial inertia. Working out with a personal trainer (or a friend) can help you stay motivated. Realize that even highly trained athletes have days when the body puts up a fight against exercise. Your attitude toward exercise is important at this point: You don't have to want to do it or enjoy every moment of it; you just need to do it! Acceptance of some discomfort and the need to overcome resistance are the dues you pay for better health.

Sometimes you may experience pain that is not threatening. A pain or "stitch" in your side while running or doing aerobic exercise is actually a cramp in your diaphragm. This is different from the pain that comes from injury. To manage it, simply slow down and focus on deep breathing and relaxing until the stitch goes away. You need to learn the difference between tolerating the natural discomfort that can come with exercising and pain that warns you to stop exercising. Pain that says "stop" is pain from an injury.

COPING WITH INJURY

Occasional injury is a normal risk of exercise, and it need not signal the end of your exercise efforts. Injury usually occurs because of lack of flexibility, muscle imbalance, or simple overexertion. Flexibility injuries—muscle pulls, ankle sprains, Achilles tendinitis, and shin splints—account for 90 percent of exercise-related injuries. You can usually prevent such injuries by warming up properly. Injury in general can be prevented by taking care to work opposing muscle groups, varying your exercise routine, and not attempting too much too soon. See Table 5.4 to learn more about when you need to stop.

Table 5.4
WARNING SIGNS TO STOP EXERCISING

◎ Pain in the chest, shoulders, arms, or abdomen

◎ Irregular heartbeat

◎ A sudden, very fast heart rate

◎ Shortness of breath when you aren't exercising very hard and you haven't been completely sedentary

◎ Unexplained dizziness

◎ Fainting

◎ Nausea

◎ Leg cramps

◎ Incoordination, confusion, or visual disturbances

◎ Pale, blue, or clammy complexion

If you do experience an injury, apply the RICE principle: Rest, Ice, Compression, and Elevation. Take it easy for a while and rest while your injury is healing. Immediately apply ice to the injured area, avoiding direct contact of ice to skin by using a towel or other material as a barrier. Cold causes damaged blood vessels to constrict, which in turn limits swelling. Continue to apply ice for 20-minute periods (followed by 20-minute rest periods without ice) a minimum of three to four times a day (more often is better) for two or three days after sustaining an injury. If possible, keep the injury wrapped lightly with an elastic bandage; compression constricts and pinches off damaged blood vessels. Just don't wrap it too tightly. Finally, keep the injury elevated, if possible, to slow the flow of blood to the area and minimize swelling. You can also use an anti-inflammatory medication to reduce irritation in the area. If an injury is severe or pain persists, consult your doctor or a physician who specializes in sports medicine. Whatever you do, don't keep using the injured body part.

Walking for Health and Weight Loss

A great way to begin exercising is to walk. Walking can be fun as well as health-enhancing. Although walking is not an exercise that necessarily elevates the heart rate, it still provides many benefits, including calorie burn. Hiking is another form of walking. It takes place on trails and involves walking hills and on uneven ground rather than just walking in the neighborhood or on a treadmill, and as a result it can burn a lot of calories, especially if your hikes last several hours.

STARTING FROM ZERO

Start walking around the neighborhood or on a high school track. Try several short walking sessions of 10 minutes each if you have been sedentary. Work on extending this time until you can walk at least 20 minutes at a time three days a week on a regular basis. Then begin to add days and extend time so that you are exercising 30 to 60 minutes a day most days of the week. As you become better conditioned, your goal is to complete 60 minutes of walking most days of the week.

If you have access to a treadmill or stationary bike, you might want to start with 10–20 minutes of walking or pedaling at a comfortable pace. Learn to use your target heart rate or perceived exertion, which was discussed earlier in this chapter, to assess the intensity of your exercise. On the treadmill you can vary the intensity by varying the angle of the machine and increasing the speed. The more vigorous (intense) your walking and the longer you walk, the more calories you will burn. Consider progressing from walking and using the treadmill to hiking. As your ability to walk is improving, you can also engage in a regular exercise program at a gym or at home.

TIP If you are a hiker, you might want to invest in the **Trails** app.[13] **Trails** is a GPS tracker that's perfectly tuned for capturing and sharing your adventures. It is ideal for casual mapping fans who take their trails seriously. **Trails** lets you review your tracks on either road maps or topographic maps, which can be downloaded to your phone so that you don't need an Internet connection while you are on the trail. The only hitch is that **Trails** has to run constantly to track your route—a big battery drain for long hikes.

To systematically increase your walking or hiking activity, it helps to use a pedometer—an instrument that attaches to your belt and measures the distance you walk or the number of steps you take. Pedometers are also available on many smartphones.

TIP A great app, and one that is simple to use, is **iTreadmill**.[14] It helps runners and walkers measure pace and distance using the motion detector of an iPhone or iPod. The device also turns into a pedometer that counts the number of steps you take. Start, stop, and pause buttons trigger **iTreadmill** to start measuring your run or walk and tracking your pace, distance, or steps. You can even enter your weight to have it estimate the number of calories you've burned. Before starting, tap the "cal" button on the top right to calibrate your stride. Then set your pace using the dial at the top right. If you turn the pacer on, the app makes a ticking, rhythmic sound to pace your footfalls.

KEEPING TRACK OF YOUR PROGRESS

You can make a fun and rewarding game out of tracking your progress as you increase your daily mileage or number of steps. First obtain a pedometer (you can buy an inexpensive one at a sporting goods store or invest a small fee for a smartphone app for this purpose) and set it for your stride. Be sure the pedometer is measuring accurately by wearing it a known distance and checking its results. Then simply wear it daily and record your progress. Always wear the pedometer correctly; usually it is designed to be worn on your hip over the side seam.

After your pedometer has been adjusted for your stride and you are sure it is measuring reasonably accurately, determine your "baseline"—that is, the distance (miles or steps) you normally walk in a day. The best way to do this is to wear the pedometer over the course of a week or over several *representative* days (days in which you do not walk much more or less than normal). Each day during the baseline period, wear your pedometer and record the distance displayed at the end of the day. Using graph paper such as that shown in the sample graph in Table 5.5a (or use the blank graph in Table 5.5b), determine how much each block or square represents. For example, if your pedometer measures number of steps, you might decide that each square represents some number of steps. If your pedometer measures mileage, you might set each block to a quarter-mile, or if digital, .2 mile (as shown on the sample graph). Divide the graph into seven-day blocks to represent each week. Note that on the graph shown, quarter miles walked is on the left-hand scale; on the right-hand scale, digital miles are shown. Then total up your miles or steps for each week (all seven days). You can even take an average of those seven days by dividing the total by 7 at the end of the week. Your goal is to increase either your total miles per day, per week, or your average mileage or steps over time.

Each week, set a new goal for the next week that is a little above the average or total miles or steps for the current week. Strive to increase your walking each week. Be reasonable in setting your goals. Don't overestimate how much and how fast you can increase your walking. Remember, the idea is to increase your walking gradually at a pace that will allow you to sustain your progress.

Aiming for 10,000 Steps per Day

The concept of walking 10,000 steps per day for health and weight loss was popularized originally in Japan and later was the subject of several research studies. Eventually the research on

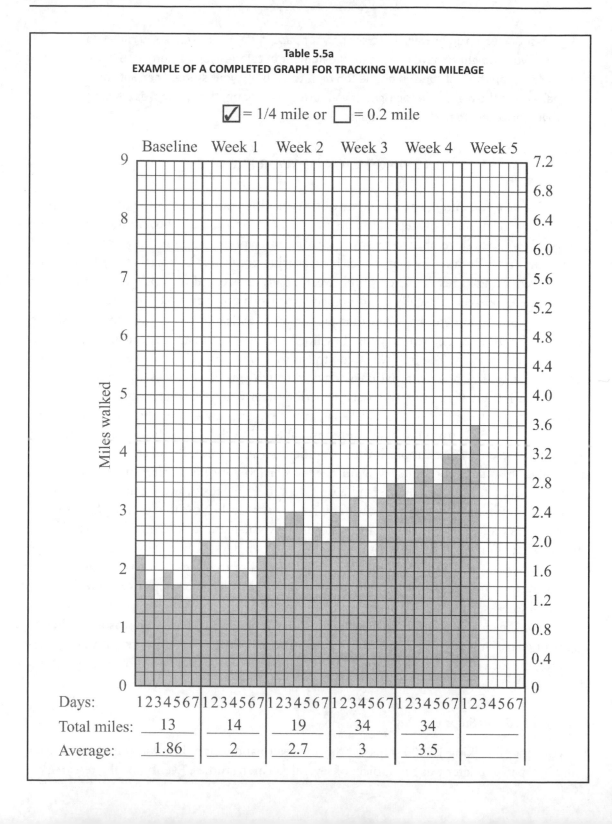

Table 5.5a

EXAMPLE OF A COMPLETED GRAPH FOR TRACKING WALKING MILEAGE

☑ = 1/4 mile or ☐ = 0.2 mile

Miles walked

	Baseline	Week 1	Week 2	Week 3	Week 4	Week 5
Days:	1234567	1234567	1234567	1234567	1234567	1234567
Total miles:	13	14	19	34	34	
Average:	1.86	2	2.7	3	3.5	

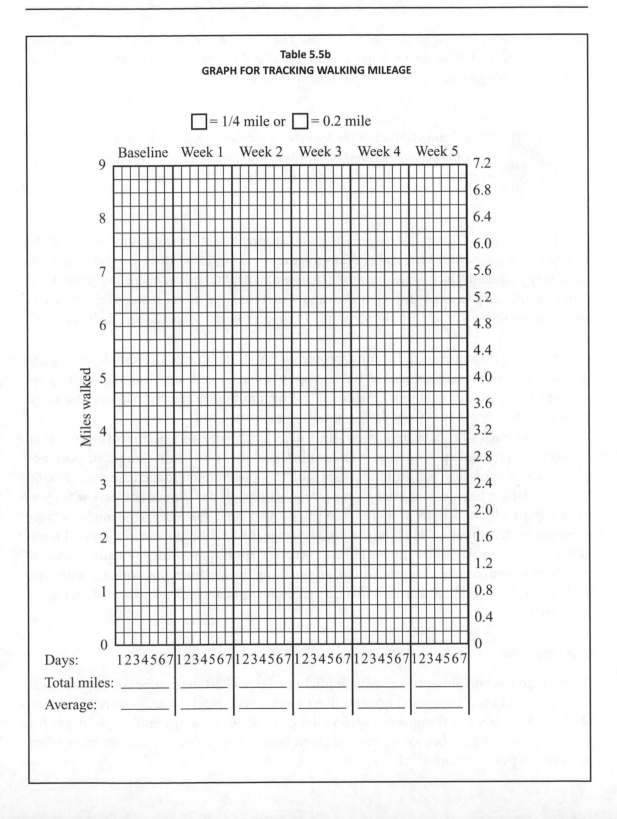

Table 5.5b
GRAPH FOR TRACKING WALKING MILEAGE

□ = 1/4 mile or □ = 0.2 mile

Baseline   Week 1   Week 2   Week 3   Week 4   Week 5

the effectiveness of this approach led to a book, *The Step Diet*, by Dr. James O. Hill and associates.[15] However, 10,000 steps per day is a high goal and might better be seen as an ideal. A more achievable goal may be to strive for your personal best.

TIP More information about *The Step Diet* is available through the website **www.thewalkingsite.com/10000steps.html**. This is a good program to motivate you to use counting steps to increase walking exercise.

For most people, 10,000 steps per day totals around five miles worth of walking, or the equivalent of a 2-hour hike. (It takes the average adult about 2,000 steps to cover a mile.) A sedentary person likely averages far fewer steps a day, depending on his or her profession. (For example, as you might expect, nurses and waitresses average more steps than psychologists or bookkeepers.) More steps pay off in greater health benefits and help subtract weight!

It is now recommended that most people do 30–60 minutes of dedicated walking per day in order to approach the goal of 10,000 steps per day. Of course, you should start by assessing where you are (what your baseline is) and then work to gradually increase your steps, aiming eventually for 10,000 per day, or some other personal best.

As you track your daily steps, note how you feel, how your body is improving, or other changes you are making to improve your health. Get in the habit of checking your pedometer at midday to see how you are doing, then look for opportunities to increase your walking if you are falling behind your usual distance for that time of day. Notice any days when you naturally get a lot of activity or those when you get very little. Consider what might be contributing to that situation and how you could change it. Use this information to build more activity into every day. Some tips for increasing daily steps include using the stairs instead of the elevator, walking the dog more often, and parking further from the store or, better yet, walking to the store. Use your imagination and come up with your own ways of getting in more steps.

Tracking Time

Rather than tracking distance walked, you might prefer to chart the number of minutes each day you spend on planned walking. You don't need a pedometer for this—only a watch or clock. Or keep track of the time you spend hiking or walking on a treadmill or pedaling on a bike. Tracking progress helps you feel good about how you are doing and lets you know when you need to put out more effort.

Selecting a Gym or Health Club

Fitness facilities vary considerably when it comes to the equipment they have available, the programs and services they offer, the atmosphere and experiences they provide, and the cost for use or membership. Some facilities are minimalists, providing nothing more than the basics, while others are more "high-end" establishments that cater to a clientele that can afford to pay for amenities such as child care or a juice bar. Increasingly, workplaces and apartment buildings are providing workout facilities for employees or tenants.

Some facilities define themselves as "serious" gyms and cater primarily to bodybuilders, while others provide social interaction as well as workout opportunities. Other facilities, such as many YMCAs, are family-oriented. Still others provide access only with a personal trainer to guide you. Some gyms have a pool or sauna, while others offer onsite massage or nutrition counseling. Fees are typically commensurate with the extent of offerings.

In choosing a gym or fitness facility, consider your own needs and preferences. In particular, take into account the ease or difficulty in commuting to the gym from your home or workplace. Having to travel more than 20 minutes is likely to decrease your motivation to go to the facility. To decide on a gym, locate the fitness facilities nearest you and arrange for a tour of each—preferably a tour that includes a trial workout or gives you a free pass for a later trial workout. Ask about hours, vacation closings, and fees, and whether the gym employs certified personal trainers. Also ask about classes and programs available for beginners or special programs such as spinning classes or kickboxing. Talk to patrons to assess their experiences.

Notice the type of equipment and its condition. Is there a variety of equipment, as well as duplicates of popular equipment such as treadmills and Stairmasters? Are there time limits on the machines? How many "Out of Order" signs do you see? Do seats and padding of machines have tears or worn places? Is the free weights area littered or tidy, cramped or roomy? Check out the floor space. Avoid gyms where machines are jammed together, taking up most of the floor space and leaving little room for floor exercises. Do you notice any personnel whose job it is to keep the place clean? Does the pool water seem appropriately treated? Is the club well lit, and is the temperature set at a comfortable level for exercise? Are the locker rooms clean and spacious? Are there telltale signs of overuse or poor maintenance, such as burned-out lights, broken lockers, torn or soiled carpets, dirty floors, or peeling paint? Refer to Table 5.6 for more questions to consider when you tour a facility.

When you settle on a gym or club, read the contract carefully if one is required. You should have the right to cancel membership within a few days of first signing. Find out what your rights are for terminating membership if you move or are permanently disabled. What is the refund policy? Can you extend your contract to make up time if you become sick and cannot work out for an extended period? Make inquiries about the financial health of the club and avoid facilities that may be experiencing economic difficulties, especially if there is an up-front membership fee. Remember that fees may not be refunded if the club or gym ceases operations.

Table 5.6
QUESTIONS TO ASK CURRENT MEMBERS ABOUT A CLUB OR GYM

Ask patrons or members how they feel about the facilities and about their experience using different aspects of the club:

◎ Are the showers temperature-controlled, or does the water temperature fluctuate when others are taking a shower or flushing the toilet?

◎ Are there enough lockers and other amenities?

◎ Is working with the trainers a positive experience?

◎ Is it easy to get an appointment with a trainer?

◎ When is the club most crowded?

◎ What is the longest wait to use a piece of equipment?

◎ Are other patrons friendly?

◎ Is there adequate parking, especially at peak hours?

◎ Is the club's vacation schedule convenient? Is it open when you want to work out?

Working with a Personal Trainer

Personal fitness trainers work one-on-one with clients, usually by appointment. Clients may exercise at the trainer's studio, or they may work out with the trainer in a gym or health club. Some trainers will come to your home and bring their own equipment, usually handheld free weights.

Some trainers offer nutrition information in addition to exercise training. Care should be taken to make sure a trainer who offers such advice and services is qualified to do so—that is, he or she has done more to work toward advanced nutrition certification than just having read a book on nutrition or taken a seminar. Some trainers or others who call themselves nutritionists attempt to implement nutrition advice given in books written by other unqualified "experts." Others may have simply taken a single course, which offers a "certificate" for completion, and subsequently call themselves nutritionists. In fact, the term "nutritionist" is unregulated and does not imply any special qualifications; anyone can use this label. But you should ask what sort of training any person who claims to be a nutritionist has—he or she should have a degree in a food science field. A sure tip-off to a bogus expert is an attempt to sell you vitamins or supplements as part of your "nutrition" program.

A good trainer will do an assessment of your flexibility and your current fitness before you start a program of exercise. The assessment should cover your flexibility, cardiovascular fitness, gait, strength, and ability to push and pull. Protocols for flexibility assessment are readily available, but the trainer needs to be trained and supervised in the use of these protocols. Similarly, some trainers do body composition assessments using a tape measure or skin calipers. This requires adequate training to avoid errors that could contribute to serious mismeasurement. Do not hesitate to ask the trainer you are considering where he or she received training and whether he or she is certified to do such assessments.

TRAINER CERTIFICATION

A variety of organizations provide certification for trainers. These include the American College of Sports Medicine (ACSM), the National Strength and Conditioning Association (NSCA), and the Aerobics and Fitness Association of America (AFAA), among others. Preferably a trainer has a B.S. in exercise and sport science or kinesiology. Another important level of experience would be having worked in a rehabilitation facility or as an assistant to a physical therapist. Beware of those who are doing personal training as an avocation (a hobby), in addition to another job, or whose only qualifications are that they play or played sports. Not all health and fitness clubs require certification or prior relevant experience. Once you obtain names and contact information, take time to interview and assess each person before making your selection.

> **TIP** For referral to a certified trainer, contact the Aerobics and Fitness Association of America at **www.afaa.com**. Or to find a certified personal trainer in your area, go to **www.personaltrainercentral.com/abouttrainers.htm**. This website is aligned with the International Sports Science Association, or ISSA, and is a training organization for personal trainers.

CHOOSING A POTENTIAL TRAINER

Ask a potential trainer questions about motivation, education and training, certification, and fees. This will help you get to know the person better and help you decide whether you want to work with him or her. Table 5.7 gives some questions you might ask a potential trainer.

Table 5.7
QUESTIONS TO ASK A POTENTIAL TRAINER

◎ Why are you a personal trainer? Is this your profession, or is it a second job or a hobby?

◎ What is your education with regard to health and fitness assessment and instruction?

◎ Have you worked in a rehabilitation facility or as an assistant to a physical therapist?

◎ By what organization, and at what level, are you certified to be a personal trainer?

◎ How many years of experience do you have?

◎ Are you trained in CPR or first aid?

◎ What are your fees?

◎ How long is a session, and to how many sessions must I commit?

◎ What is your cancellation and refund policy?

TIP   A good source of information on how to choose a personal trainer can be found at **http://exercise.about.com/cs/forprofessionals/a/choosetrainer. htm?p=1**. Also, the WebMD website has helpful information about finding and choosing a personal trainer. For more information, go to: **www.webmd. com/fitness-exercise/guide/finding-personal-fitness-trainer**.

Warning Signs in Selecting or Working with a Trainer

Heed the warning signs that indicate trainers who may not be a good choice for you. If the trainer promotes or sells supplements, protein drinks, or nutritional products as part of his or her fitness recommendations, understand that he or she may have an agenda that could conflict with your personal needs. Beware of a trainer (or fitness facility) that wants to sell you multiple advance sessions that are nonrefundable. Don't work with a trainer who is, or has been, a professional or semi-professional athlete unless he or she has other credentials as well. Avoid clubs that don't require certification for their trainers. Most especially, don't work with a trainer who seems distracted while working with you or fails to explain to you the reason for doing particular exercises. Trainers should be able to describe which muscle groups are involved in an exercise and why you are doing that exercise. Personality is important, too; you will be working closely with this person. Make sure you get along with your trainer and feel safe and comfortable asking questions. See Table 5.8 for qualities to look for in a personal trainer.

Table 5.8

QUALITIES TO LOOK FOR IN A PERSONAL TRAINER

Look for a personal trainer who exhibits certain behaviors; the trainer should:

◎ Spend time at the introductory session getting to know you and your exercise goals

◎ Do an assessment of your current flexibility and fitness status

◎ Be able to design a program to achieve the goals you specify while taking into account your physical abilities and personal preferences

◎ Introduce you to the gym and locker room and make sure you feel comfortable and relaxed, helping instill a sense of belonging

◎ Ask for emergency contact information for you

◎ Ask you about your medical history and conduct a health risk appraisal

◎ Be enthusiastic and personable

◎ Support your training efforts with positive feedback while still correcting your form

◎ Counsel you on proper exercise apparel (shoes *and* clothing) as necessary from a functional (not fashionable) standpoint

◎ Talk to you in terms you can understand

◎ Suggest exercises to do in between training sessions

◎ Avoid gossiping or talking about non-relevant topics during training sessions

At-Home Exercise

Some people do not use a gym for exercise, or they combine working out at a gym with exercise at home. More and more people are choosing to invest in home fitness equipment and turning one room of the house into their workout room. Some people have a personal trainer come to their home. A wide variety of home equipment options are available in the marketplace, ranging from inexpensive (and often useless) gadgets to expensive multipurpose, multistation machines. Whatever machine you choose, it must provide resistance if it is to be useful. For example, riding a stationary-type bicycle without resistance provides no fitness benefits.

Home equipment can provide fitness benefits, but these benefits may depend on how easy it is to use the equipment and how familiar you are with the movements required. One study found that, compared to a stationary bicycle, a stair climber, a rowing machine, and an Airdyne (a stationary bicycle with push-and-pull levers for the arms), the best choice for burning calories and improving cardiovascular fitness was a treadmill. Least effective in this study for producing fitness benefits were the conventional stationary bicycle and the Airdyne, but not because the machines themselves were ineffective—it was just that users preferred using them the least. Walking and running on a treadmill were movement patterns people in the study were already familiar with, whereas rowing required a level of skill that not everyone possessed. Even so, more and more people today are using rowing machines, because these machines allow for both cardiovascular exercise and muscle strength and endurance development without the impact of a treadmill.

Another reason why treadmills were "better" for some people in the aforementioned study was that people tended to exercise more vigorously and stick with the exercise longer when they were more familiar with the movement required. Intensity and duration were therefore maximized on the treadmill and users found it more enjoyable than the other options. Treadmills for the home also come in foldup versions that don't take up much room.

In choosing home fitness equipment, consider your current level of fitness, your likes and dislikes, your skill level, the space available for such equipment, your budget, and—of course—your motivation to work out on your own. To ease the strain on your wallet, check Internet sites such as eBay and Craigslist for used equipment, or shop at a store that specializes in used equipment. Or you can buy exercise resistance bands, which are less expensive—usually under twenty dollars. You can easily pack them in a suitcase for workouts on the road. Less expensive options such as these can be useful when you are first assessing your motivation for working out at home, and for people who don't want to invest in a lot of equipment or who have limited space.

Some people enjoy using videotapes and DVDs of various exercise routines in the privacy of their home. These provide convenient options when the weather is inclement or when you just want a change of pace. An important consideration in using a workout video or DVD is your own fitness limitations. Exercise videos and DVDs are available through Netflix, but you have to join to obtain them.

Fitness programs can also be viewed through the "on-demand" feature of some cable television providers, or you can record television fitness shows to play and work out with at a time that is more convenient to you. The Internet and smartphones provide programs and applications for exercise and workout routines, many of which are free. Some have instruction videos for doing different types of exercise.

Increasing Activities of Daily Living

Whether exercising outdoors, at a gym, with a trainer, or at home, you can achieve additional calorie expenditure by focusing on burning calories through activities of daily living. These include routine physical activities such as gardening or cleaning the house. Even once you have begun to do regular exercise, increasing activities of daily living will help you burn additional calories. Table 5.9 lists suggestions for increasing activities of daily living.

Table 5.9
SUGGESTIONS FOR INCREASING ACTIVITIES OF DAILY LIVING

◎ Take the stairs or an elevator or escalator.

◎ Walk instead of driving short distances.

◎ Park farther away and walk.

◎ Get off public transportation a stop or two early and walk.

◎ Ride your bicycle instead of taking the car.

◎ Take a walk at lunchtime or on your coffee break.

◎ Deliver items yourself rather than sending someone else.

◎ Stand and talk on the phone, or pace the floor if you have a handheld phone.

◎ Pedal a stationary bicycle while watching television.

◎ During television commercials, get up and walk around or march in place.

◎ Replace cocktail hour with exercise.

◎ Get things yourself instead of sending your children.

◎ Clean the house more often.

◎ Sweep the sidewalk in front of your house—and even in front of your neighbor's house.

◎ Rake the leaves, trim the hedges, and do the gardening yourself.

◎ Wash the car by hand instead of taking it to the car wash.

◎ Mow the grass with a push lawn mower or a power mower you don't ride.

◎ Play golf without a golf cart or caddy.

◎ When on vacation, take walking tours.

◎ At the sports stadium, during intermissions climb the stairs and walk.

◎ Go dancing more often.

◎ Put a pair of walking shoes in the trunk of your car and look for opportunities to walk.

CHAPTER SIX

Managing Thinking and Self-Talk

*EMILY ASSERTED THAT SHE "SHOULD" BE ABLE TO MANAGE HER WEIGHT. After all, she was effective in her job and ran a tight ship at home. "I know what to do; I just don't do it." Instead Emily kept finding excuses: "I'll start on Monday." "I'll have just one." "It's been a stressful day and I deserve a treat." When tempting food was present, she just couldn't say no. Emily was a perfectionist in many areas, and when she failed to live up to her own expectations, she saw herself as a failure. It took awhile for Emily to recognize that her thinking and self-talk were undermining her weight management efforts. She realized she had to stop believing her hindering self-talk and stop allowing herself to make unhealthy choices. She needed to take stock of her values and commit to leading a healthy lifestyle. Eventually Emily discovered a website called **www.Operation Beautiful.com**. It helped her let go of some of her "fat talk." She started reaching out to others with positive messages that increasingly helped her be more positive about herself and improve behavior.*

Thinking

Thinking is something you probably don't think much about. But thinking plays a big role in feelings, behavior, and weight management. How you think—what you say to yourself and how you process the information that your senses gather—helps you understand the world around you and decide how to act. Cognition—another word for thinking—consists of representing and transforming information from your senses into knowledge. This can be done by sensing something directly (through the five senses) or indirectly (by reasoning). Thinking includes the mental process of knowing, as well as aspects of knowing, such as awareness, perception, reasoning, and judgment.

149

What you say silently to yourself is one type of thinking, called *self-talk*. Self-talk is thinking that involves words, sentences, and phrases. You may not be aware that you talk to yourself, but everyone does. Self-talk is that little voice in your head that is chattering most of the time—the little voice that just now asked, "What little voice?"

TIP The website **www.OperationBeautiful.com** proposes a unique way to build and maintain a positive attitude. The stated mission of the creators of the website and its accompanying blog is to shift negative self-talk about yourself and your weight—what they call "fat talk"—to more generally positive thinking by taking certain actions. The idea behind Operation Beautiful is simple: post anonymous positive notes in public places for other people to find. The process of creating the positive messages helps you and whoever else reads the note become aware of how certain thoughts can produce good feelings and inspire others to participate in this positive movement. Think how good most people feel coming across a message such as "Smile, and someone might smile back." To spread the word, participants are asked to include the website URL in the messages they post. Check out the website to find daily, positive messages and blog with others about life-affirming accomplishments.

Self-talk

Self-talk can involve mulling over an idea, and talking silently to yourself to decide what you think about something: "Let's see, that choice is probably pretty high in calories. Maybe the fish would be a better idea." Usually such self-talk is internal and silent, but sometimes you may find yourself thinking out loud: "Where are those keys?"

When you have an internal conversation with yourself, you are engaging in self-talk. Sometimes your conversation can be an argument—as if one part of your mind is trying to persuade another part of your mind to accept some alternative action or idea:

"I shouldn't eat that."
"Well, why not? I've been really good in watching what I eat."
"But if I give in now, I'll hate myself."
"Maybe I can have just *one*."

The parts of you that carry on the argument are sometimes called sub-personalities, or "voices." Chapter 7, Challenging Your "Inner Voices," is devoted to identifying these voices and understanding how they can affect behavior and feelings.

At times you may have an imagined dialogue with another person; it could be mentally reviewing a previous, real interaction or going over an encounter you anticipate. Can you recall a time when you had an argument or sharp words with someone and later kept reviewing it in your mind? You were using self-talk to think—that is, ruminate—about what happened. (You probably also imagined what you could have said instead.) Another example is when you think about what you want to say to another person and you rehearse it first in your mind.

Often self-talk is an internal, verbalized stream-of-consciousness thinking—the continuous, disconnected flow of thoughts through your mind: "Nice car; wish I had one of those. I feel fat. Maybe I should get to the gym. I wonder if he'll call tonight. How long do I have to wait for this light to turn green?" This is an example of mind chatter—random thoughts that come as if from nowhere, more or less all the time. Another example of thinking is when you hear a jingle that keeps repeating in your head and you mutter to yourself, "Why can't I stop that?" The jingle can sound like a track of a CD that keeps repeating; sometimes repetitive, unwanted thoughts come unbidden into your head in the same way.

Feelings, or emotions, are another function of the mind, and can be influenced by—and contribute to—self-talk. Feelings are products of the mind and are another way of "knowing" the world; they are nonverbal signals that tell the rational mind to pay attention to something—and to decide what to do. They can range from being mild to strong, helping you gauge how important something is to you. They sound the alarm when there is a threat, and trigger your attention if something is positive. Emotions and cognition complement each other. Thus, feelings can trigger self-talk, and self-talk can influence feelings.

WHAT CONTRIBUTES TO SELF-TALK?

Self-talk is influenced by several components in addition to feelings: information that comes to your *awareness* and that you *focus on*; your *experiences* in life and how you *understand* or interpret those experiences; your underlying *beliefs*; and the way in which you *process information*. Although much information is always impinging on your senses, your brain's processing allows only a portion of it to come into your awareness. Once you are aware of something, you may or may not focus on it. (Or it may slip out of your mind.) When you focus on something, you use your beliefs and prior experiences to try to make sense out of the situation at hand. As a result of how you process the information, you react in some way.

Imagine that you go to a party where there is a table heaped with food. When you approach the table, your mind scans the food and focuses on the desserts. The appearance of the desserts causes you to anticipate the taste, and you imagine eating a particular dessert. Past experience with sweet taste, and an attractive item, direct your thinking to what you want to eat right now, and you feel excited. At this point, you are likely to indulge your taste buds. This is one example of how thinking works.

Take another example: suppose your friend tells you about a new diet that is working for her. You may become interested and think it could possibly work for you, too. You might ask for more details, and perhaps you buy the new diet book she recommends. If you try the new diet and you don't lose weight, you could decide that nothing you do is going to help you lose weight, and you begin to feel discouraged. Instead of deciding that the diet might have been poorly conceived or that other factors came into play to cause failure, you blame yourself, and you feel bad. This conclusion could give rise to self-talk such as "I can't do it," and reinforce an already existing belief that losing weight is too hard for you to ever do it. Failing sets up the expectation of failure in future dieting efforts, and this is reinforced by negative self-talk. Although initially you got your hopes up, eventually they were dashed.

BECOMING AWARE OF YOUR SELF-TALK

It may not be immediately obvious to you that you engage in self-talk until you reflect on— listen in to—your thinking. The best way to do this is by keeping a journal or diary and writing down your thoughts. In that way, you can not only become aware that you are talking to yourself, but also discover what it is that you are thinking most about! Keeping a record of your thoughts and the circumstances in which they occur and the emotions that accompany them is called *self-monitoring*. (You learned about this in Chapter 3, Changing Behavior, in which monitoring of cues and reinforcers was discussed.) By writing down your self-talk, you will probably discover that certain themes reoccur. For example, you may find that you frequently criticize yourself harshly, or that you have a lot of worry thoughts. Other themes may involve the ways that you think things "should" be, or the perceived unfairness of your struggling with a weight problem.

Sometimes these themes point to the use of cognitive distortions—ways of thinking that distort understanding. As a result, you end up feeling bad, perhaps choosing behaviors that are not healthy. For example, if you think someone should not have spoken to you so harshly, you could feel angry—and then get something to eat to feel better. Errors of interpretation can contribute to painful emotions that could impair your emotional well-being. Cognitive distortions and these sorts of interpretations are discussed in more detail later in this chapter. But first let's consider a new approach to thinking and therapy.

ACT: A New Therapy

One of the several new therapies[1] that are part of the "third wave" of modern psychology (which were also touched on in Chapter 3, Changing Behavior) is Acceptance and Commitment Therapy (ACT). Steven C. Hayes, Ph.D., professor of clinical psychology at University of Nevada,

Reno, and his associates developed ACT,[2] which offers a new way of thinking about therapy. The letters in ACT stand for Accept, Choose, and Take Action. ACT encourages you to

◎ **A**ccept your reactions to events and your thoughts and feelings about such events with mindfulness—that is, with an attitude of awareness, openness, interest, receptivity, and without judgment

◎ **C**hoose values that give direction to your life and goals that support these values

◎ **T**ake committed action in accordance with your values and goals

ACT is a practical approach to life. The goal of ACT is to encourage you to live life more in the present, more focused on important values, and less focused on thoughts, feelings, and experiences as being painful or wanting to avoid them. ACT is not about overcoming pain or fighting emotions; it's about embracing all that life presents, including the suffering that is inevitable in all lives. It offers a way to be with suffering without being overwhelmed by it, by encouraging you to choose to live a life based on your values and what matters most to you. Focusing on acceptance, mindfulness, and values, ACT helps people better cope with obstacles in life in order to lead lives of greater satisfaction.

Accept. The "A" in ACT refers to the idea that we get hooked into the *content* of our thoughts and feelings (that is, our reactions to events) and need to learn to accept those thoughts and feelings rather than react to them. Ordinarily, we become *fused*, or joined, with the content of our thoughts. For example, when we think, "She hurt me with her comment," we believe that this thought and the hurt feelings that accompany it represent a "literal truth" that must be believed and acted upon. Or our reactions indicate rules that must be obeyed, or important events that require our full attention, or threatening events that must be gotten rid of. The remedy is to *defuse* ourselves from our thoughts and feelings—that is, to notice them without becoming overwhelmed by them. We can view the thought "She hurt me with her comment" as "just a thought." It is not necessary to act on it. As to the feeling of hurt, we can just notice it and let it pass in due time. Defusing involves being able to step back and observe thoughts and feelings without becoming caught up in them. When we can defuse, we can recognize that thoughts and feelings are transient (that is, they come and go)—an ever-changing stream of words, sounds, and images. We can remain neutral and simply observe the event and the attendant thoughts and feelings without being drawn into them. When we defuse from our thoughts and feelings, they have much less impact and influence.

Consider a situation in which, after looking in a mirror, you think to yourself, "I'm fat." As a result, you are likely to feel bad. Soon afterward you may eat something to feel better to try and suppress the thought and forget your feelings. This is called *experiential avoidance*—trying to escape or avoid pain and bad feelings. It may be true that you need to lose weight to be healthier or because you want to feel better about yourself or to look better. Instead of trying to escape the thought and bad feeling, it is better to accept that you just had a thought about being fat, and that there were painful feelings along with that thought. The solution is to defuse—recognize that these are just thoughts and feelings triggered by an event (looking in the mirror), and what you need to do is take workable action—i.e., focus on staying mindful and adopting a healthier lifestyle.

Mindfulness is the practice of living in the present moment and observing thoughts and feelings from a neutral place, rather than getting lost in them or overwhelmed by them, or trying to control them. Acceptance means observing thoughts and feelings and allowing them to come and go without struggling with them—without fusing with them.

Return to the example of the thought "I'm fat." You may realize that you have this thought often, and it hurts when you have it. It does hurt, but trying to escape the pain of the thought is not the solution. What you need to do right now is to acknowledge the reality and take care of yourself in the present moment by telling yourself, "At this moment, to go on with my life, I need to . . . finish the laundry, . . . make dinner, . . . take a shower, or whatever. And I need to make healthier choices with food and exercise." By focusing on what needs to be done to change your lifestyle, eventually your weight is likely to arrive at a healthier place.

Some people are afraid that if they accept themselves as they are, they won't be motivated to change. Such acceptance is passive and implies giving up. Rather, you want to engage in *active* acceptance. That is, you may accept the present situation (which, after all, cannot be changed at the moment) and at the same time commit yourself to a higher value—adopting a lifestyle that may lead to a healthier weight. Acceptance of what is, committing to personal values, and taking action in accordance with these values is the essence of ACT.

Acceptance is analogous to the Serenity Prayer, which is about accepting those things (thoughts and feelings) we cannot change (like the memory of a bad experience in the past, or the reality of a painful current situation) and taking actions to change that which can be changed, like making healthier choices or getting exercise. Acceptance does not mean accepting untenable situations—for example, being in an abusive relationship. And it does not mean accepting obesity as inevitable. Acceptance in ACT relates to unpleasant private experiences—painful thoughts and feelings such as worries and anxiety (which may be prompted by current difficult situations). Acceptance in ACT is not chiefly about external situations or circumstances (although it is always a good idea to resolve unsatisfactory situations). It is not about having trouble with a micromanaging boss. It is about having *upsetting thoughts and feelings* about having trouble with a micromanaging boss. It is not about reacting badly to your reflection in a mirror; it is about having *painful thoughts and feelings* in reaction to your reflection.

Choose. The "C" in ACT refers to making a commitment to higher values and choosing goals that serve those values. Values give meaning to life. As mentioned in Chapter 3, Changing Behavior, a value is a belief or philosophy that is personally meaningful to you. Though most people don't think a lot about what their values are, every person has a core set of personal values that guides his or her behavior. Values can range from the commonplace, such as a belief in doing a good job and being on time, to the more psychological, such as a commitment to being able to take care of yourself, caring about others, or having integrity.[3] Of course, what you value is up to you, and it is important that you decide what matters to you. Values are the overarching principles that give direction to behavior, and should not be confused with goals, which are things that can be obtained.

Take Action. Finally, the "T" in ACT refers to taking action in accordance with your values and goals. It means doing what matters, even if it is difficult or uncomfortable. To do this, you need to discover what is important to your "true" self. Consider that you already have many values, some of which you are better able to articulate than others. Perhaps you value friendship and having good relationships, so you stay in touch with friends. Or you may value your general health, so you do things like brush you teeth regularly and visit the doctor as needed. You may not have given as much attention to living a healthy lifestyle. When you decide what truly matters to you, you'll focus on what you want your life to stand for, and what you want out of life. Then you will more easily act in ways that move you toward your goals, even if that means bringing cravings and urges to eat along for the ride. Of course, people can differ on exactly what constitutes a healthy lifestyle. You might consider referring to the definition of optimum fitness offered in Chapter 5, Getting Started with Exercise, as one possible description of a healthy lifestyle, adding to it the idea of making healthy food choices.

THE OBSERVING SELF

Another important concept in ACT is that of the *observing self*. There are two parts to the mind: the thinking self (the part that is responsible for all your thoughts, self-talk, beliefs, memories, judgments, fantasies, etc.) and the observing self (the part of your mind that is able to be aware of whatever you are thinking or feeling or doing at any moment without getting caught up in the content). Without the observing self, you couldn't develop mindfulness skills. And the more you practice mindfulness skills, the more you'll become aware of this part of your mind (the observing self), and be able to access it when you need it. The observing self is neutral and doesn't judge; it merely notices.

Let's go back to the thought "I'm fat." The observing self notices that this thought occurred just as you looked in the mirror, and the observer notices that you have mixed feelings of frustration and sadness—you feel bad. The observer "just notices"; it doesn't try to make the thought or feelings go away. It is your thinking and experiencing self that wants the feelings to go away. The observing self stays neutral; it acknowledges reality. When you can stay in neutral and are mindful (that is, open to whatever is happening in the present moment), you are less likely to get caught up in painful emotional turmoil. It is a good idea, then, to be an observer of your own thoughts and feelings—not to try to escape them, but to ride them out. It is also helpful to notice when you are making the interpretive thinking errors known as cognitive distortions that are covered in detail in the next section of the chapter.

> **TIP** Acceptance and Commitment Therapy (ACT) aims to help people live life more in the present, more focused on important values and goals, and less easily overwhelmed by painful thoughts, feelings, and experiences. For more about ACT, go to: **http://contextualpsychology.org/act** and click on "ACT for the public." For a long but non-technical article on ACT, entitled "Embracing Your Demons," go to: **www.actmindfully.com.au/upimages/Dr_Russ_Harris_-_A_ Non-technical_Overview_of_ACT.pdf**.

Cognitive Distortions

We tend to believe that our thinking is always correct—that it doesn't mislead us in most cases (except when we have the wrong information to start with). In fact, the mind can be a trickster. We can't always trust what we think. In obsessive-compulsive disorder (OCD), the mind tricks the person into believing certain repetitive and intrusive thoughts and acting on them as if they were the objective truth. Likewise, for all of us, the mind can develop bad habits that are referred to as *cognitive distortions*—ways of interpreting or understanding the information from our senses that are misleading. Similarly, the mind makes errors in attribution. One of these involves erroneously attributing causality to two or more events that occur close together in time—that one event caused the other. The mind can make mistakes, so it is a good idea to step back and notice your thoughts with a bit of skepticism.

> **TIP** To learn more about errors in thinking that can lead to wrong conclusions and possibly problematic behavior, learn more about attribution theory. Check out: **http://allpsych.com/psychology101/attribution_attraction.html**. To read more about fallacies in thinking, go to **www.skepticsfieldguide.net/ 2005/01/examples-of-false-cause-correlation.html**.

Researchers and clinicians have explored how the interpretive errors we call cognitive distortions negatively affect behavior. Generally people are not aware of making these errors; cognitive distortions are unconscious, bad habits that most people would probably reject if they were conscious of them. When you make these errors, you are processing the evidence from your senses in a distorted or biased way. As a result, you come to conclusions that make it harder to act in your own best interests. Learning to recognize these errors in thinking can help you avoid them.

Some common cognitive distortions are described in Table 6.1; the material that follows goes into more detail about each type of cognitive distortion.

TIP John Tagg is an educator and author of several books, including *The Learning Paradigm College*. He wrote a good article on cognitive distortions that you can find at: **http://daphne.palomar.edu/jtagg/cds.htm**.

ALL-OR-NOTHING THINKING

All-or-nothing thinking is polarized thinking—seeing things in stark contrasts—good or bad, black or white, right or wrong, perfect or failure. There is little or no room for grays or middle ground. Such thinking often points to perfectionism. Examples of all-or-nothing thinking include: "I broke my diet, so I may as well keep on eating." To avoid making the error of all-or-nothing thinking, cultivate the habit of being open to other points of view: "Okay, I wish I hadn't eaten that; now I need to refocus and make the best of the rest of the day."

CATASTROPHIZING

Catastrophizing involves thinking that if a future, negative outcome does occur, it will be terrible, overwhelming, unmanageable, or intolerable. It involves both overestimating the threat and underestimating your ability to cope. (Chapter 8, Managing Stress, talks more about this.)

Overestimating the Threat

When you catastrophize, you tend to *overestimate the threat* or the negative consequences of events that haven't even happened yet. Often catastrophic thoughts can be identified by the stem statement: "What if . . . ?" "What if I gain weight?" "What if I give in to temptation?" "What if I make a mistake?" "What if they think I'm stupid?" Often the threat is imaginary or minimal at most, but it feels like it is real and huge. Sometimes the threat is actual and serious. Often it is something beyond your immediate control. If you can't do anything about it, there is no point in worrying. (You just have to accept it.) If there is something you can do now to influence the situation, then plan to take action. Focus on what you can actually do. (Hint:

Table 6.1
OVERVIEW OF COGNITIVE DISTORTIONS

◎ **All-or-nothing thinking:** Seeing things as belonging to only two completely opposing or dichotomous categories: all or none, black or white, right or wrong, perfect or a failure. Examples of such thinking include: "If I make a mistake, it is terrible and awful, and I am a failure," and "If I make one unhealthy choice, then I'm not healthy."

◎ **Catastrophizing:** Focusing on potential problems in the future. Worry thoughts that assume that the worst will happen usually start with "What if . . .?" For example: "What if I gain all the weight back and then some?" "What if I can't do it?"

◎ **Overgeneralization:** Using a single piece of evidence from an isolated experience or a single negative event as proof that a never-ending pattern of defeat exists. "She criticized my work on that one report, so she won't like anything I do."

◎ **Jumping to conclusions:** Making an interpretation based on minimal facts or misinterpretation of the evidence. "I have nothing to do this weekend, so there must be something wrong with me."

◎ **Mind-reading:** Thinking that you know what someone else is thinking without checking it out with that person. "He hasn't said it, but I think he is bothered by my weight."

◎ **Fortune-telling:** Anticipating things will turn out badly and feeling convinced that a prediction is an already established fact. "I won't enjoy the party."

◎ **Filtering:** Picking out a single detail and dwelling on it exclusively so that your vision of reality is distorted. "I'm upset that I only lost a pound this week. I'm not succeeding!"

◎ **Disqualifying the positive:** Rejecting positive experiences by insisting that they don't count for some reason. "I was just lucky to have lost two pounds this week."

◎ **Emotional reasoning:** Assuming that your negative emotions necessarily reflect reality. "I feel bad, so I must be bad."

◎ **"Should" thinking concerning yourself:** Relying on your own (perhaps irrational) internal rules about how things "should" be in order to pass judgment, rather than being willing to accept yourself as you are. "I shouldn't have to set limits on my eating; other people don't." (Sometimes people use "should" thinking as a whip to motivate themselves with guilt, as in "I should have lost more weight by now.")

◎ **"Should" thinking concerning others:** Applying your personal rules to others, which often results in frustration or anger and resentment for one or both of you. "Things should be fair." "You should not feel that way." "People are wrong to act like that."

◎ **Taking things personally:** Seeing yourself as the cause or source of some negative external event that is not entirely about you. "It's all my fault."

◎ **Discounting the positive:** Overlooking your successes and casting thoughts in a negative or pessimistic way. "Losing a pound this week doesn't count."

◎ **Labeling:** Describing a person or situation in a narrow, derogatory, or negative way. Labeling is simplistic and judgmental and prevents further analysis. It is dismissive and suggests that little can be done or nothing more needs to be understood. "She's an idiot." "He's a workaholic."

If you can't put it on a to-do list, don't worry about it.) For example, instead of worrying about losing weight, pay attention to changing your eating and getting regular exercise.

Worrying is usually an attempt to control or feel in control of something beyond your control—the future or someone else's behavior. When worry thoughts do occur, it is best to recognize them for what they really are—worries about future threat or coping ability, not something in the here and now. Rather than attaching to them—getting fused with your worry thoughts—simply notice them. Think of thoughts as waves that continuously wash up on the shore—and wash out again. Like someone sitting on the beach, you can watch them come and go without getting caught up in them.

Underestimating Your Coping Ability

Another part of catastrophizing is the tendency to *underestimate your ability to cope*. In this case, you worry that you won't be able to handle the problem or cope with the projected consequences of the threat. The overestimation of threat, coupled with an underestimation of your ability to cope, usually results in emotional overload and an attempt to retreat from the problem—often by eating to avoid thinking about the problem and to squelch feelings of anxiety or other emotions. Examples of this thinking include: "If I don't lose weight this time . . . then I couldn't stand what people would think," ". . . then I'd be too ashamed to even try again," or ". . . that would mean I really can't ever control my eating." The problem is, the worry thought you are trying to forget keeps coming back again and again. So the best thing to do is just let the thought be there—defuse from it—without letting it overwhelm you. Don't try to make it go away. Accept it for what it is—just a worry thought—and realize that you don't need to do anything but let it be.

The more you deem a threat to be catastrophic, the less you are likely to feel you can cope. In most cases you are more capable than you give yourself credit for. In fact, people almost always do cope. In the very worst situations—tsunamis, hurricanes, bankruptcy, deaths in the family, divorces—people find a way to cope and survive. You might think that you should plan ahead: "If such-and-such happens, how will I cope?" But too often you think about what you would do over and over again. You obsess about what you would need to do, trying on different scenarios and potential solutions. Don't do this. You are trying to control the future and your feelings of anxiety with such misdirected planning. Such thinking leads nowhere except to more anxiety. Instead, acknowledge to yourself that whatever the catastrophe, you will handle it at the time. In the meantime, figure out what you need to do at this moment to live your life.

OVER-GENERALIZATION

People sometimes decide what something means based on one seemingly relevant piece of evidence, the importance of which they then exaggerate. Deciding that you can't lose weight because you tried once and didn't succeed—and then acting as if this means that it will always be that way—is an example of over-generalizing. To avoid making this interpretive error, check all the facts and make an informed decision. Separate facts from feelings. Try to be even-handed in evaluating the facts, and take into consideration evidence for and against the conclusion you came to. For example, before you decide that it is impossible for you to maintain regular exercise because you joined a gym once and then never went, consider that there are other ways you might successfully make exercise a regular part of your lifestyle.

JUMPING TO CONCLUSIONS

When you jump to a conclusion, you decide what something means by relying only on intuition or suspicions, with no concrete evidence to support your conclusion—or you believe and rely on unreliable sources. You may be making unwarranted connections between ideas or events that are unrelated, or that are related in a much different way. Take, for example, the person who says, "I have the feeling he's cheating," or "I just don't think I have what it takes to lose weight."

Sometimes intuition can be right, but sometimes it misleads you. Before you accept a thought as "fact," consider that the mind can play tricks that make you feel bad. Ask yourself what is coming through to my intuition? Is there any evidence to suggest that you could be right? Or is it perhaps fear, anxiety, or a concern that *you* are not okay in some way? Check out the facts, and keep an open mind to the situation until you have more reason and evidence to support a conclusion.

MIND-READING

Like jumping to conclusions, mind-reading also involves making assumptions. In the case of mind-reading, the assumptions are about another person's thoughts or feelings. "I think she is mad at me and that I don't like her friend." Mind-reading is assuming that you know what is in someone else's mind or what he or she is feeling without checking it out, and then going ahead and acting as if what you think is true. Stop and check yourself when you think you already know what someone's behavior means. What is the evidence for your assumption? Ask yourself whether you are engaging in mind-reading—and thus possibly reaching an erroneous conclusion. What have you done to check out your conclusions?

FORTUNE-TELLING

Fortune-telling involves predicting the future, usually with little or no evidence to support the prediction, such as, "I won't enjoy the party." But it is not possible to know the future. When you try to foretell the future, you may anticipate the future in a self-protective but potentially damaging way, relying on your feelings about a future event to predict its outcome. Deciding ahead of time that you won't enjoy a party virtually assures that you won't. It becomes a self-fulfilling prophecy. It is better to be open to future possibilities and consider how your behavior can influence your feelings about an outcome. Having a bad time at the party isn't a foregone conclusion unless you decide it to be so. Likewise, predicting that you won't be successful in losing weight increases the chances that you won't.

Those who have failed at losing weight or keeping it off are vulnerable to fortune-telling because of their past experiences. However, weight management is possible for everyone when they make permanent changes in their food choices and exercise. The National Weight Control Registry (NWCR), established in 1994, is conducting the largest, ongoing investigation of long-term successful weight loss. So far they have tracked and examined weight loss strategies of over 5,000 people. They have reported that although there is a wide variety of ways that people lose weight, most succeed in keeping it off by maintaining a low-calorie, low-fat way of eating in conjunction with high levels of physical activity. NWCR provides concrete evidence that many ordinary people can take off weight and keep it off.

You need to maintain hope that the future brings new possibilities and be open to them. Rely on real evidence and facts to anticipate what the future will bring. In the meantime, bring your focus to the here and now, and be open and receptive to your experience. Remember that if you eat less and exercise more each day, you will be closer to achieving your healthy lifestyle goals.

FILTERING

Filtering is a thinking error that involves paying selective attention to information. When you filter information, you notice only certain things and ignore other information. Filtering can cause you to miss data that you need in order to cope more effectively. For example, you may notice all your faults, what you did wrong, and how you failed, but at the same time filter out what you did right and whatever successes you may have had.

You may be able to recite examples of how you failed and reasons why you don't have what it takes to succeed with weight management, but then you fail to pay much attention to the many times you made healthy food choices, managed your behavior well, or achieved other small successes. To overcome the error of filtering, you need to become aware of this bias in your thinking and give credit to your accomplishments.

Many people don't realize that weight loss is not linear; it generally takes a longer time than expected for changes to show up. You need to take care not to lose sight of the fact that what counts are not small slips, but rather the overall trend of positive behavior change. As healthier choices are made more often and exercise is increased gradually, adjustments in weight will follow. Weight change follows sustained, long-term, healthy behavior, not occasional, short-term deviations. This is why the focus needs to be on behavior change, not weight.

DISQUALIFYING THE POSITIVE

Disqualifying the positive is about interpreting successes in a negative light. "It was just luck that I won the race." This cognitive error turns success on its head. It leads you to decide that anything positive that happened had little or nothing to do with your effort or commitment. Be sure to take credit for the smallest successes. Keep a positive attitude; it is not about losing weight quickly—it is about changing your lifestyle over time.

EMOTIONAL REASONING

Emotions are important sources of information. They are usually the first alert system that tells you to pay attention to something. Emotions, however, are most helpful when used in conjunction with rational thinking. When emotions drive action, trouble can result. You may recall a time when you acted out of emotion and later regretted it. People who use emotional reasoning may also reach conclusions about themselves based exclusively on feelings. For example: "I feel bad, so I must not measure up." "I feel guilty, so I must have done something wrong." These conclusions are based on nothing more than feelings, and they subsequently generate painful thoughts. Remember that feelings are not facts. They are only one tool you have for understanding and behaving.

"SHOULD" THINKING

"Should" thinking occurs when you want things to be different from the way they actually are. Usually you think that the way things are is wrong-headed, and that your way of thinking is right. People who engage in "should" reasoning seem to have a little rulebook in their heads: "The World According to Me." They operate on assumptions they make about right and wrong, and they don't want to accept the realities that exist. As a result, they often feel angry and protest when their assumptions are violated: "Things should be *fair!*" "Should" reasoning is often used by people who need to be right and who refuse to entertain contrary points of view. As a result, their relationships often suffer.

Adopting mindfulness—which is an open and receptive attitude that does not include judgments of right and wrong, is an antidote for "should" thinking. It allows you to stay present in the moment and not get sucked into right/wrong thoughts and arguments, which often create discomfort or pain.

Empathy—seeing the other person's point of view, without necessarily agreeing with it—is required to overcome "should" thinking. Even if you are convinced that the other person is wrong, you can generally find a way to validate his or her right to his or her opinion. Don't get into a struggle over who is right. "Should" thinking is about control—of knowing the rules and upholding standards. People who indulge in "should" thinking try to control by deciding and acting on what they declare to be "right." Such thinking is inflexible and unproductive.

Not getting caught in "should" thinking makes it possible to take reasonable or realistic steps to change the situation at hand. The challenge is to set aside anger and "should" reasoning and think of another approach to solving the problem.

TAKING THINGS PERSONALLY

Sometimes you may erroneously interpret other people's behavior as being all about you. A woman who was about 20 pounds overweight was having lunch with a large group of people when one person at the table made a comment as a very overweight person passed by: "How can people let themselves go like that?" The woman interpreted the remark as meant for her. She had fallen victim to the interpretation error of personalization—taking things personally. As a result, she felt bad.

People who take things personally tend to have doubts about their own worth. As a result, they expect others not to value them very highly. Others' remarks and behavior are regarded with suspicion, and they react with hurt feelings, indignation, and withdrawal to perceptions of their being devalued. They usually nurture feelings of anger about the perceived slight or insult, not realizing that their own misunderstanding and negative self-view are the real cause of their emotional upset.

If you tend to take things personally, feeling that other people are putting you down or mistreating you on purpose, you need to examine your beliefs about yourself. Low self-esteem and self-critical beliefs create the expectation that others are out to hurt you. In most cases, this is not true. The tendency to take things personally also arises from the belief that being loved and respected by everyone is a dire necessity. If you find yourself feeling hurt by others' remarks, consider what beliefs you hold that may be giving rise to these feelings.

Even if an unkind remark or act is meant for you, you don't have to take it personally. To preserve your self-esteem, learn how to hear and use criticism but not let it hurt you. Perhaps the person is just being insensitive. Not every personal remark or comment made by another is meant to be hurtful. But it could contain some truth that would be worth considering. Consider the often-painful situation of undergoing a job review. You may hear critical things that hurt your feelings. You may feel that these comments are unfair or biased. Try to evaluate feedback for what it is—just information. It may or may not be fact. If there is some truth there, use it. If not, disregard it.

LABELING

Another interpretive error is labeling. This involves making a quick judgment about another person and applying a negative label such as "jerk," "idiot," "narrow-minded," or "hypersensitive." Making a sweeping conclusion about someone is also labeling. Deciding that someone is "always so defensive" or "impossible to get along with" causes you to form an expectation and to see them and treat them in a particular way. Once you label, you find evidence to support your conclusion, and you overlook any information to the contrary. Often the impetus to label comes from the arousal of some emotion, perhaps by a negative interaction with the person being labeled. Sometimes labeling takes the form of a catty, offhand remark. Even so, labeling biases your thinking about another person.

Consider the man who made a judgment about each person he encountered immediately upon meeting them. In many cases these judgments kept him from taking seriously any information that did not confirm his original unfounded opinion. When he moved from an artistic section of a large city to a small academic community, he decided that the people in his new neighborhood were too "linear," and he just couldn't relate to them. He missed his old friends and made few efforts to make new ones. Having labeled the people around him in a negative way, he missed the opportunity to learn more about them and perhaps come to like some of them. Feeling isolated and lonely, he ate himself into a weight problem.

Labeling does not recognize the nuances of people's personalities or take into account all the evidence. Often labeling is used to shift blame to another person or entity and is accompanied by feelings of anger or upset. To avoid labeling, first notice when you are doing it—it is usually signaled by pejorative words such as, "stupid," "selfish," or "idiotic." When you find yourself labeling, ask yourself whether this is a way of feeling superior to another person. Remember that it is easy to find fault with anyone—no one is perfect.

HELPING AND HINDERING SELF-TALK

Identifying your cognitive distortions is one way to begin adopting thinking that can help you manage your weight. Learning to recognize and promote helping self-talk is also a good way to further your weight management goals. Attaining your goal weight and maintaining it over time remains the biggest challenge for weight management. Many variables have been investigated in the hope of shedding light on what predicts success. Researchers agree that there are multiple causes of obesity, and that obesity is probably not a unitary phenomenon. Increasingly obesity is being conceptualized as a chronic, prevalent, and refractory disorder. Research has suggested that self-talk is one of many factors that plays a role in weight management.

It is known that self-talk can fuel emotions, and emotions can in turn produce more self-talk. Research has shown that people who are depressed have a hard time thinking anything other than depressing thoughts. What's worse, such thoughts lead to even more intense feelings of depression. Likewise, ruminating over angry thoughts can make a person even angrier, just as thoughts of being alone, without social interaction, can increase feelings of loneliness. A person with a positive outlook on life generally experiences pleasant thoughts, and his or her actions tend to reflect those of a person with a positive attitude. But the person who is a pessimist tends to have gloomy thoughts, and sees things in a negative light.

Some scientists have been able to demonstrate that the ratio of positive to negative thoughts characterizes various mood states and the ability to cope.[4,5] This doesn't necessarily mean that one should try to get rid of negative thoughts and replace them with more positive ones, although some experts recommend this. However, recognizing the difference between helping and hindering thoughts can be helpful. The concept of "negative" or "positive" self-talk suggests that some thoughts *feel* bad and others *feel* good—that is, this way of conceptualizing self-talk implies that the emotional valence of thoughts is what counts. A more useful way to characterize self-talk is to ask what the *function* of the thought is. Does the self-talk help to achieve a goal or impede reaching the goal? Is it consistent with guiding principles and values, or does it contribute to hindering action?

For example, some research has shown that certain kinds of self-talk—*helping* thoughts—characterize those who succeed in managing weight, whereas other types of self-talk—*hindering* thoughts—typify those who do not succeed. An example of a helping thought would be: "Just stay away from the food table and focus on talking to friends." This is a helping thought that gives a self-instruction about what to do. Alternatively, a hindering thought might be: "Oh, it's a party, after all; and how often do I get a chance to go to a party with such great food?" This is a thought that gives you permission to overeat by making an excuse and giving a rationalization.

SELF-TALK OF UNSUCCESSFUL DIETERS
VERSUS THAT OF THOSE WHO SUCCEED

Research has demonstrated that people's self-talk can influence their coping ability when it comes to depression.[6] In one study, when people exhibited more positive self-talk than negative self-talk, they were less prone to depression and were better able to cope, especially as the ratio approached 2:1—two positive thoughts for every one negative thought.

In terms of weight management, other research has shown important differences in helping and hindering self-talk between those who succeeded in losing and maintaining weight loss versus those who still struggled with losing weight.[7] This research looked closely at how much helping self-talk versus hindering self-talk characterized those who were successful at losing weight and keeping it off and those who were not.

TIP To understand more about self-talk, check out **www.youtube.com/ watch?v=n0L1-fTC7F8**. Here you will find a video by Dr. Bill Lampton, communication expert, entitled "Support Yourself with Upbeat Self-talk."

In this research, people who were able to maintain weight loss showed a relatively healthy ratio of two-thirds helping to one-third hindering self-talk, whereas dieters tended to have lower proportions of helping self-talk. That is, they engaged in relatively more hindering self-talk than helping self-talk. However, the exact ratios of helping to hindering self-talk for both maintainers and dieters depended on several factors. Situation was one of these; for example, socializing with friends often led to excuses to overindulge (hindering self-talk) for both those who succeeded and those who didn't. Another factor was how far from goal weight the dieter was at the time of the study. Those who had more weight to lose exhibited more hindering self-talk. Those who were closer to goal but who were still dieting showed better ratios of self-talk than those who were further away. Likewise, the longer maintainers had been at goal weight, the better their ratios were. Early maintainers (those with less than six months at goal weight) had slightly less healthy ratios.

Hindering self-talk of dieters took many forms: excuses and rationalizations, self-blame, blaming others, losing sight of goals and guiding life principles and values, looking for immediate gratification, feelings of deprivation, feeling deprived or resentful, deliberately abandoning goals and guiding life values, or simply ceasing thinking (i.e., going blank or spacing out).

In contrast, helping self-talk of those who succeeded was characterized by using self-instruction, acknowledging personal accomplishments, maintaining an optimistic attitude and positive expectations, keeping sight of and staying mindful of goals and guiding life principles and values, staying mindful of long-term consequences, focusing on immediate rewards for "doing the right thing," and remaining conscious, aware, and mindful. For examples of hindering and helping self-talk, see Table 6.2.

Of course, it is not possible to know whether self-talk caused maintainers to succeed or dieters to struggle with weight, or whether success or failure caused a particular type of self-talk. We just know that those who had been at goal weight longer had healthier self-talk than those further away from their weight goal. What is important here is to take notice of the kind of self-talk that characterized each group and determine which kinds of self-talk you engage in.

Like most people, you probably combine several kinds of thoughts at any given time. See Table 6.3 for examples of combined hindering self-talk statements. It is helpful to tease apart the types of self-talk you use and ascertain your ratio and proportions of helpful versus hindering self-talk. Doing so will help you recognize which thoughts are distressing and hinder your weight management efforts, and which thoughts keep you focused on your goals and values.

Table 6.2
COMPARISON OF HINDERING AND HELPING SELF-TALK

Hindering Self-talk	Helping Self-talk
Using excuses, rationalizations, and justifications. *Examples:* "Just one won't hurt." "I may as well eat it now and get it over with." "I'd better eat it so it doesn't go bad in the refrigerator." "I need to rest today instead of trying to exercise." "I'll start tomorrow." "I can't ask others to change their way of eating just because I need to lose weight."	**Using self-instruction.** *Examples:* "Wait 10 minutes before eating, and focus on doing something else right now." "Stay out of the kitchen. Enjoy reading your book." "Stop. Don't do that. Do something else." "Let's get going to the gym now." "Just drink some water and go back to bed."
Engaging in excessive self-blame, self-criticism, or self-denigration. *Examples:* "I'm ashamed of myself." "I hate my body." "I'm disgusting." "I'm a failure." "There is something wrong with me." "No one could like anyone as fat as I am."	**Providing acknowledgement of personal accomplishments.** *Examples:* "I've worked hard to lose all this weight." "I can stay in control." "I'm pleased that I'm getting stronger." "It's okay to give myself pats on the back for small successes." "Yes, I bought a whole box—but I only ate one, and threw away the rest."
Blaming others or external circumstances. *Examples:* "I have to take clients out for lunch almost every day, so I can't control my calories." "They keep bringing food to work; I can't help eating it." "With my schedule I just can't fit in time to exercise." "She insisted that I eat. I didn't want to offend her."	**Having an optimistic attitude and positive expectations.** *Examples:* "I think I can do it this time." "If she can do it, I can do it." "I feel empowered about managing my weight in a way I have never felt before." "I can handle this." "I'm going to complete a 5K race next month even if I have to walk part of it."
Losing sight of goals, values, and guiding life principles. *Examples:* "What's the use?" "Who cares?" "Why bother?" "Why keep trying?" "What's the point?" "It won't matter."	**Attending to future consequences of proposed actions and staying in touch with goals, values, and guiding life principles.** *Examples:* "If I eat this, I could lose control." "I want to maintain my success." "I want to be healthy, and this won't help." "If I eat it, I'll probably eat more, and then I'll feel bad."
Focusing on immediate gratification. *Examples:* "It would taste so good." "What looks good to eat?" "I'll feel better if I eat." "I love chocolate."	**Attending to long-term consequences to avoid making unhealthy choices.** *Examples:* "I'll keep gaining weight if I keep binge eating." "If I want to be healthy, I have to stop using excuses to eat inappropriately."

(continued on next page)

Table 6.2
COMPARISON OF HINDERING AND HELPING SELF-TALK
(CONTINUED)

Hindering Self-talk	Helping Self-talk
Focusing on being deprived and resentful. *Examples:* "Why can't I eat like other people?" "Why me?" "I hate having to change what I eat." "Why can't I eat what I want?" "I wish I didn't have to do this." "I hate exercise." "Low-calorie food doesn't taste good." "Poor me, I have to give up everything I like."	**Focusing on immediate rewards of making a better choice.** *Examples:* "I'll feel better about myself when I choose something healthy to eat." "Making good food choices makes me feel good." "I feel like I've accomplished something every time I finish my exercise routine."
Deliberately abandoning goals, values, and guiding life principles. *Examples:* "I know I should stop, but I don't want to." "I just need something to nibble on, so I'm going to eat." "I want something sweet."	**Maintaining a single-minded focus on goals, values, and guiding life principles.** *Examples:* "I've worked too hard to blow it now." "I'm taking it one day at a time." "Is this what I really want?" "Does this accord with my values?"
Not thinking and just eating. *Examples:* Going blank, numb, or spacing out. Choosing not to think. Going into a trance. Not thinking.	**Remaining conscious, aware, and mindful of values and guiding life principles.** *Examples:* "A healthy lifestyle is important to me." "I want to be healthy." "Exercise is what I do." "I make healthy food choices."

ASSESSING YOUR GOAL-RELATED SELF-TALK

A good first step in attempting to improve your self-talk is Self-Test 6.1, Inventory of Goal-Related Self-Talk, which was developed and validated as part of the research project mentioned earlier.[8] This self-test helps you identify the ratio of your helping to hindering types of self-talk. Complete the questionnaire and follow the scoring instructions provided. If your ratio of helping to total self-talk is less than 0.5, your self-talk may be undermining your weight loss efforts. After you complete the self-test, look at Table 6.4, Key to Goal-Related Self-Talk, which is a key to the types of helping and hindering self-talk that each item of the inventory represents. Refer back to Table 6.2, Comparison of Helping and Hindering Self-Talk, for more examples.

Table 6.3
COMBINING TYPES OF HINDERING SELF-TALK

It is not uncommon for people to combine several types of hindering thoughts at once. Here are some examples:

◎ "It was Super Bowl weekend *(blaming external circumstances)* and I was bad *(self-blame)*. I ate and drank too much."

◎ "Someone brought doughnuts to the meeting *(blaming others)* and they were just there in front of me *(rationalization)*. Before I knew it I had eaten several *(abandoning conscious control)*."

◎ "I decided that it had been a rough day and I deserved a treat *(excuse and rationalization)* so I ate one of the cookies offered *(abandoning conscious control)* and afterwards I couldn't stop thinking about how good they were *(focusing on immediate gratification)*. I just had to go to the store and buy some more *(deliberately abandoning goals)*. Afterward I felt terrible for eating the whole bag *(self-criticism)*."

Dimensions of Helping and Hindering Thinking

The sixteen types of self-talk described in the Comparison of Helping and Hindering Self-talk table and assessed in the Inventory of Goal-related Self-talk were subjected to a statistical procedure called factor analysis in the research study mentioned. Results suggested that these types of self-talk tapped into four important dimensions of helpful versus hindering problem thinking.[9]

Five of the hindering self-talk items (#1, excuses and rationalizations; #3, self-blame; #9, immediate gratification; #13, deliberately abandoning goals and life principles; #15, not thinking, blanking out, going numb) loaded on one factor, suggesting that people who used these types of thoughts function at the level of *program control*. That is, the behavior of people having these sorts of thoughts was more or less automatic and required minimal conscious control. These hindering thoughts reflected inadequate self-vigilance, selective or misdirected attention to information, or the intentional neglect of information that could be helpful in attaining a goal. Program control thoughts seemed to characterize dieters in the study.

Two items of hindering thoughts (#5, blaming others or external circumstances; #11, feeling deprived and resentful) and one inverse of a helping thought (#6, not having an optimistic attitude) loaded on another factor and seemed to reflect a kind of dimension of *peevishness*. That is, taken together, blaming others or circumstances, focusing on feeling deprived or resentful, and not having an optimistic attitude suggested ill humor, a querulous temperament, obstinacy, and difficulty in being pleased that is likely to be goal-hindering.

SELF-TEST 6.1
Inventory of Goal-Related Self-Talk

Instructions: Put a check mark by each of the statements that is true for you.

___ 1. I find excuses for eating what I know I shouldn't, or I rationalize that I will start all over again later.

___ 2. I tell myself what to do and how to cope so that I can stay or get back on track.

___ 3. I get down on myself and become self-critical because of my weight or my eating.

___ 4. I periodically remind myself that at times I have been able to do well managing my weight or my eating.

___ 5. I often think that others, or circumstances beyond my control, are the reason for my eating or my weight management difficulties.

___ 6. I try to stay optimistic and have positive expectations for succeeding.

___ 7. When the opportunity to eat something presents itself or I want something good to eat, I avoid thinking about the long-term consequences of eating—such as gaining weight or feeling bad later.

___ 8. I frequently remind myself of why I want to lose weight or maintain weight in order to stay motivated and avoid overeating.

___ 9. I get to thinking about how good something will taste, and I forget about everything else.

___ 10. I focus on how bad I'll feel if I do something unhelpful—such as overeat or skip my exercise.

___ 11. I often feel deprived, tired of doing without, or annoyed with having to manage my eating or my weight.

___ 12. I usually focus on how good I'll feel for doing what I need to do now to manage my eating or my weight.

___ 13. I often don't care about what I "should" do, and I focus more on what I want to do.

___ 14. I use mindfulness to stay present in the moment.

___ 15. Sometimes I stop thinking altogether and just eat; only afterwards do I think about what I've done.

___ 16. I want to be healthy, and I value regular exercise.

Scoring:

Count all the check marks in the even-numbered statements: _____

Divide your total checked number of even-numbered statements by 16: _____

Interpretation: If your result is 0.50 or less, your self-talk is hindering your weight loss efforts.

Table 6.4
KEY TO "INVENTORY OF GOAL-RELATED SELF-TALK"

1. I find excuses for eating what I know I shouldn't, or I rationalize that I will start all over again later. **(Excuses, rationalizations, and justifications)**

2. I tell myself what to do and how to cope so that I can stay or get back on track. **(Self-instruction)**

3. I get down on myself and become self-critical because of my weight or my eating. **(Self-blame)**

4. I periodically remind myself that at times I have been able to do well managing my weight or my eating. **(Acknowledgment of accomplishments)**

5. I often think that others, or circumstances beyond my control, are the reason for my eating or my weight management difficulties. **(Blaming external circumstances)**

6. I try to stay optimistic and have positive expectations for succeeding. **(Optimistic attitude and positive expectations)**

7. When the opportunity to eat something presents itself or I want something good to eat, I avoid thinking about long-term consequences of eating—such as gaining weight or feeling bad later. **(Losing sight of goals and values)**

8. I frequently remind myself of why I want to lose weight or maintain weight in order to stay motivated and avoid overeating. **(Attending to distant consequences; reminding self of goals)**

9. I get to thinking about how good something will taste, and I forget about everything else. **(Immediate gratification)**

10. I focus on how bad I'll feel if I do something unhelpful—such as overeat or skipping my exercise. **(Attending to distant consequences)**

11. I often feel deprived, tired of doing without, or annoyed with having to manage my eating or my weight. **(Deprivation, resentment)**

12. I usually focus on how good I'll feel for doing what I need to do now to manage my eating or my weight. **(Focus on immediate reward)**

13. I often don't care about what I "should" do, and I focus more on what I want to do. **(Deliberate abandonment of guiding life principles)**

14. I use mindfulness to stay present in the moment. **(Maintain single-minded focus on goals and guiding life principles)**

15. Sometimes I stop thinking altogether and just eat; only afterwards do I think about what I've done. **(Dissociating, not thinking)**

16. I want to be healthy, and I value regular exercise. **(Aware/conscious of life values)**

Peevishness can produce thoughts such as, "Why me?" and "No one is going to tell me what I can and can't eat." Many who struggle with a weight problem also struggle with the seeming unfairness of it: "Others have it easy; they don't have to watch their weight," they think. Resentment can lead to feelings of entitlement. You may refuse to set limits on yourself regarding food, or you may avoid regular exercise. This kind of attitude can even produce internal quarrels between that part of you that wants to lose weight or be healthy and the part that declares, in essence, "I don't care." When the latter sentiment wins, attention narrows to the idea of eating. Making healthy choices is ignored. Some dieters also exhibited peevishness.

Two hindering thought types (#7, losing sight of goals and guiding principles or values, and the inverse of #16, not staying in touch with goals for a healthy lifestyle) loaded on a third factor and appeared to involve *avoidance* of thinking about one's behavior or the future consequences of that behavior, which dieters also exhibited. These findings are supported by other research,[10] which found that those who are obese reject notions of self-control, avoid placing limitations on themselves, and doubt the possibility of change.

The struggle of unsuccessful dieters appeared to be hampered by poor information management in the form of cognitive distortions, fluctuating and poorly defined values, and attention directed at immediate gratification. The hindering self-talk typical of failure showed a bias toward distorting or selectively considering information, blaming external circumstances, avoiding self-discipline, failing to refer to guiding principles, and neglecting to notice the rewards associated with goal-facilitating behavior.

Six of the helping thoughts (#2, self-instruction; #4, acknowledging accomplishments; #8, attending to future consequences of proposed actions; #10, attending to consequences to avoid hindering behavior; #12, focus on reward for doing the "right" thing; #14, maintaining a single-minded focus on goals and guiding life principles) loaded on the fourth factor and reflected thinking guided by principles and values. These helping thoughts indicated the use of *principle control.* Those whose thinking was guided by principle control—the maintainers in this study—were consciously directing attention to observable elements of the situation as part of the cognitive processing, and were comparing intended action with beliefs about the healthy way to behave. There was a high level of self-vigilance and consciousness, and the use of cognitive strategies to delay gratification. (For example, maintainers reminded themselves of their weight loss goals and, when faced with temptation, tended to delay the decision to eat and then got involved in another activity.)

This research suggested that those who succeeded in losing and maintaining weight loss tended to use higher-order values and standards of comparison to guide their behavior, and they kept their attention on their goals, which promoted better self-regulation.

Taken together, this research suggested that those who succeed in losing weight and keeping it off stayed in conscious control of their behavior, kept sight of their goals, and valued life principles, whereas those who struggled with their weight were more likely to operate on automatic, to feel resentful about having to engage in weight management efforts, and often avoided thinking about the consequences of their behavior. In other words, those most likely to succeed exhibited principle control thinking, and those who struggled were more likely to be under program control. In the material that follows, you will read more about program control and principle control and how to be more successful in managing your thinking.

PROGRAM CONTROL

When you are under *program control*, you lack clarity about your personal life values or guiding life principles, or you lose sight of them. In its simplest form, program control means functioning on automatic without reference to your overriding values. It points to seeking immediate gratification and disregarding long-term goals. Program control involves getting caught up in hindering thinking so much that it obliterates other useful sources of behavior regulation—that is, your values. When you are under program control, you lose touch with what you want out of life in the long run, and this allows you to give in to immediate temptations.

The combination of hindering self-talk and cognitive distortions can make it hard for people to make positive long-term changes. Recall that the behavior of people experiencing cognitive distortions is often automatic and not under conscious control. Hindering self-talk also tends to be automatic, as well as dismissive of goals and values. This mindless kind of thinking is characteristic of program control. You are experiencing program control when hindering self-talk, avoidance (choosing not to think about consequences), and peevishness cause you to lose sight of, or deny, your values and guiding principles as related to health and weight management. When you are under program control, you seek only short-term positive or feel-good experiences and attempt to avoid negative or feel-bad ones in the here and now. Experiential avoidance, a concept from ACT, which was discussed earlier in this chapter, involves trying to control or alter private events (such as thoughts, feelings, sensations, or memories) in a way that is harmful in the long run to your personal well-being.[11] Eating is one way of avoiding the experience of a painful reality and the thoughts that this might generate. Giving into eating lets you forget about the need for self-discipline for weight management.

Consider a feel-bad thought like "I don't measure up" or "I'm fat." You could attempt to suppress such thoughts by trying to think of something else. Such experiential avoidance doesn't work very well. Usually the thought you are trying to suppress keeps coming back. And when suppression doesn't work, the thought can lead to more feel-bad emotions such as increased anxiety or sadness. In an attempt to escape the unpleasantness that the thought and the feeling engender, you might go get something to eat or have a few drinks to numb yourself. Unfortunately, trying to control anxiety just evokes more anxiety, and that leads to more attempts to escape. It is better to simply be aware of the unpleasantness and tolerate the feelings until they pass on their own. As one person put it, "I guess I have to learn to be comfortable with being uncomfortable."

Storytelling

Often those under program control are attached to a story that sets a context for their thinking and behavior. Here's one person's story: "I'm so busy at work that I sometimes forget to eat lunch. I have an open-door policy and anyone can come in for my assistance. Unfortunately, I often can't get everything done during working hours, so I have to stay late. Sometimes I don't leave work until 8 o'clock. Fortunately, my husband cooks, but I'm so hungry by the time we eat that I often have second or third helpings. After dinner I'm exhausted so I just go right to bed." Another story went something like this: "I am a binge eater. I started eating this way when I was in college, and whenever things get really stressful, I binge. I've tried therapy but nothing helps. I am now fifty pounds overweight, and I can't stop bingeing."

While everything said in each of these stories could be absolutely true, the person telling each story is fused, or joined, with his or her story and is trying to solve his or her problems from within the story—without giving it up. The problem is that real solutions may not exist for the story—at least not for the story being told in this particular way. The storyteller has created a conceptualization of herself that is narrow and cagelike, and inflexible behavior patterns are the unavoidable result. Many of us are fused with stories that limit our options. Consider, instead, transcending the story you tell of yourself by choosing to define and live a life in a meaningful way by clarifying and making contact with larger principles and values. These larger principles and values can serve as the chosen standard by which other things and behavior can be evaluated.

TIP Author and columnist Mike Bellah has written an article about the stories we tell ourselves. To check it out, go to: **www.bestyears.com/storieswetell.html**. To read an excerpt from Don Miguel Ruiz's book *The Voice of Knowledge*, on how to stop telling hindering stories, go to: **www.newliving.com/issues/may_2004/articles/ruiz.html**.

Let's consider the people in the stories shared here. In the first story, the person defines herself as available to anyone at work at any time they wish to call upon her. She fails to even consider setting limits that allow her to get her work done in a timely fashion. She regards herself as a nice and giving person. By defining herself in such a way, she has allowed herself no options—thus there is no way out. Choosing to adopt firmer boundaries is necessary for her to find a way out of her story. She has to revise her values—and her story—so that she takes care of her own needs before the needs of others.

The second story is about a person who is stuck in the avoidance of pain (stress) by engaging in bingeing, and as a result, she does not have the ability to behave effectively. What if she were to accept that stress is an inevitable part of life that everyone must address, and that binge eating is simply her personal means of escaping stress? What if she could make contact with a higher value—wanting her life to be about more than food or weight, wanting her life to be about healthy living despite the stresses she faces?

Changing or abandoning your victim story is a first step to defusing or separating from your story. Defusing allows you to step back and observe the story without becoming stuck in it. By taking the point of view of the observer of your thoughts and behavior, you may be able to see other choices. What function does the caretaking in the first story serve? What other options are there? What function does the binge eating serve in the second story? How can the binge eating be overcome? Only when you can see that you are telling yourself a story and are willing to let go of it can you write a new ending. In so doing, it is necessary for you to confront your underlying, core beliefs and reconsider them.

Core Beliefs

Core beliefs are underlying and deeply rooted assumptions. They are called *core beliefs* because they are so central to the core of your self-concept. Such beliefs can be very emotionally loaded and can give rise to thoughts that cause emotional distress. For example, a thought like "I am a fraud" or "I can't succeed" emanates from a core belief such as "I'm weak" or "I'm can't make it on my own."

For more information on core beliefs and false beliefs by Gary van Warmerdam, who promotes audiotapes on self-mastery, go to: **www.pathwaytohappiness.com/writings_falsebeliefs.htm.**

Frequently core beliefs are formed as children. They may reflect your family's—and especially your parents'—viewpoints, which eventually become adopted as your own beliefs. This happens unconsciously; when it is happening, you do not realize that you are absorbing these ideas and making them your own. Take the person who has been overweight since childhood, and whose siblings and parents constantly picked at her about her eating. She probably developed a core belief about herself, her weight, and her eating that may sound something like: "I don't measure up." Or a person who as a child was frequently criticized for all manner of things may have the core belief: "I'm not lovable."

For an example of how core beliefs are formed, listen to Dr. Shad Helmstetter's "The Story of Self-talk" on YouTube at **www.youtube.com/watch?v=rvzfnm9uk-0.**

Beliefs have a powerful impact on many of your attitudes, moods, and behaviors. The woman mentioned previously who was picked at when it came to her weight and eating feels pessimistic about ever changing and today resents anyone commenting about her eating. The person who was severely criticized as a child is likely to struggle with depression and may use food to escape feeling sad and down.

People who let others walk all over them, or who feel they have to please others to be liked, may have a core belief associated with feeling worthless or undeserving. They become caretakers of others to cover up the feelings that these core beliefs generate. Those with low self-esteem, fear of rejection, and fear of failure may believe, "I need others to accept me" or "I can't deal with rejection." Some other core beliefs that can lead to hindering behavior include

◎   I don't count

◎   I'm not lovable

◎   I'm worthless

◎   I don't deserve

◎   I'm defective

All people have core beliefs that are basic to their self-definition, and not all of these are self-hindering. "I'm an intelligent person" or "I'm good with people" are core beliefs that usually facilitate good performance in a job. Core beliefs can be life-enhancing; some people view themselves as personable, trustworthy, honest, reliable, or good-natured. But some deeply held core beliefs reflect fears about the self, such as "I'm different; I don't fit in," or "I'm weak and need support from others."

Destructive core beliefs often give rise to automatic thoughts—painful ideas that come into your head almost without forethought. They may seem to materialize for no reason. The obese person may have the automatic thought "I hate myself." Or the person who is on a diet again might have the sudden thought "I just can't do this." Such thoughts often stem from some deeply held, self-hindering core belief. These thoughts can be so automatic and familiar that they are very difficult to pinpoint unless you listen in on your self-talk and keep a record of your thoughts. Once you do that, you may be able to "hear" the thought and identify the underlying core belief. As with thoughts, beliefs are constructions of the mind. They are not facts. When you uncover a hindering core belief, you can recognize it for what it is—a false belief that is left over from an earlier time or experience that does not have to be believed or acted upon any more. You need to defuse yourself from destructive core beliefs.

Once you identify your damaging core beliefs, you can recognize them for what they are—just tricks your mind is playing on you. Refuse to let such beliefs define you any more. It may be painful to acknowledge your fears about yourself, but doing so allows you to rise above the fears and define the direction you now want your life to take.

PRINCIPLE CONTROL

Principle control is very different from program control. When your behavior is under program control, it is like you are operating on autopilot. When your behavior is under *principle control*, you are in touch with guiding principles and personal values that provide direction for your behavior. You are mindful, and are able to stay in touch with the present moment more fully as a conscious being. You are flexible, able to change or persist based on what the situation affords in service to overarching values.

Values

As discussed in Chapter 2, Getting and Staying Motivated, values are not ends in themselves. Rather, they are directions without a destination. They are about living in a chosen and meaningful way. Values provide the compass heading for your life. Values guide the process of living, but are not themselves outcomes to be achieved. A value should not be "to lose weight." (That is a goal.) The value is to make healthy choices that contribute to a healthy lifestyle.

There are those who have never defined socially acceptable personal values. The values these people embrace may simply be self-serving. Some people who were taught good values by their families or their religion may have consciously forsaken those values. But most people have just forgotten or lost touch with what is important to them, or have never taken the time to think about it. To move forward and address hindering self-talk and core beliefs, it is important that you define your values, stay mindful and present in the moment, accept life's difficulties and suffering, and take action based on your guiding principles.

When you are guided by principle control, you can be aware of hindering self-talk without giving in to it. You are able to simply notice a hindering thought for what it is, without being overwhelmed by it. In order to do this, you need to recognize that thoughts and feelings are transient and need not dictate behavior—that values provide direction for behavior. With principle control, you can let go of the struggle with the inevitable pain of life and do what is necessary to live according to your stated values. It is not necessary to eliminate hindering self-talk so much as it is more important to recognize thoughts that hinder you and not give in to them. Then bring your focus to helping thoughts. Helping thoughts are guided by values. You can accomplish this by staying focused on the larger values of your life and listening to the helping self-talk that points the way to your goals.

Hindering self-talk defeats goal achievement and leads to neglect of guiding principles and life values. Helping thoughts are those generated with values in mind—thoughts that help you to live your life according to chosen principles. Thoughts and feelings are transient; they come and go. An example might be, "This is too hard." If you attach to this idea, you might quit. But if you recognize that this is just a thought that popped into your head, probably because you were stressed, you need not act on it. In other words, you need to keep moving toward your goal.

A good analogy would be that of climbing a high mountain. It isn't easy to climb up over boulders hour after hour, and if you look too far ahead, you can get discouraged by the thought "I have so far to go." On the other hand, if you take it one boulder at a time, in due time you will reach your destination.

The Funnel of Awareness

To succeed in managing food temptations, you need to stay in touch with your values so that you can win arguments with those other inner voices of yours that advocate giving in. If you can stay in touch with your values, you have a better chance of winning the argument for healthy behavior. Alternatively, you may be persuaded by the inner voice that argues, "It's too hard," and give up. If you do, you are likely to lose touch altogether with your values and fall into mindless behavior.

Awareness or consciousness can range from being very broad to being quite narrow. When awareness is broad, values and guiding principles are easily accessible to conscious thought. When awareness gets narrower, values may recede to a distance in your mind and parts of your consciousness can actually argue with one another over what actions to take. At its most narrow, awareness constricts so that thinking is at a minimum. When awareness reaches this point, thinking can actually stop. At such times, eating exhibits a stimulus–response pattern of behavior: food-eat-food-eat. Food is consumed as if the eater were in a trance. This is what happens to many binge eaters.

To illustrate this, imagine an upside-down triangle, a funnel, divided into unequal thirds. At the top, in the widest third, are "values." In the middle third there are "arguments" between inner voices or parts of yourself. And in the bottom third is the "trance," the stimulus–response state where thinking no longer goes on. This concept is illustrated in Figure 6.1.

The key is to stay mindful and in touch with your goals and values—the top of the funnel. If you find yourself slipping down the funnel to the middle and having arguments with yourself about what to do, be careful not to believe the hindering self-talk. Don't let yourself give in to such thoughts. They just come from one part of you, albeit a part that resists conforming to your value of living a healthy lifestyle. Chapter 7, Challenging Your "Inner Voices," focuses more on identifying and defying these internal voices. Let's consider that next.

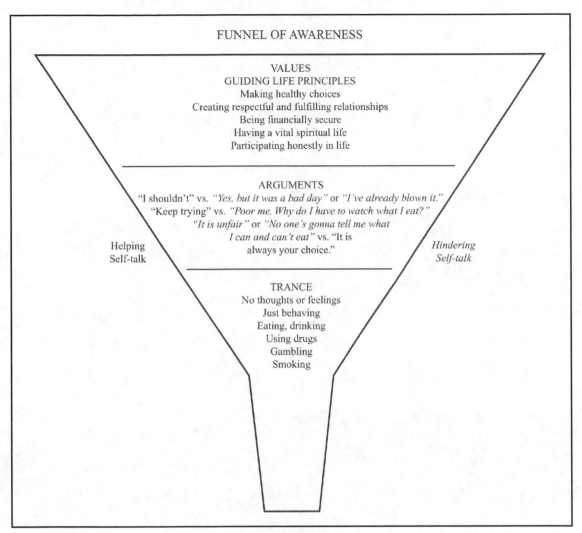

Figure 6.1
FUNNEL OF AWARENESS

CHAPTER SEVEN

Challenging Your "Inner Voices"

SOPHIA'S MOTHER DIED WHEN SOPHIA WAS ONLY 15. *For years before her death, Sophia's mother insisted on weighing Sophia once a week and lecturing her on the perils of getting fat. Between weigh-ins, Sophia's mother was always watching and commenting on what Sophia ate. Now, as an adult, Sophia had a serious rebellious side when it came to food or eating. "I don't want anyone telling me what to eat or what to weigh." In spite of the presence of that strong, internal rebel, Sophia wanted to lose the extra 30 pounds she had gained during her pregnancy. "I think I would just feel better if I dropped these extra pounds. The problem is, I start losing weight and my rebel pulls success out from under me." Once Sophia recognized that she had an internal "rebel voice"—what is sometimes called a subpersonality—she was able to identify that voice and her other inner voices and make better choices.*

Automatic Thoughts and "Inner Voices"

Sophia is not alone in having to face and come to terms with her subpersonalities. An academic journal included this description of a case of emotional eating: a young female college student described an inner voice that often "put her down" by saying things like, "You're not good enough." These thoughts seemed to occur automatically, and they attacked her self-esteem or her abilities to do well. Another voice worried that her boyfriend did not find her attractive or that she would do poorly on her exams and not get into graduate school. Such thoughts happened most often after she ate so much that she felt uncomfortably full. After overeating she would feel guilty and worthless and become even more self-critical. Her inner voices included "the Critic" and "the Worrier."

TIP An article entitled "The Inner Dialogue," written by Remez Sasson, an author of several books on positive thinking, advises visitors how to become mindful of the mind's incessant chatter, which is often negative, and to encourage a more positive voice. The article can be found at: **www.successconsciousness.com/index_00002b.htm**.

Voice Dialogue

A helpful way to understand inner voices or subpersonalities is a method called Voice Dialogue.[1] Developed by Hal Stone, Ph.D., and Sidra Stone, Ph.D., clinical psychologists in Marin, California, Voice Dialogue is a way of contacting, understanding, and working with the many selves that make up your personality. The idea behind this method is not to try and change selves, get rid of them, or help them grow up and be more sensible.[2] Rather, the aim is to allow you greater choice in your behavior by helping you identify which parts of your personality you are fused with and which parts you have disowned—denied, ignored, put aside, refused to allow to emerge. The Voice Dialogue technique allows you to unhook from those selves that have dominated your behavior and begin to explore and become acquainted with their opposites.[3]

Chapter 6, Managing Thinking and Self-Talk, introduced the concepts of the *thinking self* and the *observing self*. Recall that the thinking self is the part of the mind that is responsible for all your thoughts, self-talk, beliefs, memories, judgments, fantasies, and so forth. It has a strong influence on behavior and emotions. The observing self is that part of you that is able to be aware and mindful of whatever you are thinking or feeling or doing at any moment without getting caught up in the content. In Voice Dialogue, the *ego* is the equivalent of the thinking mind, and the *aware ego* is the same as the observing self. For our purposes here, we will continue to use the terms *thinking self* and the *observing self*, rather than the terms used by Voice Dialogue.

SUBPERSONALITIES

According to Voice Dialogue, the thinking mind (ego) is comprised of various parts or subpersonalities, which may also be referred to as selves or inner voices. One of these parts starts developing at birth. Voice Dialogue calls this part of the thinking mind the Protector/Controller. This self learns what behaviors are safe and what behaviors bring rewards. It also notices what behaviors bring pain and which are punished. Early on, the Protector/Controller subpersonality figures out the world from a child's perspective and over time adopts a code of conduct. Eventually this self matures, and by adulthood it becomes what Voice Dialogue calls the Operating Ego—the mature version of the Protector/Controller. It still has the job of protecting the individual and trying to control the environment. However, it shares space with other subpersonalities that have developed as we mature.

As time moves on, and depending on how the child is cared for and the child's environment, other parts of the personality develop.[4] These are additional subpersonalities or inner voices. Voice Dialogue calls these additional subpersonalities the primary selves because they dictate behavior. For example, a Pusher voice may develop to make sure we get done what needs to be done. If it pushes hard enough, we graduate from school or become successful in our career. A Pleaser subpersonality generally develops that causes us to be polite and behave in socially beneficial ways. A Critic develops to keep us living according to our own personal code of conduct or our expectations for our own behavior. The Rulemaker is the subpersonality that decides how things should be and how people should act. Sophie, from the chapter opening vignette, had a Rebel voice that refused to be bound by other people's expectations.

DISOWNED VOICES

The subpersonalities that are primary—the main selves that govern present behavior—have opposite or disowned parts that are not always conscious. So, for example, the Pusher may drive a person to be a workaholic, but the disowned and opposite part of the Pusher is associated with playfulness or relaxation, even with laziness.

Consider the surgeon who refused to take vacations because he had so much work to do. His Pusher wouldn't let him consider taking time off. This was the primary self that he identified with. When he was at home, he spent his time reading medical journals or writing articles for publication. He ignored his family and refused to give himself time off for relaxation. He didn't even realize how this part of him was robbing him of his personal life. He embraced his Pusher and rejected his Relaxer, his disowned self. This man was so fused with his thinking self and not in touch with his observing self that he didn't even realize he had a choice in his behavior.

There are other common examples of opposite selves. Some people have a Procrastinator inner voice, and disown their Proactive self. Other people have a Self-Distrusting voice, and they spurn the part that is Self-Confident. Those people who are rational and intellectual types have often lost touch with their Experiencing or Emotional Self.

Conflicting Selves

The observing self is able to notice and accept both the primary inner voices and the disowned selves, without identifying with either. Your observing self is functioning when you are being mindful. (Remember that mindfulness is a process, not a destination.) The results of becoming more mindful are that you gain access to, and acceptance of, more of who you are. When you are mindful of your inner voices, you realize that it is okay if they are in conflict or disagree with one another. When this happens, your thinking self can also feel conflicted. Sophie wanted to lose weight, but she also resisted implementing self-discipline, which she regarded as coming from the demands of others. However, you can make a decision, even though there is another part of you that prefers some alternative. By embracing more of your inner voices and their often conflicting needs, you are able to make more conscious decisions rather than acting out of habit or compulsion.

TIP   An interesting introduction to the concept of subpersonalities and the practice of Voice Dialogue can be obtained by going to: **www.youtube.com/watch?v=4UvrAQaDGg4**. In this video the presenter describes how inner voices view the world differently from one another. This video provides an introduction to the work of psychologists Hal and Sidra Stone, who in the 1970s developed the concept of the personality as having many individual parts or "selves." Additional videos on Voice Dialogue are associated with the introductory one. A good article on the concept of various selves or subpersonalities can also be found at: **www.delos-inc.com/articles/Embracing_All_Our_Selves.pdf**.

Inner Voices

The notion of inner voices applies to weight management as well. A number of voices can chime in when you want to lose weight or are faced with changing a habit or behavior. Let's consider these inner voices now.

Each inner voice or subpersonality has its own type of self-talk. It also has its own set of beliefs and prescribed ways of behaving. A common inner voice is that of the Critic. It is this voice that is self-critical and can precipitate emotions such as guilt or shame. Another commonly heard voice is that of the Worrier. The Worrier frets about real and imagined threats and whether you can cope; it spins up anxiety. The voice of the Caretaker (or "people pleaser") advocates anticipating the needs of others and meeting them, often at the sacrifice of your own needs. It makes you assume responsibility for other people. Some people have a Victim voice that expresses self-pity or complains about unfairness. The Blamer lays the fault at the feet of others and can elicit anger. The Enforcer (also called the "Rulemaker") talks about the rules and what needs to be done according to your rules, which it holds dear (though many of these rules are not universally held). The Rebel, on the other hand, rejects rules and setting limits. The Perfectionist urges you to set high goals for yourself as a measure of your self-worth. And sometimes your perfectionism is applied to others. If others don't meet up to your standards, the Perfectionist can become critical. Alternatively, perfectionism can be driven by believing that others will value you only if you are perfect. The voice of the Pessimist sees things in bleak terms, engendering expectations of failure.

TIP A spiritually based answer from a Hermetic philosophy point of view regarding subpersonalities is provided at: **www.plotinus.com/what_are_subpersonalities.htm**. The authors provide exercises for you to do to access and recognize your own subpersonalities.

THE CROWD

There are many internal voices. In Voice Dialogue, the multiple inner voices are called the Crowd. In 12-step programs, participants call these multiple voices the Committee. These names ring true, as several inner voices talking at once sound like a crowd or committee that can't make decisions or get along. Members of the Crowd get into arguments with one another. One voice may express one opinion while another voice disagrees and argues back. Some of the voices of the Crowd or the Committee can sound quite rational, while others employ emotional arguments. "I feel so stressed I just have to get something to eat."

Some voices collude with each other. The Critic and the Perfectionist often go hand in hand, as do the Caretaker and the Victim. In certain situations, the Enforcer can call in the Blamer for help. Similarly, the Blamer and the Victim are often partners. Voices can form coalitions against other voices in the crowd. The Victim and the Blamer get together and argue against the good advice of the Healthy voice and the Responsible voice:

"My boss was really rough on me today. He stresses me out."

"Well, go for a walk to reduce your stress. After all, it's your reaction to your boss that is causing the stress. Maybe there is a better way to interact with him."

"Yes, but I shouldn't have to put up with his antics."

IS HEARING VOICES BAD?

Everyone has a set of inner voices, but some people worry about what it means to have internal voices. Some people ask, "Aren't crazy people the only ones who hear voices?" Actually, no. Everyone "hears" his or her own thoughts. The difference between those who are seriously mentally ill and other people who "hear" and act on voices is that the mentally ill don't realize that the voices belong to them and they find them seriously disruptive and disturbing. They think someone or something outside themselves is telling them what to do, inserting thoughts into their head, or whispering behind their backs.

It may come as a surprise, then, to hear that many people who "hear" voices in their head experience some of them as positive. Some voices are adaptive in life, contrary to those voices like the Blamer and the Critic that can foster goal-defeating behavior. Some people believe they can use their inner voices to share a conversation with God through prayer, or to connect with some higher power for good. Many people describe some of their inner voices as being a positive influence in their lives, comforting or inspiring them as they go about their daily business. Others believe they are guided to do "the right thing" by an inner voice for good. Those who are tuned into their healthy voice hear thoughts about the need to get regular exercise and make healthy food choices.

The experience of childhood trauma can give rise to destructive voices such as that of the Victim or the Pessimist, while those who have had more positive life experiences and have formed healthier beliefs about themselves and other people are more likely to develop voices with a more helpful perspective. The Self-Confident voice provides self-talk that is assured, positive, and secure: "I'm training to run a 5K race in a few months; I'm excited about it." The person who has suffered severe trauma may even develop a Paranoid voice.

TIP   Brigham and Women's Hospital, an affiliate of Harvard Medical School, posted a good article on inner dialogue on its website entitled "Listen to Your Head." The article discusses self-talk and weight management. To check it out, go to: **www.brighamandwomens.org/healtheweightforwomen/ emotions/listen_to_your_head.aspx?sub=2**.

WHERE VOICES COME FROM

Early experiences with family and caregivers contribute to the formation of each person's various selves or inner voices. What individuals have heard said to or about themselves or others becomes internalized and integrated into their thinking and their inner voices, as well as being expressed in their behavior. People learn what to expect from others and what others expect of them by the way they were treated growing up. These expectations shape each person's sense of self-worth and self-esteem. Different selves develop as we mature, and these selves influence feelings and behavior in the present moment.

Parents and family are important role models for children. If a parent is a worrier, the child is likely to develop an anxious attitude toward life and internalize the parent's worrier voice. If a parent is critical of a child, the child will internalize the parent's criticisms and eventually develop an internal critical voice of his or her own. Children who are told repeatedly that they are fat and lazy and who are treated as if they can't manage themselves come to see themselves as not measuring up—and may act accordingly. They may develop a pessimistic internal voice or try to compensate by becoming a caretaker of others. Criticism from parents, teachers, coaches, or others is often internalized as true statements about the self. A person who hears negative feedback may try to compensate by becoming a perfectionist. The child who is teased or bullied by peers or siblings is likely to internalize beliefs of being inadequate or unacceptable. Such persons might find themselves saddled with a victim internal voice in adulthood.

Take the example of Sophia, whose mother took her to doctors and enrolled her in programs to lose weight when she was a child and early adolescent. As a result, she developed the idea that she was not okay, and that in order to be loved she needed to be thinner. Kids at school bullied her, and she didn't have many friends. Eating was a way of escaping the pain of being ostracized. As she grew older, when her mother commented that she shouldn't be eating, she became angry and belligerent. "Don't tell me what to do." To escape her mother's criticism, she would sneak food into her room. As an adult, she still had a strong "rebel" internal voice. But she also had a Guilt voice for having been angry with her mother when she had actually wanted to please her all along.

On the other hand, children who are told "You can do it" are more likely to believe in themselves and to try new challenges. Being praised or acknowledged for good achievements, even if the achievements aren't perfect, contributes to higher self-esteem and greater self-confidence. Children absorb not only what parents say, but also what they do. Parents who are supportive when a child's actions fall short boost the child's self-esteem. Such a child probably has an inner voice that may offer messages of self-confidence and promote a positive, take-charge attitude.

In a similar way, the child who has high-achieving parents may internalize the nonverbal message that it is important to set high expectations and do well, even if the parents never actually say so. The father who gets into arguments easily and acts aggressively toward others may influence his son to behave in a similar way. A parent who defers to others and is meek and unassertive teaches a child to do the same. The mother who models taking care of others first and being a people-pleaser is likely to raise a daughter who also becomes a caretaker and a people-pleaser.

This is what happened to Nita, mentioned in the opening vignette in Chapter 1, Understanding the Relationship between Weight and Health. Her mother was a caretaker, and Nita adopted caretaking behaviors as a teen and, later, as an adult. So she took on responsibility for other people's thoughts, feelings, and behaviors. Saying no was difficult for her. And like her mother, she rarely let others know when she was upset. Those few times that she expressed her anger, she "took back" her feelings and quickly apologized. After even minor conflicts, she would eat to forget about her negative feelings. Nita's Caretaker voice reflected lack of assertiveness and the need for the approval and love of others.

Another woman realized that she was always confronting anyone who she thought did not treat her well. When she was growing up, her mother had demanded that she fight back both physically and verbally in such circumstances. She learned to be vigilant for any transgressions people might make. Being always on the alert kept her stirred up. Eating, especially at night, let her relax and provided relief from needing to watch out for people who might offend her. Anger was a prevalent emotion for her and was often hard to control. Hers was a Blamer voice.

Some children adopt behavior that is the opposite of one of their parents and identify instead with the other parent or with an admired person outside the immediate family, such as a teacher or coach. One man who had an angry father became a caretaker like his mother, eschewing conflict as she had always done. Another person whose mother was highly critical of others adopted the more forgiving attitude of her father. Another had a friend whose mother was very supportive of her, and whom she thought of as a "second mother." This support offset the criticism she experienced at home.

In general, the comments and attitudes expressed by parents, caretakers, peers, and significant others eventually become incorporated into a person's own set of inner voices, each of which can be characterized by its own kind of self-talk.

> **TIP** The **www.Kellevision.com** website, produced by a licensed therapist, provides articles and a blog on mental health issues. A good article on self-talk is "The Voices in Your Head: Tuning in to Your Self-talk." It gives examples of healthy and unhealthy self-talk. Check out the article at: **www.kellevision. com/kellevision/2009/11/the-voices-in-your-head-tuning-in-to-your-self-talk.html**.

Identifying Your Inner Voices

It is usually possible to name each of your voices according to the kinds of things each one says, and by its perspective and beliefs. In this section you will find descriptions of some common "voices" that characterize self-talk for many people. Some voices are more prominent at times than others. Each voice reflects some subpersonality or part of your personality. Identifying your most primary and perhaps troublesome voices allows you to figure out the disowned voice that is its opposite. In doing so, you can have greater choice in your behavior and thinking.

It is unlikely that these voices will disappear altogether or change significantly, but in any case that is not the aim. Voice Dialogue however, suggests that a helpful strategy can be to introduce more healthy self-talk to your Operating Ego. Your Operating Ego, according to Voice Dialogue, is the more mature part of you that was originally the Protector/Controller self. This self, armed with healthy self-talk, speaks from your internalized understanding of what is best for you. You may choose to give this self/voice a different name, such as Best Friend or Wise Self or Healthy Self. For now, consider which of the following voices give you trouble and which voices are their possible healthy opposites.

THE CRITIC

The Critic is judgmental, faultfinding, and self-critical. At times this voice may sound like a scolding parent, pointing out your faults and commenting on shortcomings. It may discount achievements and is likely to attribute successes to luck, timing, or an accident of fate. In your head, you may hear the Critic make "you" statements: "There must be something wrong with you that you're not losing weight." "You are so stupid." Or the Critic may use "I" statements: "I should know better." "I hate my fat thighs." "I'll never measure up." "I hate myself for being fat." "I don't deserve to eat anything."

The Critic steals your self-confidence, undermines your self-esteem, and makes you feel demoralized. It promotes shame and guilt. The Critic can prevent you from making an effort, or ensure that you give up your efforts prematurely by calling upon your Procrastinator voice to join in. "I'll start my diet tomorrow." At its worse, the Critic can create or exacerbate depression by saying, "I'm the problem. I'm never going to change. My life is a mess."

The Critic's judgments may extend to others as well, finding fault with their behaviors, ideas, and accomplishments. The Critic can be self-righteous, or envious of others: "Why don't people just mind their own business and leave me alone?" "She thinks she's so great because she's lost weight." The Critic may join hands with your Perfectionist voice that holds others to high standards: "She doesn't measure up."

The Critic wants to be "right" in all matters of opinion. To be right, the Critic believes the other person must be wrong. As a result, the Critic can be argumentative and unreasonable. Here is where the Critic joins forces with the Blamer: "She's wrong."

The opposite of the Critic, the disowned self, is that part of you that is accepting, understanding, and forgiving. It has self-compassion and compassion for others. The disowned self readily feels empathy for others and is kind-hearted. Its manner is soft, gentle, and easy. It pardons the self and others when something doesn't go well, and encourages learning from mishaps. A good name for the self that is the opposite of the Critic is the Compassionate Self.

 To view a video made by Colleen, a layperson rather than an expert, as she talks about her own inner critic, go to: **www.youtube.com/ watch?v=82jWzDfuhNI**.

THE WORRIER

The Worrier voice whispers thoughts that make you fearful and anxious. It predicts dire events. The Worrier voice often starts thoughts with, "What if . . ." "What if I gain weight?" "What if they don't like me?" "What if I make a mistake?" "What if I say something stupid?" "What if I have a panic attack?" With these catastrophizing thoughts, your Worrier voice makes you feel upset, anxious, fearful, inadequate, even panic-stricken at times.

Other Worrier thoughts take the form of "if/then" predictions. "If a man were to see my body, then he wouldn't love me." "If I make a mistake, I'll get fired." "If I lose my job, I'll never get another one as good." "If I have a panic attack, then I won't be able to cope."

The Worrier voice ruminates about scary events that haven't happened yet, and that generally have a low probability of happening. One man worried that he would lose his job if he made even a single mistake, even though his job reviews were consistently good. A college student worried that if she did poorly on a single test, she wouldn't be admitted to graduate school. A woman worried that she would regain the weight she had lost if she made a single high-calorie food choice. Worrying cannot control any of these possible events; only actions count.

Some Worriers worry about problems that may not exist or that are highly improbable. One person worried that he might have married the wrong person, even though he admitted that he mostly was happy in his marriage. A woman worried that she would run out of money even though she lived frugally and had a substantial portfolio. Yet another woman, who was promoted to a high-ranking job, worried that if anyone found out that she came from a blue-collar family, she would be removed from her position.

Often the Worrier worries about situations that cannot be changed or influenced. One woman worried that her son might never marry, even though he was only 31 and was dating some women. Another worried that others would think badly of her, even though she had no way of knowing what they were thinking. As a result, she avoided social situations. With such worrying, anxiety increases—and getting something to eat can help reduce anxiety and provide a distraction from worrying for awhile.

The Worrier is hypersensitive to threat, whether real or imagined. The Worrier may expect others to be critical and disapproving and fears being the target of disapproval, criticism, and rejection. The Worrier compares your performance to that of others and worries, "I don't measure up." As a result, the Worrier voice can lead you to avoid situations in which you think someone else will find fault with or criticize you. By trying to anticipate and avoid problems, the Worrier actually creates problems by causing anxiety that can spiral out of control.

If you are a Worrier, you can get caught up in a swirl of worried thoughts, like so many dry leaves being kicked up by the wind. One worried thought leads to another worried thought, and then another, on and on—seemingly without end.

The part of you that is the opposite of the Worrier thinks rationally about the reality of threat and your ability to cope. It discerns what can be influenced and what cannot, and accepts the latter with equanimity and calmness. If anxiety appears, this Equanimity voice is cool and steady. It knows that anxiety is just a feeling that can come and go, and to fight it is to make it worse. Equanimity is self-confident and self-assured. Fears may present, but

Equanimity exhibits the ability to use common sense and maintain the necessary presence of mind to handle situations that can be handled.

Dr. Beverly Potter, a psychologist who specializes in self-management, has written a helpful article about the worrywart in all of us, and about how thinking can be like an elephant running wild and out of control. To check out this article, go to: **www.docpotter.com/ww_self-talk.html**.

THE CARETAKER

The Caretaker voice tells you to put the needs of others first, and to take responsibility for others. This voice is sometimes known as the People-Pleaser. It advocates that you nurture other people or try to make them happy, often at your own expense. The Caretaker hopes that if you are nice to others, they will like you better or overlook your faults. The Caretaker says things like, "I can't ask my children and my family to change their way of eating for me." "It's not right to make others go without treats and suffer because I need to lose weight." "It's not polite to ask that the hostess change the menu for me." "I don't want to hurt her feelings." "I would rather suffer than see someone else suffer."

The Caretaker tells you not to risk hurting or disappointing others, even if that means getting hurt or disappointed yourself. The Caretaker is afraid to take assertive action in relationships, even when assertiveness is called for. It says yes when it really should say no. It instructs you to curry the approval of others by being nice, polite, agreeable, and undemanding. The Caretaker reminds you that, to be liked and loved, you must defer to others. If you heed all the Caretaker's demands, you are likely to end up feeling unappreciated and resentful, as well as exhausted. Getting something to eat serves as a quick reward, and "grazing" on food throughout the day can dismiss such feelings from your mind, at least temporarily.

An example of someone whose behavior was governed by her Caretaker voice was the woman who insisted on carrying bundles for others, even when they were not overburdened: "But I want to help." She said she felt good when she was helping. She did everything for her husband, including fetching him a beer when he was watching football on television. However, she quietly resented his apparent helplessness and insensitivity to her needs. She ate to feel better, and over time she gained 40 extra pounds.

The opposite of the Caretaker is the Caregiver. The Caregiver gives without strings attached—without hoping for a hidden bargain. The Caregiver understands that taking care of yourself first enables you to better take care of others. The Caregiver self doesn't assume responsibility for others (except children, who can't take care of themselves), but rather offers assistance to responsible adults as needed. The Caregiver respects another's right to be responsible for his or her own thoughts, feelings, and behavior. This self has good boundaries, and is able to say no without guilt.

> **TIP** A good article on how to stop being a people-pleaser, written by author Laurie Pawlik-Lienlen, can be found at: **http://psychology.suite101.com/article.cfm/boundaries**. She discusses the need for good boundaries. An additional article on setting healthy boundaries is also available on this website. Another article on boundaries by psychotherapist Glen Gibson can be found at: **www.counselling-london.org.uk/psychotherapy-camden-issues/resilience-boundaries/**.

THE VICTIM

The Victim voice expresses feelings of helplessness and sometimes martyrdom. It may complain, "Poor me! Why can't I be normal?" "It's not fair that others can eat what they want and I can't." "I can't help myself." "No one is there for me." "I can't get what I need." "I do so much for others, but I don't get anything in return." Sometimes the Victim voice expresses despair and expectation of failure: "I've been fat all my life. There's no hope for me." Because such thoughts are based on wrong assumptions, they lead to more bad decisions that are likely to lead to still more pain, failure, and discouragement. The Victim voice can keep you from trying to change your lifestyle. It reminds you that you feel bad, and that eating helps you feel better—for awhile.

In some cases, the Victim complains of being different, of not belonging. The Victim tells you to expect to be excluded by others and advocates avoiding situations where this could happen. One man explained: "No one would want to go out with me. No woman is attracted to a bald, fat man." A woman described her predicament: "I'd like to make friends, but I don't know how. I had one friend once, but she stopped calling. Even people at work don't seem to like me." Both of these people relied on food to distract themselves from these bad feelings.

Of course, some people have suffered at the hands of others or have been dealt blows by the events in their life. But even if this is so, allowing yourself to feel like a Victim and pitying yourself can become a bad habit that interferes with creating future happiness. Some people even embrace being a Victim, because they feel it proclaims to the world how badly they have been treated. They fear that giving up their victim story would allow others to think the situation couldn't have been so bad after all. One divorced woman said, "If I were to get on with my life and maybe even date again, it would mean I wasn't so hurt by all he did to me."

Allowing your Victim to prevail can cause you to feel like you are owed something, that you are entitled to compensation.[5] This can be where the Victim and the Rebel join forces. "If it weren't for my mother harassing me about what I ate as a child, I'd be able to have more self-discipline. Now I feel like I should be able to eat whatever I want and when I want it."

The Victim can also join with the Critic and reveal feelings of anger or bitterness. One man felt betrayed by his own body and punished himself repeatedly with angry binges. His voices said things like, "I hate myself. I can't control my eating. I'm disgusting. I have a lousy family and a lousy life." Or the Victim and Blamer may together voice complaints such as: "Doctors' offices should have bigger chairs without arms. After all, large people have to wait for doctors, too." "I'm sick and tired of seeing all those magazines at the checkout stand showing skinny women." "Obesity is a handicap; airlines should offer larger seats without additional charges for handicapped people like me."

The opposite of the Victim is the voice of Responsibility. This part of you thinks that you are responsible for your life and for what happens to you—not that you cause pain and misfortune, but rather that you have to cope with it. It acknowledges that there is pain in life, and that no one gets through life without some disappointment. The Responsibility voice promotes self-esteem and confidence. It questions negative thoughts and doesn't become fused with them. When Responsibility joins with Optimism, life goes better.

 To learn more about the Victim Mentality, go to: **www. more-selfesteem.com/victim_mentality.htm**. The author, Karl Perera, offers a subscription newsletter on self-esteem and an e-book for sale.

THE BLAMER

The Blamer voice shifts responsibility for behavior to others or to external circumstances. The Blamer believes, "It is not my fault." It doesn't let you take responsibility for whatever role you played in the outcome of events. The Blamer constantly is blaming others, the past, or something else for life's being difficult: "It's not my fault I can't lose weight." "Nobody cares." "If it weren't for my (children, stress, schedule, etc.), I'd be able to (exercise, stick to a diet, lose weight, etc.)." Often the blaming and defensiveness are only to cover up feelings of defectiveness or failure. The Blamer encourages feelings of helplessness and anger.

Sophia from our chapter opening vignette had a strong Blamer voice as well as a Rebel: "My mother dragged me to weight control programs when I was a kid. That's why I hate dieting." Another woman shifted responsibility for her overeating to her spouse. "He always wants to go out for fast food. He makes it too hard for me to control my weight." When someone else or something else is seen as the source of problem, the Blamer fails to notice his or her own responsibility and thus sees little point in trying to change his or her behavior.

The opposite of the Blamer is the voice of Accountability. This voice enables you to be accountable for the part you played in some outcome, or to see things from a more neutral place without placing blame. In essence it says: "What are the facts? Give me just the facts." Instead of negativity and criticism, Accountability sees both sides of things: "When he criticized my work, I knew he was under a lot of stress from his boss. I do need to take more care when I send e-mails." Accountability enables you to be objective and to do what you can to improve a situation. It helps you reach your full potential and avoids the pitfall of blaming. "Losing weight takes self-discipline; I need to do better with this."

TIP To view a video by Dr. Brian Walsh, author of *Unleashing Your Brilliance* and speaker at the Walsh Seminars, about stopping blaming and becoming empowered, go to: **www.youtube.com/watch?v=SHhq_skecRI**.

THE ENFORCER

The Enforcer voice (sometimes called the Rulemaker) has a penchant for orderliness, perfectionism, and rigid control. The Enforcer demands that you pay attention to rules, details, procedures, lists, and schedules at the expense of flexibility, openness, and efficiency. It tries to reduce uncertainty and control circumstances by making and enforcing rules. The Enforcer often requires that you pay extraordinary attention to detail and repeatedly check for possible mistakes. It says things like: "I have to exercise every day." "I have to be doing something productive." "If I have a dessert, I have to do extra exercise." "I must avoid eating all fat."

The Enforcer feels that rules are necessary to get things done. It wants a rule for every situation. It is uncomfortable when there are no rules, and shocked when someone breaks the rules, no matter their justification.

The Enforcer tells you that you "must" do certain things in a certain way. It tells you to do more, even when you are already doing too much. One person's Enforcer told him that he must guard against making a mistake. If that meant working overtime to get something just right, he did it. As a result, he often felt exhausted from working long hours and fretting about doing things perfectly. For this man, eating something provided temporary relief from the expectations of the Enforcer.

The disowned opposite of the Enforcer is more relaxed, flexible, and laid back. It can go with the flow of things and adapt to circumstances. It argues that rules should not be followed blindly, and it may allow you to follow the spirit of a rule instead of following every rule to the letter. This voice might be called the Easy voice. It is aware of and comfortable with guidelines but doesn't need rules to feel safe. Fun is part of this voice, but Easy never takes fun too seriously. It can have a sense of humor. "Whoa . . . I think I blew that one." Easy is flexible in matters of authority and procedures while still being conscientious. "I really feel like having Eggs Benedict, even though it's not one of my usual selections. It's on my 'rarely chosen' list, and I don't have it often . . . so once in a while is okay."

THE REBEL

The Rebel voice displays a strong sense of entitlement. It tells you that you should have what you want when you want it, and that self-discipline with regard to eating is a bother and an infringement on personal choice. In the guise of self-acceptance, it can relieve you of the responsibility for doing something to curb your eating or your weight. It may even put down those who delay gratification or exercise moderation in their food choices.

Kirstie Alley is an actress who rose to fame on the late 1980s television show *Cheers*. Subsequently, she gained more than 100 pounds over her healthier weight. Despite admitting that she doesn't like how she looks, she has been quoted as saying, "I haven't worked out for three years. I'm just going for the stuff that looks yummy." She says that she tends to eat the most when she's really happy. The actress rebelliously acknowledges a taste for what she calls "abundance"—she says she would have "20 cake domes" in a row if she could.

Another woman who also had a strong Rebel voice was often touchy and easily annoyed by others who made suggestions about anything to her. Others found her touchiness and her bitter complaining about dieting and weight to be off-putting. Her unwillingness to use self-discipline to control her eating urges made it difficult for her to follow a diet for very long.

Sophie's Rebel voice conflicted with her Healthy voice, which kept telling her she would feel better if she lost some weight. She had a tough time resolving the conflict. Her Healthy voice won her over as it kept reminding her of her value of feeling good about herself and having the ability to move around more easily. Even so, her Rebel voice kept up a constant barrage of hindering thoughts. Sophie recognized that a part of her didn't want to exercise self-discipline, but she chose to listen to her Healthy voice instead.

THE PESSIMIST

The Pessimist focuses on how bad things are and sees everything in a negative light. "Life is boring." "The job is boring." "Life is not fair." "Something is bound to go wrong." "Things will never get better." This voice ruminates about what went wrong in the past and uses this as evidence that the future will be bleak. The Pessimist engenders expectations of failure. It is the voice of doom and gloom. The Pessimist is demoralizing. It whispers thoughts, "I've tried before and failed, so why should things be different now?" "No one else really cares, so why try?" "Bad luck is the story of my life."

If you have an internal Pessimist voice, others may think of you as having a negative attitude. The Pessimist in you can keep you from beginning a weight management effort, or can cause you to quit prematurely. If you expect to fail, your ability to sustain effort is diminished. When your outlook on life is negative, food and eating may be the only bright spots in your day.

The Optimist is the obvious counterpart to the Pessimist. Research has shown that an optimistic worldview carries certain advantages.[6] Optimists live longer and experience less stress. The Optimist sees hardships as "learning experiences." The Optimist voice tells you to believe in yourself and your abilities, and to expect good things to happen. Negative events are minor setbacks to be overcome and learned from, while positive events are evidence of further good things to come. The Optimist sees events as short-term, changeable, and mostly under his or her control; the Pessimist sees events as long-lasting, out of his or her control, and subject to luck or other external forces.

To hear Dr. Martin Seligman, author of *Learned Optimism*, discuss optimism, go to: **www.youtube.com/watch?v=8-rMuJW-UKg**. Additional videos by Dr. Seligman and others speaking about optimism can also be found at YouTube.

THE EXCUSE-MAKER

The Excuse-Maker finds excuses, provides justifications, and offers spurious rationalizations to make it okay for you to take actions that deviate from healthy behavior. The Excuse-Maker argues, "Yes, but . . ." It says things like, "With my schedule, it's impossible to eat right." "I deserve a little treat now and then." "No one will see me now, so why not?" "I've blown it already today, so why not eat what I want?" The Excuse-Maker undermines motivation, hinders coping behavior, and defeats efforts to manage eating or weight. It's easy to come up with excuses for letting your impulses get in your way: "I'll have just one."

The Excuse-Maker says things like "I'll start tomorrow" and "I'm not ready yet." It ignores or minimizes facts about the health effects of disordered eating, or attempts to convince you that it's okay to delay taking action. "Yes, I'm overweight, but my blood pressure and cholesterol are fine." "Just because I have an extra 30 pounds doesn't mean I'm not fit." "I'm only 40; I don't have to worry about heart disease yet."

Excuse-making keeps you stuck, wanting change, but not doing anything to achieve it. Granted, it helps you avoid the pain of taking action, but it also keeps you from getting what you say you want.

The opposite voice to the Excuse-Maker is the voice that reminds you to take personal responsibility for your actions. The Responsibility voice tells you to remember your values and goals and act accordingly. It calls you out when you are making excuses and spurious rationalizations in order to justify behaving in ways that undermine your health and weight management effort. The voice of Responsibility knows that you are in charge of your own behavior; no one and nothing can make you do what you need to do except yourself. Responsibility reminds you that it is your choice. Taking responsibility for your life is that extra ingredient that makes taking action a natural thing. Your Responsibility self reminds you to be proactive, not passive.

TIP Susan Heathfield, a human resource expert, has written an interesting article entitled "Success in Life and Work." Check it out at: **http://humanresources. about.com/od/success/qt/responsible_s5.htm**.

Working with Your Inner Voices

The first step in working with your inner voices is to develop a greater awareness of which voices are the most salient in your thinking and most affect your eating behavior. When you read the descriptions in the previous section, did any of these voices sound familiar to you? If so, which ones most influence you? You probably don't have all of the voices listed in the chapter, and you may have others not described here. Some of your voices are likely to be more prominent or troublesome than others. Use your Observing Self to notice which voices and thoughts run your life.

TIP An interesting video on YouTube by Mary Lore, author of *Managing Thought: How Do Your Thoughts Rule Your World?*, talks about watching inner thoughts and observing them rather than acting on them. To view this clip, go to: **www.youtube.com/watch?v=yHuejVXNxaU**.

HELPING YOUR SUPPORTIVE VOICE

After identifying the voices that make up your Crowd or Committee, you can learn to recognize and to listen more closely to what Voice Dialogue calls your Operating Ego voice—your supportive and protecting voice. You can give this voice a new name if you wish—one that means something to you. You might call it your Wise Self, your Best Friend, your Healthy Self, the voice of your Aware Self, or the voice of your Coach.

The Coach is a particularly good metaphor for a supportive voice. If you have ever participated in a sport and had the benefit of a good coach, you know that such a coach is always on your side. Even when he or she offers criticism, it is never cruel or disparaging. A good coach is willing to show you how to improve and is truthful about your problems, encouraging you when things get rough, and always able to guide and inspire.

To help your supportive voice, you need to find thoughts that will counterbalance—oppose or offset—the negative and hindering thoughts expressed by some of your subpersonalities. It is unlikely that you will ever entirely rid yourself of a few particular inner voices, but you can moderate their effect on you by creating and rehearsing counterbalancing statements or self-talk. These may sound like the thoughts of the disowned, opposite voices that were described in the previous sections, or your Operating Ego voice.

Creating Counterbalancing Statements

We all need help to learn how to pay attention to thoughts that will help us and not hinder our efforts at living a lifestyle that is consistent with our guiding principles and values. The following list details some helpful guidelines for constructing counterbalancing self-talk. Following the guidelines you will find some examples of hindering thoughts and counterbalancing statements you can use to counter such negative self-talk.

1. If there is some truth to the negative or hindering thought, create a compound sentence in which the first part of the compound sentence acknowledges that truth.

2. In the second part of the compound sentence, create a thought that opposes or offsets the idea expressed in the negative or hindering thought.

3. Use the conjunction "and" (not "but") to connect the two sentences. (The conjunction "but" negates the sentence that goes before; instead, to be believable to you, the negative or hindering truth needs to be acknowledged and validated.)

4. If the hindering thought doesn't contain a truth and instead expresses an opinion, attitude, conclusion, worry, or other kind of hindering thought, create an opposing thought that expresses a truth or a preference or gives a self-instruction.

5. Make sure that you can believe the counterbalancing thought that you create, and that it is relevant and soothing to you.

6. Encourage your observing self to notice the hindering self-talk of some of your negative voices, and also to notice what the opposite voice might think.

Examples of Hindering and Counterbalancing Thoughts

The following are examples of counterbalancing thoughts created to offset or balance self-defeating or hindering thoughts. Notice how they use acceptance and refocus behavior according to values and goals.

Hindering thought: "Poor me! Why can't I eat like other people?"

Counterbalancing thought: "Some people do seem to be able to eat what they like, and I can't if I want my weight to be healthy."
This counterbalancing thought acknowledges the truth of the complaint and redirects thinking to long-term health goals. Notice that this thought accepts a truth and reiterates a goal.

Hindering thought: "I should do better."

Counterbalancing thought: "I'd prefer to do better; I need to focus on what I need to do right now."
This counterbalancing thought replaces a "should" thought with a preference thought and links it to a self-instructional thought. This is a thought that directs you to take action based on goals.

Hindering thought: "What if they think I'm stupid?"

Counterbalancing thought: "I can't control what people think, and worrying about it just makes me anxious."
This counterbalancing thought states a fact that refutes the worried thought and reminds you of the consequences of worrying about something that can't be controlled. Again, this is an accepting thought.

Hindering thought: "I feel fat."

Counterbalancing thought: "Feeling fat is not a feeling; it is a perception. I'm my worst critic, and I need to focus on making healthy choices instead of berating myself."
This counterbalancing thought states a fact and redirects the focus of your thoughts to managing behavior. This thought directs you to remember your values.

Hindering thought: "I've blown it; I may as well give up."

Counterbalancing thought: "Okay, I made a poor choice. I need to learn from that mistake and start again right now to get back on track."
The first sentence in this counterbalancing thought acknowledges the conclusion you reached; the second sentence is a self-instruction

that tells you what to do instead of giving up. This thought accepts a truth and redirects you to your goals.

Hindering thought: "I can't control my eating."

Counterbalancing thought: "Sometimes I don't control my eating; other times I do. I need to stay focused on doing the best I can."

This counterbalancing thought shifts the all-or-nothing evaluation to one that reflects an accurately moderate position. It then provides an instruction that can motivate appropriate action. This is an accepting thought that redirects your behavior.

> **TIP** Life coaches Robert and Christine Gerzon discuss their "Three Steps to Creative Inner Talk" at **www.gerzon.com/resources/three_steps.html**. According to them, inner talk consists of mind chatter, mental pictures, and physical feelings; they advise listening in on your "Chatterbox" and finding your "Inner Guide." (The Inner Guide is analogous to the Voice Dialogue's Operating Ego.)

CHAPTER EIGHT

Addressing Stress

*MADISON JUST COULDN'T SAY NO TO OTHERS' REQUESTS. Madison worked as a personal cook, and she planned all the meals five days a week for the family of her employer. Planning ahead and managing menus was stressful. Occasionally Madison's employer would ask her to cater a weekend party for 20 to 30 people on short notice. Madison was afraid to decline for fear of losing her job. She nibbled as she cooked and often ate the leftovers. Her weight kept climbing, and she worried that her employer might begin to object to her appearance. Then she found **www.ehow.com/how_5169934_increase-assertiveness-skills.html**, a webpage that helped her learn to be more assertive. She also learned how to elicit the relaxation response and use deep breathing to relieve stress. As she learned to take better care of herself, her anxiety eased and her nibbling diminished.*

Stress and Thinking

We experience stress when we perceive a threat and view this threat as taxing or exceeding our resources for coping. Events or problem situations do not themselves produce stress. Rather, the way we understand an event determines our personal reaction to it. As the philosopher Epictetus once said, "Men are disturbed not by things, but by the view they take of them." Echoing this sentiment, Shakespeare wrote, "Nothing is neither good nor bad, but thinking makes it so." When you encounter something that you feel threatened by and you aren't sure you can handle it, you feel stressed. Another person facing the same situation who believes that he or she can handle this event is not as likely to feel stressed.

For example, if you are unable to meet a deadline for a project at work and you decide that this is a "terrible" turn of events, you will be quite upset. You might even put off starting or working further on the project to avoid thinking about the project and feeling anxious about the deadline. Someone else might not see this same situation as being so terrible and would simply negotiate a new deadline with the boss. That person is unlikely to feel as stressed as you, either because he or she sees the situation as less threatening or because he or she feels it can be handled. How you appraise, or assess, a perceived threat, and your ability to cope, determine your stress level in a particular situation.

TIP If you would like to find out your perceived stress level, a self-test developed and validated by Sheldon Cohen,[1] a psychologist, and his associates can be found at **www.mindgarden.com/docs/PerceivedStressScale.pdf**. The Perceived Stress Scale (PSS) is a widely used psychological instrument for measuring the perception of stress. It is a measure of the degree to which situations in one's life are appraised (thought about) as stressful. Download the PDF from this website to get the PSS. Follow the instructions for scoring. A score of 15 or more indicates higher stress levels.

Appraising Stress

Stress appraisal is a two-stage process. In the *primary appraisal* stage, you first decide whether a threat is real or imagined, and how dangerous you believe it to be. Sometimes it is hard to tell whether the perceived threat is real. In that case, further investigation is needed to determine the accuracy of your perception. Likewise, if a perceived threat is thought to occur in the near future, rather than at a distant time, it will be experienced as more stressful. It is helpful to consider the probability, versus the possibility, of the threat's being real. (Theoretically anything is possible; the real question is how probable is it?) For instance, it is not very probable that you will become obese from a single overindulgence, and your fear that you will is likely imagined. Of course, repeated indulgences can lead to weight gain.

If you decide the threat is real and probable, you must then decide whether the threat is significant, and how immediate it is. How much is it likely to hurt you physically or emotionally? It could be that the threat is real but that you are overestimating how bad it really is. It may be true that a single small indulgence might lead to some weight gain, but it will probably not result in large, sudden weight gain. Sometimes people perceive threats where there are none. For example, you aren't likely to develop diabetes just from eating a little sugar, though eating lots of sugary foods *will* put you at greater risk for diabetes if such eating leads to obesity in the future.

What if the threat is significant and highly probable—like having a bad outcome from visiting a nonlicensed physician or therapist? Of course, the best thing is to avoid exposure to any threat that is avoidable. If a threat is unavoidable, like the car breaking down on a dark road, you just have to cope with it as best you can. It may be helpful to have a contingency plan at the ready for coping—perhaps having a cell phone with you at all times.

The *secondary appraisal* stage has to do with evaluating your options for coping. If you think you can cope with the threat, you are likely to be less stressed, though you will still be alert to taking necessary action. If you decide you can't cope, regardless of whether or not the threat is actually real and significant, you will feel stressed, and you may try to avoid or escape the thoughts of a perceived stressful situation.

TIP The American Institute of Stress is a nonprofit organization that serves as a clearinghouse for information on a variety of stress-related subjects. Its article "Stress Reduction, Stress Relievers" discusses a variety of coping strategies for stress management. To access it, go to: **www.stress.org/ topic-reduction.htm**.

Stress and Coping

Stress demands coping.[2, 3] That is, it requires that you make some sort of response to the demand or set of demands that are perceived as stressful. Responses to stress fall into three broad components—the brain and body's response to stress, the cognitive or thinking response of the mind to stress, and how you have learned to respond to stress.

The body has its own way of coping with stress. Any threat or challenge that an individual perceives in the environment triggers a chain of neuroendocrine events. One of these is the secretion of catecholamines (hormones) such as epinephrine and norepinephrine, which stimulates the "fight or flight" response—which in turn leads to elevated heart rate and a rise in blood pressure. This is followed by the release of cortisol, the stress hormone. Prolonged secretion of cortisol will lead to health problems such as the breakdown of the cardiovascular, digestive, musculoskeletal, and immune systems. When a person cannot recover from ongoing or chronic stress, physical and psychological exhaustion results.

The cognitive component of stress is based on how the individual appraises the situation. According to Lazarus and Folkman,[4] the person's appraisal of threat and the unique coping strategies that he or she uses determine his or her level of stress. In Chapter 6, Managing Thinking and Self-Talk, we discussed the overestimation of threat, which causes anxiety and stress, and the underestimation of coping ability with regard to catastrophizing.

The learned component of coping with stress includes a wide range of stress management techniques that have been found to help ease stress. These include changing the way you think about a situation (e.g., become better at appraising threat and your ability to cope), and using techniques such as eliciting the relaxation response, using deep breathing, engaging in meditation, using guided imagery, and doing exercise to reduce stress. There are also failed strategies for stress management, which result in even more stress. One is the phenomenon of learned helplessness—giving up without trying hard to survive.[5] This phenomenon has also been linked to depression.[6] (The opposite of learned helplessness is learned optimism, which was discussed in Chapter 7, Challenging Your "Inner Voices".)

Both the mind (the cognition and learning components) and the brain/body play a role with regard to stress and coping. Once threat is perceived and coping initially evaluated cognitively, the body experiences arousal. Coping is clearly a complex process influenced by both personality characteristics of the person experiencing the stress, and by the social and physical characteristics of the setting. A strong-willed person who has good social support is likely to be better at coping with stress. And there is an optimal level of stress that actually facilitates good performance. Up to a point, stress stimulates action. But when coping strategies are overwhelmed by demands of the environment, or coping strategies fail, stress becomes unhealthy.[7]

Consider the example of the woman with an open-door policy at work. She made herself available to anyone who needed her advice or who wanted even just to talk. There were times, however, when she couldn't get her own work done because of the intrusion of others. Gradually others started stopping by her office a lot, causing her stress level to rise (and performance of her duties to degrade). To set appropriate boundaries meant having to be assertive and reverse her open-door policy. She was unwilling to do that. The result was that she overate when she got home to deal with her high stress level at work.

 TIP For a comprehensive article on stress management entitled "How to Reduce, Prevent, and Cope with Stress," go to: **http://helpguide.org/mental/ stress_management_relief_coping.htm#top**.

Coping Skills for Managing Stress

Coping is any cognitive or behavioral effort you make to handle stress, and some are more effective than others. Coping involves learning new skills for coping and using them regularly. Coping skills for managing stress can be either problem-focused or emotion-focused.

PROBLEM-FOCUSED COPING

Problem-focused coping involves problem-solving and other active attempts to change a problematic event or stressful situation. This type of coping is helpful for making positive changes in lifestyle. It is best used when a situation or event can be influenced or changed in some way.

Many people with an eating or weight problem don't use problem-focused coping. They often believe it is better to avoid a problem than to confront it directly. They may use eating as a way of distracting their attention from problems or difficulties. Or they may just give up trying to make a change because they don't know how to go about it, or because they think their efforts will be in vain.

Take the example of attempting to incorporate exercise into your life. Two approaches might be that you join a gym or hire a personal trainer to come to the house at times that are convenient to you. One of these solutions might work, but what if you have one or more small children or a career to manage, and there appears to be no time in your schedule for exercise? Now the question is, how can you modify this situation to make time for regular exercise, given that you have limitations? Perhaps you can exchange time with another parent, work out during your lunch hour at work, or get your spouse to watch over the kids while you take time for exercise. It helps if your spouse or employer is willing to work with you to find a solution. The core problem is "making time to exercise." An associated problem is how to find someone to watch the children while you exercise, or how to balance your need to exercise with the demands of your career. When you practice problem-solving coping, you work to address the problems that are stopping you from exercising.

Some people don't use problem-focused coping, because they think there is no easy or available solution, or perhaps they think they have no right to ask someone else to change if the solution to the problem involves another person. Thoughts such as "I don't want to inconvenience my spouse or coworker" or "What if she gets upset because of my request?" may prevent the person from taking action. Once the decision is made that the situation cannot be changed, they simply give up and find some means—usually eating—of forgetting about the problem.

Hannah had a husband who snacked in front of the TV every night. His snacking made it hard for her to resist snacking, too. She thought it was not fair of her to ask him to change his behavior just because she wanted to change her eating. This belief kept her from broaching the subject with him until her therapist urged her to bring it up for discussion. To her surprise, he agreed that he, too, shouldn't eat "junk" food, and they talked about healthier alternatives.

In a similar but more difficult situation, the wife of a man needing to lose weight did most of the shopping and the cooking. She, too, was overweight, but she wasn't motivated to do anything about it. She bought sweets and snack foods for the children and herself, which thus were readily available to tempt him as well. He had to find other ways to cope. Sometimes he could do the shopping and cooking, but mostly he had to decide for himself to use portion control at mealtime. When snacks and goodies were available, he had to decide what foods to eat. His value of good health was the guiding principle he used when faced with temptation.

Sometimes it is somewhat easy to influence a difficult situation with problem-focused coping, but more often it is necessary to find creative solutions to make something happen.

When a difficult situation is not amenable to influence, the problem becomes how to make the best of it. Suppose in the situation first mentioned, Hannah's spouse had refused to change his snacking while in front of the television. Hannah then would be faced with finding another way to solve her problem—perhaps going to another room to watch television or read. She would also, in all likelihood, have had to manage her hurt or irritation about his lack of cooperation. In that event, she would need to employ effective emotion-focused coping strategies as well.

EMOTION-FOCUSED COPING

Emotion is defined by the dictionary as a strong, subjective feeling often accompanied by a physical reaction. The emotional "knowing system" is like the cognitive knowing system and is another, separate way of experiencing ourselves and the environment. Emotions alert the mind to evaluate the situation and take some kind of action.

Effective emotion-focused coping helps mitigate the negative thoughts and feelings that accompany a stressful situation. Such coping is most needed when there is little chance of changing or influencing a difficult situation. Even if the situation can be changed, good emotion-focused coping skills are often needed to manage residual upset or stress.

Emotion-focused coping strategies can be either effective or ineffective and unhelpful. Ineffective emotion-focused strategies include avoiding, distancing, minimizing, or discharging. Examples of avoidance strategies include overeating, drinking too much, gambling, overspending, or abusing drugs. These behaviors divert your attention from the problem and its associated thoughts and feelings. Distancing is an emotional escape strategy that involves emotional detachment or denial. The person using this strategy stops caring or insists that there really is no problem at all. With minimizing, the person acknowledges there is a problem but discounts its importance. Emotional discharge strategies are verbal or behavioral expressions of unpleasant emotions that serve to reduce tension, especially anger-related tension. Examples of discharge strategies include yelling, cursing, hitting, throwing things, or slamming doors.

These emotion-focused coping strategies may temporarily divert attention from painful feelings or provide the appearance of a solution to a problem, but in the long run they create a worse problem. These strategies do nothing to change the existing stressful situation. Furthermore, reliance on avoidance, distancing, or minimizing interferes with the accurate assessment of the problem and delays the adoption of more effective coping strategies. Unfortunately, people who are prone to stress tend to fall back on ineffective emotion-focused coping because they have not been good problem-solvers in the past. In particular, those with an eating or weight problem tend to rely on ineffective emotion-focused coping strategies.

Effective emotion-focused coping uses the observing self to notice the thoughts and feelings that are occurring, and rather than struggling with them or trying to avoid them, the observing self simply notices and does not become embroiled in what the mind and emotions are doing. Other emotion-focused strategies include the learned strategies mentioned earlier. More on emotion-focused coping is provided later in this chapter. First let's consider how to improve your problem-focused coping.

TIP Elizabeth Scott, M.S., has written an interesting article, "How to Develop a Stress Relief Plan That Works." To access it, go to: **http://stress.about.com/ od/understandingstress/a/relief.htm**.

Improving Problem-Focused Coping

Effective problem-focused coping involves assessing and defining a problem accurately, generating possible solution alternatives, deciding which to try, and evaluating how effective your choices are in influencing the situation. If none of the solutions work, you may not have defined the problem accurately. Then you must go back to the first step and redefine the problem.

DEFINING THE PROBLEM

Defining a problem correctly is a crucial part of good problem-solving skills. It involves seeking out available and relevant facts, describing these facts clearly, separating facts from assumptions, and identifying obstacles and conflicts. Some people may have difficulty defining a problem due to a tendency to describe problems in overly vague, general, exaggerated, or negative terms. For example, you may lump several problems into one and feel overwhelmed or unable to find a solution. Feeling overwhelmed should be your first clue that several problems are being lumped together with others; you need to tease apart the problems and tackle each one separately.

Take the example introduced earlier of the man whose overweight wife was not particularly supportive of his weight management efforts. He had to break the big problem down into more manageable pieces: How do I handle meals? How do I handle tempting goodies? What do I do when the wife and kids are snacking in front of the television? And so forth.

In defining a problem, it is important to be concrete and focus on behavior. For example, rather than defining the problem as "I need to lose weight," break it into specific component problems: "I need to reduce calories by cutting back portions," "I need to eliminate sweets," "I need to avoid snacking after dinner," "I need to schedule in times for exercise." Although the objective is to lose weight, the problem definition focuses on the specific behavior changes that need to be made.

Self-monitoring can be helpful in defining a problem. This technique was introduced in Chapter 3, Changing Behavior. Self-monitoring is a means of gathering information about behavior patterns by identifying the antecedents and consequences of a particular behavior. One way to self-monitor is to record information: time of day, food eaten and location, level of hunger, thoughts, feelings/emotions, physical sensations, and feelings afterward. Once you have this information, decide where you can make changes in your behavior patterns.

BRAINSTORMING ALTERNATIVE SOLUTIONS

Brainstorming involves generating lots of ideas without screening or evaluating them first. This invites creativity and encourages you to see a problem and possible solutions in different ways. After defining your problem or problems and coming up with a list of alternative solutions via brainstorming, you will want to evaluate each solution for merit. For example, one person who saw lack of enough exercise as a problem generated the following list of alternative solutions: (1) contact a friend to walk with on a regular basis, (2) hire a personal trainer, (3) join a gym, (4) purchase or rent workout DVDs or videotapes to do at home.

IMPLEMENTING AND EVALUATING A SOLUTION

Once you have generated a number of possible solutions, consider how practical, as well as how effective, each alternative is likely to be. Then choose one (or more) and try it out. Be sure to give each alternative a fair chance to work.

Then after you have implemented your solution, evaluate it. If a solution you have tried results in partial success, consider how you might improve on this, or decide whether partial success is good enough. Be sure you aren't being unrealistic in your expectations. For example, if you try brushing your teeth to interrupt an urge to eat and it works some of the time but not all of the time, it is still a good strategy to use. If the solution you try doesn't work at all, try another. There are always solutions that could be workable even though you might not like any of them. In all likelihood, there is more than one problem subsumed in the initial definition. Go back and start again. Table 8.1 summarizes the steps involved in problem-solving.

Improving Emotion-Focused Coping

Successful emotion-focused coping strategies include eliciting the relaxation response; using mindfulness, deep breathing, imagery, and meditation; learning distress tolerance and emotion regulation skills; learning to be assertive; and managing interpersonal conflict effectively.

Table 8.1
HOW TO PROBLEM-SOLVE EFFECTIVELY

1. Isolate and identify in concrete and specific terms each of the problems involved. Define each problem in terms of behavior to be changed.

2. Treat "feeling overwhelmed" as a signal that several problems are being seen as one big one.

3. Brainstorm as many possible solutions to each problem as you can.

4. Choose one or more solutions and try each out.

5. Evaluate the effectiveness of the solutions you have tried; be sure you have given them a fair chance of success.

6. Review the results. If one solution doesn't help, try another. Return to step 4 and repeat the next steps until you find a workable solution. If you do not find a solution, go to step 7.

7. If none of the solutions you try work, go back and reassess the problem. Look for several problems masquerading as a single problem.

Stress and the negative emotions that accompany stress are often the precursors to overeating. Using relaxation to cope with stress and subsequent urges to eat is helpful. Learning to be more relaxed in general, not just when the urge to eat is present, helps control anxiety and reduces your vulnerability to stress and episodes of overeating. One of the best ways to begin your relaxation training is with progressive deep muscle relaxation. Learning this basic skill will allow you to move on to master the more immediate method of using deep breathing to relax. Focusing on breathing followed by guided imagery is another way to find relaxation. Meditation is like a mind relaxation technique and teaches you to not attach to thoughts as they come through your head.

TIP

Herbert Benson, M.D., of the Benson-Henry Institute for Mind Body Medicine at Massachusetts General Hospital, provides guidelines for an easy way to elicit the relaxation response at this website: **www.instituteoflifestylemedicine.org/file/doc/tools_resources/ ElicitingTheRelaxationResponse.pdf**.

PROGRESSIVE DEEP MUSCLE RELAXATION

If you do not know how to relax, progressive deep muscle relaxation is an important place to start. You can purchase audiotapes, videotapes, and DVDs that can introduce you to progressive relaxation techniques. Check your local bookstore or use the Internet to find a suitable tape. Do a Google search on "relaxation tapes" for options. YouTube videos on the topic can be a resource as well.

It is also possible to teach yourself progressive deep muscle relaxation. The aim of the process is to learn the difference between muscle tension and relaxation, and it has three phases. The first phase involves learning how a tense muscle feels. The next involves discovering what tension release feels like. Finally, you learn to recognize the difference between tensed and relaxed muscles. It is a great technique for reducing overall body tension. Once you learn the long version, you can progress to a shortened version and use it to elicit the relaxation response more quickly.

To begin learning progressive deep muscle relaxation, find a quiet, relaxing place where you will not be disturbed for at least fifteen to twenty minutes. Then sit or lie down, remove your contact lenses or glasses, and loosen any tight clothing. Start with your right hand. Make a fist as if you were having blood taken from your arm. Notice how it feels. Your muscles will be taut and strained, maybe even trembling. (Never tense so hard that it hurts.) Hold the tension for a few seconds, and then let go. Relax your fist, and let the tension slip away. Notice the warmth that comes with relaxation. Repeat the tensing and relaxing of your right hand a few times, and notice the difference between the two phases. Does your hand throb or feel tight when tensed? Does your hand tingle or feel warm when relaxed?

Now progress to the other muscle groups. Move up the right arm to include the forearm with the hand, then the whole arm. Complete that arm, and then do the same sequence—hand, hand and forearm, whole arm—with the left arm. Next focus on your legs: first the right foot, then the foot and calf together, then the whole leg, followed by the left leg. (Do not include your arms when you are tensing and relaxing your legs.) After each tensing and each relaxing, notice the difference in sensations. Pay attention to physical changes.

Continue up your torso, tensing the buttocks, then the abdomen, then the chest and shoulders and neck. For your head, tense and relax first the jaw only, then your forehead. Then tense all the facial muscles at the same time. Finally, tense and relax your whole body at once, including arms and legs. Notice the difference between feeling tense and feeling relaxed.

After you have tensed and relaxed your whole body at once for several repetitions, allow yourself to enjoy total relaxation for a few minutes before continuing with your daily activities. The feeling of warmth and relaxation tells you that you have elicited the relaxation response. Remember what relaxation feels like, and when you are totally relaxed, remind yourself that you can achieve this state of relaxation again whenever you choose by simply focusing on where your body is holding tension and thinking to yourself, "Relax, let go." Do the progressive deep muscle relaxation exercise several times until you can easily slip into relaxation by bringing your attention to the idea of relaxing. (Eliciting the relaxation response with progressive relaxation is also good for helping you fall asleep.)

After you are proficient at eliciting the relaxation response with the long procedure, you can do a shortened version that includes just four main muscle groups. The first step is to tense and relax both legs, feet, and buttocks at once. Then move up to the abdomen and chest for the second step. Next do the arms, shoulders, and neck at once. Finally do the face and head. You can do this sitting at your desk or at home, almost any time.

DEEP (DIAPHRAGMATIC) BREATHING

To elicit the relaxation response through deep breathing (also known as diaphragmatic or belly breathing), inhale slowly and deeply through your nose and allow your lungs to breathe in as much air as possible. Let your abdomen relax and expand, so that you take in more air. Hold your breath for a few seconds once you have filled your lungs. Then exhale slowly through your mouth until your lungs feel almost empty, focusing on letting go of muscle tension throughout your body as you do so.

You may be able to learn to do this more easily by lying down on your back on a firm bed or carpeted floor and placing a pillow on your stomach. You should be able to observe the top of the pillow as it moves up and down with your breathing. As you breathe more deeply, observe the difference in how high you can make the pillow rise. Recall the sensation of relaxation you had when you did the progressive deep muscle relaxation exercise. Repeat the deep breathing cycle several times until you feel more relaxed. Remind yourself that you can attain this state of relaxation again, anytime you choose to do so, just by breathing deeply. And you can do this anywhere—in a meeting, at a movie, sitting with friends—without others really noticing what you are doing.

TIP

The **Breath Pacer** is a smartphone app that helps you breathe at slow, measured intervals to reduce stress. The app suggests breath intervals based on your height (a good indicator of your body's cardiovascular demands), but you can change settings depending on how long you want to inhale and exhale. It also gives you simple audio and visual cues for pacing your breathing. A bar on the screen rises as you inhale and drops as you exhale. The sound of rain rises and falls in sync with the bar and your breathing, which means you don't have to watch the screen. You can tune out and breathe in response to the sound of rainfall.

IMAGERY

Imagery can also be used to evoke the relaxation response and improve your mood. Imagery involves allowing yourself to "see" in your mind's eye scenes or action as in a movie. Everyone has the ability to call up mental images, even if they think they don't. Dreams are one example of unconscious "mental movies." When you visualize a scene in your mind, you are consciously directing the imagery process. You can use imagery to evoke the relaxation response by visualizing a pleasant or relaxing scene. The scene can be based on a memory of some place you have actually been, or you can invent a place. The steps for doing imagery are listed in Table 8.2.

 You may find it helpful to download free audio tracks for muscle relaxation, deep breathing, and imagery from **http://cmhc.utexas.edu/mindbodylab.html** created by the Counseling Center at University of Texas at Austin. This website provides a forest guided imagery exercise at: **http://cmhc.utexas.edu/mbl_audio9.html**. There is also a guided imagery for a tropical island cove at: **http://cmhc.utexas.edu/mbl_audio7.html**.

MEDITATION

Meditation is relaxation for the mind. The aim is to quiet the mind by simply watching or observing thoughts. During meditation the observing self listens to mind chatter as if from afar and without attaching to any of the thoughts as they come and go. Meditation starts by finding a quiet, comfortable place—though you need not sit on the floor in a "lotus" position; it is okay to sit on a chair or on pillows, just so long as you are comfortable. Choose a time and place when you will not be interrupted. It helps to have a bell to ring to start your session, but this is not necessary. It also helps to have a clock to check your time—but don't set an alarm.

 There is a nice smartphone app called **White Noise** (by TMSoft) that provides background sounds for meditation, including that of a Tibetan singing bowl, and that also provides a timer for turning off the sound and ending the meditation session. The app is available for a number of smartphones, as well as for the iPod Touch and the iPad.

Once you get settled, start your meditation session by paying attention to your breathing. The practical effort needed to focus completely on your breathing takes your mind away

Table 8.2
USING IMAGERY TO ELICIT THE RELAXATION RESPONSE

1. Relax.

It is best to find a private place where you will not be interrupted for a period of time—usually ten to fifteen minutes. However, if necessary, you could do this anywhere (for example, on a park bench or a bus) during whatever time you have available. Get as comfortable as you can. Close your eyes, and using the deep breathing technique described previously, allow yourself to relax. Turn your focus inward, and allow an image to arise, without trying to control it or "do it right." Remember, there is no right or wrong way to do imagery, and with practice it becomes easier.

2. Picture a relaxing scene.

Allow a relaxing or pleasant scene to come to mind. Examples of such scenes might include a lovely beach, a sunny lake, a picturesque hiking trail, or the green grass of a quiet meadow. Direct your attention to the sensory details—the sounds, colors, smell, touch, and temperature. Notice the enjoyable aspects of the scene and give yourself permission to become more involved and relaxed.

3. Bring the imagery to a close when you are ready.

Continue until you have enjoyed the mental imaging sufficiently and are feeling relaxed and satisfied. Tell yourself you can return to this place (the enjoyable scene) anytime you wish, simply by taking several deep breaths. Without opening your eyes, allow the mental images to fade. Then gently bring your consciousness back to the present. Open your eyes, stretch your muscles, and continue your day with an improved perspective.

4. Write out and record your relaxing scene ahead of time.

You may find it easier to do imagery if you write out the details of the scene that you want to imagine. Then read aloud what you have written and record it on an audiotape to play back while you are relaxing. When you are recording your scene, take care to speak slowly and use a relaxing tone of voice.

5. Practice doing imagery.

Do imagery at least once a day, repeating steps 1 and 2 each time, until you feel confident in your ability to improve your mood by using imagery. If you wish, try different kinds of images to alter your mood.

from the mind chatter that constantly goes on in your head. It also allows feelings to settle into a time of calm. At first, plan to do a fifteen-minute meditation session. Just focus on your breathing and allow yourself to think of nothing. When thoughts do come into your mind, just gently bring your focus back to your breathing and allow the thoughts to float away. Do the same thing with any sounds that may be intrusive, or any more thoughts that may come. Gradually the process of meditation takes on its own energy, bringing feelings of peace and calmness, and opening you to new insights.

A video demonstrating one way to meditate is available at: **www.youtube.com/watch?v=e0rSmxsVHPE**.

KEEPING A STRESS DIARY

Another helpful tool for managing stress and improving your emotional coping is keeping a diary of stressful events in which you record stress events as you experience them. You can use the diary to identify and rate your feelings during the event from 0 to 10, least stressful to most stressful. Write down the fundamental cause of the event, your physical symptoms during the event (e.g., flushed face, increased heart rate), and how well you think you handled the event. Writing also allows you to collect your thoughts and feelings and make more rational decisions about how to react. Use this diary to problem-solve how to better handle such events in the future.

An Internet source for a stress diary to fill out online can be found at: **www.mindtools.com/pages/article/newTCS_01.htm**. Click on "template" partway down the page. This will get you to the free stress diary form.

Managing Stress with Mindfulness

Dr. Marsha Linehan, a clinician and a professor of psychology at the University of Washington, teaches mindfulness, distress tolerance, and emotion regulation skills for coping with emotional distress. She has developed an effective approach to therapy known as Dialectical Behavior Therapy (DBT). Dr. Linehan first teaches her patients mindfulness skills, which she regards as the basis for balancing rational thinking (the "rational mind" in her terms) and emotional experiencing (the "emotional mind"). According to Dr. Linehan, the wise mind is that part of you that holds both reason and emotion at the same time and draws wisdom from both. Mindfulness skills can help you to tolerate emotional distress better and cope more successfully with painful feelings.

 A good Internet resource for learning more about Dr. Linehan's work and Dialectical Behavior Therapy (DBT) is: **www.dbtselfhelp.com**.

Mindfulness lies at the core of Buddhist meditative practices but has a much broader application as well. It is universal in that it has to do with the ability to pay attention in the here and now, to sustain penetrative awareness, and to achieve insight that is not available from simply thinking. Recall that the definition of *mindfulness* is "an open, receptive, and nonjudgmental attitude." Mindfulness allows the person using it to see thoughts as thoughts and events as events, independent of their content and emotional "charge." That is, thoughts and feelings come and go; they are transient. A mindful person, using his or her observing self, can experience these thoughts without trying to change them, replace them with other thoughts, or "fix" them. Rather, thoughts, feelings, and events can be simply observed with relative calm or serenity. In this way, it is possible to achieve greater self-knowledge and self-acceptance.

According to Zindel Segal, Mark Williams, and John Teasdale, in their book *Mindfulness-Based Cognitive Therapy for Depression,* "mindfulness is not a technique or method, although there are many different methods and techniques for its cultivation. Rather, it is more aptly described as a way of being, or a way of seeing, one that involves 'coming to one's senses' in every meaning of that phrase." Another way of describing mindfulness is systematic self-observation that involves suspending the impulse to judge, characterize, or evaluate experiences. Mindfulness focuses on awareness of inner sensations, perceptions, impulses, emotions, thoughts, and the process of thinking itself, as well as outer manifestations, such as speech, actions, habits, and behaviors. Mindfulness helps you to focus your attention in a way that can be very helpful for coping more effectively with difficult emotions.

Mindfulness involves learning to observe, describe, and participate with awareness. It also involves taking a nonjudgmental attitude, focusing on one thing at a time, and taking action at that moment that is in alignment with your values and guiding life principles. When you actively observe, you attend to events, emotions, and other behavioral responses, even if the emotions are distressing, without trying to avoid or escape. To do this, a part of your consciousness must step back from the event itself and act as an observer of whatever is happening. This "observer" part of you is alert and watching whatever is going on without getting caught up in the experience or reacting to it. When you participate with awareness, you let yourself experience events and feelings without judging or trying to escape them by thinking of something else.

Dr. Linehan describes three "What to Do" and three "How to Do It" skills for achieving mindfulness. Practice these six mindfulness skills, adapted in Table 8.3, at every opportunity—not just when things get stressful. Begin with the simple technique of "just noticing" the pressure of your foot on the floor or the pressure of your back against the chair. If you are walking, "just notice" that you are walking and what it feels like to walk, without judging whether you are "doing it right." When you are eating, be aware of the sensations of eating, and "just notice," without judging the thoughts, feelings, and experience associated with eating at that time. These small steps are the beginning of becoming mindful. Eventually, you will be able to adopt the observing self position even when you are in a stress-producing situation.

MANAGING DISTRESS WITH MINDFULNESS

Mindfulness is an important approach to stress management that can be easily used by a wide range of people. Practitioners of mindfulness report that they actually enjoy the cultivation of greater awareness and self-knowledge. They say this even though it is sometimes painful, because it does not allow them to avoid unpleasantness. However, when unpleasantness is there, they do not struggle with it or try to push it away. Mindfulness is a way of dealing skillfully with both inner experience and external events. It provides a way of "being with" a problem and letting go of the need for an instant solution. Becoming aware of a difficulty and holding it in awareness can provide a time out from the mind getting caught in old mental routines and ineffective habits. It paves the way for "doing what works" in the moment.

Distress Tolerance Skills

According to Dr. Linehan, who has done years of research on managing negative emotions, mindfulness forms a foundation for coping with painful feelings. In addition to becoming mindful, it is necessary to learn distress-tolerance skills, as well as skills for emotion regulation.

The ability to tolerate stress and deal effectively and appropriately with it is necessary for good mental health. Stress and pain are parts of life and cannot be altogether avoided or removed. Personal growth and change inevitably result in some discomfort, at least in the short term. Distress tolerance involves being able to accept, in a nonjudgmental fashion, both yourself and your current situation. It is the ability to perceive your environment without demanding that it be different, to experience emotions without attempting to escape, and to observe your own current thoughts and actions without attempting to stop or control them.

Table 8.3
MINDFULNESS SKILLS

"What to Do" Skills for Achieving Mindfulness

1. **Observe your experience**. Just notice your experience or what is happening without getting caught in it. Step aside from yourself and observe, but don't attach your attention to anything. Become a self-observer. Use your observing self to notice your thinking self and its mind chatter. So—for example—notice that you are reading while you read.

2. **Describe what is happening**. Put words to the experience. Acknowledge and describe to yourself what you are feeling or what you are doing. Objectively describe the facts. When a feeling or thought arises or an action occurs, simply acknowledge it and describe it to yourself. For example, the observing self might say, "I am reading this book."

3. **Participate in the experience**. Let yourself experience the feelings or event in the moment, while acting in each situation as needed. Let go of ruminating and stay in the moment. If you find yourself thinking of other things from the past or in the future, bring your attention back to the present. For example, if your mind wanders while reading this, just gently bring your attention back to reading. Let your observing self notice that your thinking mind wandered away.

"How to Do It" Skills for Achieving Mindfulness

1. **Be nonjudgmental**. Separate your opinions from the facts. Stay away from notions of "fair" or "unfair," "right" or "wrong," "good" or "bad," "should" or "shouldn't." When you do find yourself judging, simply release your judgments and return to observing the facts. Your observing self does not make judgments.

2. **Stay in the moment**. Focus your attention on the present moment. Don't escape by letting your mind think of things in the past or the future. Do one thing at a time. Let go of distractions—again, and again, and again.

3. **Focus on what works at that moment**. Do what needs to be done at the moment. Meet the needs of the situation you are in—not one you wish you were in, not one that is more comfortable, not one that allows you to ignore your feelings in the present situation. Let go of vengeance, useless anger, self-pity, unwarranted worry, blame, rebelliousness, and righteousness. Stay in touch with your values and guiding principles.

However, acceptance need not lead to complacency. The idea is to accept your present circumstances and work toward changing them if they need to be changed—and, if they cannot be changed, to make the best of the situation.

There are a number of things you can do to help yourself tolerate painful events and emotions. Soothe yourself by engaging one or more of your senses—sight, touch, taste, smell, and hearing. Buy yourself some flowers. Light a scented candle. Apply perfume or lotion. Drink a cup of fragrant herbal tea. Take a bubble bath. Go to an art museum. Engage in healthy activities such as gardening, hiking, and biking. Check the newspaper or Internet for groups and activities that you might participate in. Choose activities that provide opportunities to experience positive emotions—joy, happiness, satisfaction. Do something nice for someone else—volunteer your services to a charity, for example. And when you do these things, call a friend and ask him or her to join you. Finally, do something nice just for yourself: read a book, go to a movie, listen to music.

TIP Check out the website **www.meetup.com** for social groups and activities in your area. Meetup is the world's largest network of local groups. It makes it easy for anyone to organize a local group or find one of the thousands already meeting up face-to-face. This is not a dating website (though it might lead to meeting someone for that purpose); it is for finding fun things to do.

EMOTION-REGULATION SKILLS

The ability to manage overall emotional health also requires the application of mindfulness skills. It is most important that you remain nonjudgmental when you observe and describe your current emotions. By stepping back from, and becoming more mindful of, your emotional experiencing, you become less at the mercy of your emotions. Dr. Linehan describes a number of specific emotion-regulation steps, which are listed in Table 8.4.

Assertiveness

Assertiveness, aggressiveness, passive/aggressiveness, and passiveness are four styles of interpersonal behavior. Most people use a mix of styles but have one preferred or most frequently used style.

If you behave *assertively*, you express how you feel and assert your rights while still respecting the rights of others. When communicating assertively, you express your wants, ideas, opinions, and feelings directly and honestly, without having to make excuses or apologize.

Doing so allows you to feel self-confident and good about yourself, because you increase the likelihood of being heard and getting what you need. Other people are likely to feel that you respect them, and are more likely to respect you in return.

Some people confuse assertiveness with *aggression*. In fact, an aggressive interpersonal style is used to overpower, intimidate, or manipulate another for the purpose of achieving a desired end. By definition, aggressive behavior disregards the other person's rights in a situation. Aggressive verbal communication is the outright expression of anger—yelling, cursing, name-calling, making sarcastic comments, criticizing, blaming. Other examples of aggressive nonverbal behavior include slamming doors, giving "dirty" looks, and retreating into silence. Aggressive physical behavior includes pushing, shoving, hitting, or blocking another's way. The person who is treated aggressively may feel hurt, afraid, angry, intimidated, belittled, and humiliated. Targets of abuse may come to believe they deserve no better treatment, or may retaliate with passive/aggressive behavior.

Passive/aggressive behavior is used to express dissent while hopefully avoiding outright conflict. Since the behavior is subtle, the perpetrator can deny her intentions if the target of the passive/aggressive behavior does react negatively. Passive/aggressive behavior is intended to look innocent, but is in fact covertly aggressive. It can involve little acts of sabotage, such as "forgetting" something important, withholding something of value, making sarcastic comments under the guise of joking, or doing mildly annoying things—like not being ready on time. At times, overeating can be a passive/aggressive behavior used to irritate others or show defiance. In other cases, overeating is an outright aggressive behavior aimed at punishing oneself or another.

Passiveness is another style of interpersonal behavior that one can adopt to avoid conflict with others. The passive person does not assert his or her rights in order to preserve the peace and avoid making waves. Passive behavior says, "You count; I don't." Passiveness may point to codependency—excusing or enabling another's unhealthy behavior. All too often, passiveness characterizes those who don't know what they want or feel or what their rights are in an interpersonal situation. Sometimes the overweight person who takes a more passive role is looking for a "hidden bargain"—hoping that if she is nice to others, they will like her despite her perceived shortcomings. Unfortunately, this hoped-for benefit is not always forthcoming, and she pays a significant personal price for it—her health and her self-respect.

TIP If you would like to take an online test of your assertiveness, go to: **www.queendom.com/tests/access_page/index.htm?idRegTest=675**. You can get your overall score for free, but if you want the detailed report, you have to buy it. After you go to "Let's Get Started" near the bottom of the page, just click "No, thanks" when it asks if you want to save your test results. If you might want to buy the report, you need to register.

Table 8.4
EMOTION-REGULATION STEPS

1. **Identify and label emotions**. The first step in emotion regulation is to identify and label your emotions. Many people with an eating problem have never learned to differentiate one emotion from another. They often lump all negative emotions together into an undifferentiated mass they call "feeling bad." They are like artists who have only one or two colors to work with, instead of an entire palette. Having a whole palette of emotions is necessary for good mental health. Being able to identify and label a range of emotions and emotional responses is important. You can more easily identify an emotion if you observe and describe the events that prompt the feeling, understand the meaning or interpretation you assign to the event, and notice where in the body you experience the feeling and how you express it.

2. **Identify obstacles to emotion management**. Emotions have functions. Generally, emotions function to stimulate your rational mind to take action. But rational thought is not needed for all action. For example, you don't have to decide to jump out of the way of an oncoming bus; you just do it. Emotions also communicate information about you to others. When you show anger, others may become quiet. Emotions can be used to influence or control the behavior of others, and they validate your own perceptions and interpretations of events. Emotions motivate your behavior. Feeling anxious can make you want to eat—or it may ruin your appetite. When there is a "payoff" for an emotion—for example, getting others to feel sorry for you or take care of you because you are suffering—this becomes an obstacle to emotion management. If you stop suffering, you must give up the attention you get for having problems. Likewise, because emotions often trigger a knee-jerk reaction, you may need to catch the emotion earlier in the process to interrupt the automatic reaction. The first step in doing this is to become an observer of your own experience.

3. **Reduce vulnerability to stress**. Stressful situations, thoughts, or memories make most people more emotionally reactive. People with eating problems are hypersensitive to threat and are very reactive to stressors. If you become a better problem-solver, you are more likely to keep stress under control. Take care of yourself physically—eat properly and get adequate exercise and sleep—to increase your tolerance for stress. Vulnerability to stress is increased when you are tired, hungry, in pain, or otherwise physically compromised. Restrictive dieting or not getting enough exercise increases your vulnerability to stress.

4. **Change your circumstances or change your attitude**. When you are in a bad situation, take action to get out of it. For example, if you are in an abusive relationship, decide what you need to do to change it or leave it. Perhaps marital counseling will help. If not, consider the possibility of leaving, particularly if children in the relationship are also targets of abuse. (Remember: abuse can be verbal, physical, or emotional.) If you cannot change a stressful situation—for example, if you must take care of your ill and aging parent—make the best of it. Change your attitude from one of suffering to acceptance. Remember that it may take time for some circumstances to change. And, sadly, it is true that no one is happy all the time.

Table 8.4
EMOTION-REGULATION STEPS
(CONTINUED)

5. **Increase positive emotional experiences**. Take action to get involved in experiences that produce good or happy emotions. People usually feel bad for good reason. They are unhappy about their circumstances, and dwell on how awful it is. To compensate for painful emotions, you need to increase positive experiences and to notice and take advantage of any when they do occur. Find activities that help you to feel better.

6. **Increase mindfulness of current emotions**. To increase mindfulness of your current emotions, you must be willing to experience distressing emotions in the moment without judging them or trying to inhibit them, block them, or seek distraction from them. If you feel angry but think you shouldn't be angry, you are likely to feel guilty as well as angry. This makes distress more intense and tolerance more difficult. It is better to just notice, put into words, and experience your anger and the distressing situation without judging yourself for feeling angry, trying to distract yourself from your anger, or losing sight of what is the most effective course of action to take at that moment.

7. **Take opposite action**. One way to change or moderate an emotion or mood is to act in a way that is inconsistent with that emotion or mood. Do something that seems contrary to how you feel. For example, when you are stressed, you might listen to soothing music or watch a funny TV show—that is, find something to do that is the opposite of how you feel when you are upset. This would be doing what works in the moment. If you feel unhappy, go to the zoo or the gym. Alexis felt depressed because a number of people in her family and circle of friends were ill or suffering from various misfortunes, so she started training to run a marathon. Having a goal and training for the race elevated her mood and helped her overcome depression, even though the plight of some of her friends and family members had not changed.

8. **Apply distress tolerance techniques**. It is important to be able to tolerate painful emotions without trying to avoid or escape them. Earlier in this chapter a number of techniques were given for tolerating distress. These included using self-soothing, engaging in healthy activities that promote positive emotions, accepting present circumstances without fighting the emotions that they bring, and taking the best action in the moment to cope. By using these, you will discover that the intensity and duration of these emotions fade sooner than you may expect. When a distressful event happens, acceptance is the only way out. Avoid judging things as good or bad; it is best to acknowledge and accept that which cannot be changed. Make a commitment to accept reality as it is and work with it.

LACK OF ASSERTIVENESS AND WEIGHT PROBLEMS

People who are overweight or obese may resort to an aggressive style of communication as a defense against feeling vulnerable to criticism. Some defend their size, claiming that obesity is not a health problem, and rather that dieting is. (Dieting does cause its own problems.) More often, those who are obese feel they are not entitled to speak up, and instead act passively. Lack of assertiveness is a problem for many who are overweight. This passivity shows up when the overweight person puts others' needs first—becomes the caretaker of others—or when he or she acts the part of a doormat and lets others walk all over them. Although those who lack assertiveness may be assertive in some circumstances, such as at work or with strangers, they may fail to be assertive in other situations, like with their significant others. To avoid conflict, they do not stand up for their rights in the hope that others will not bring attention to their weight. They tend to accommodate others excessively or keep quiet about feeling hurt. They may fear displeasing others, hurting another's feelings, or losing the relationship. Often they ignore their own anger or upset. If emotions do surface, they may minimize or rationalize the actions of others that contributed to hurt feelings. In all likelihood, they don't know their personal rights. They then turn to food to avoid or suppress painful feelings. Table 8.5 provides a list of some of the basic rights that every person has.

BECOMING MORE ASSERTIVE

Even though you may have one preferred interpersonal style (assertive, aggressive, passive/aggressive, or passive), there are times when another style is called for. It is unreasonable to expect that you will never communicate in an aggressive or a passive fashion, even if your preferred style is assertive. If a robber holds you at gunpoint, it may be better to cooperate passively rather than to react in either an aggressive or an assertive fashion. Usually it is better not to meet aggressive communication with aggression, but if you are attacked it is often better to fight back. When someone is overly emotional, it is better to wait for things to cool down before asserting yourself. Likewise, you need to choose the right level of assertiveness. For example, "Please don't do that" is a low level of assertiveness. "Don't do that" might be an intermediate level, whereas "Stop" is a high level of assertiveness.

 TIP A good Internet source for learning to be more assertive, operated in partnership with **www.Livestrong.com**, can be found at: **www.ehow.com/ how_5169934_increase-assertiveness-skills.html**.

Table 8.5
EVERYONE'S PERSONAL RIGHTS

◎ To be treated with respect and dignity

◎ To have your own values and standards

◎ To make your own choices and decisions

◎ To make mistakes and not be perfect

◎ To have and express feelings appropriately

◎ To ask questions and seek clarification

◎ To negotiate for change

◎ To say "no" and refuse requests

◎ To make a request

◎ To change your mind

◎ To have your own personal space

◎ To refuse to take responsibility for someone else's thoughts, feelings, or behaviors

◎ To refuse to live in a verbally, physically, emotionally, or sexually abusive environment

---

Making a Refusal

To be successful in weight management, you must be able to say "No" and stick to it. You must first believe that you have the right to refuse. Instead of just saying "No" or "No, thank you," it is tempting to add on an excuse or justification for refusing. People often invent or embellish an excuse so that the refusal will be more easily accepted. Sometimes you do it to soften the "blow" of saying no to another person or so that you appear to be a "nice" person. Or you may make an excuse to take yourself "off the hook." Unfortunately, you can get so wrapped up in inventing an excuse to go along with the refusal that you feel even more awkward saying no, or make yourself vulnerable to the other person's counter to your refusal. Table 8.6 provides some guidelines for making an effective refusal.

Table 8.6
GUIDELINES FOR MAKING AN EFFECTIVE REFUSAL

1. Be direct and avoid making excuses.

An example of a refusal with an excuse is, "No, thanks. I'm trying to cut down on my sugar intake, and I don't think it is a good idea to have any cookies." Then the other person may say, "Oh, one won't hurt you. Here, share one with me." A refusal without explanation is less likely to invite counterarguments.

2. Acknowledge the other person's good intentions.

For example, "I know you made the cookies yourself, and I'm sure they are excellent, but no, thanks."

3. If necessary, offer a compromise.

"I see you have gone to a lot of trouble to make this lovely dessert. I'll have a bite of my husband's portion, but don't give me my own serving, please."

4. Avoid people who won't take "no" for an answer.

If every time you go to lunch with a friend, she orders a dessert and insists you share it, avoid going to lunch with her. Suggest you and she take a walk instead.

Using "I" statements

Assertive communication means using "I" statements instead of "you" statements. A "you" statement is usually a blaming statement: "You make me mad when you leave dirty dishes in the sink all day." An assertive "I" statement communicates from your perspective and your experience: "I feel so frustrated when I come home and find dirty dishes in the sink." By using an "I" statement, you take responsibility for your feelings and don't assign responsibility to someone else. In addition, "I" statements, because they may more neutrally describe the facts of the situation, can be more effective when asking for a change in behavior.

> "I've noticed several evenings now when I've come home that dirty dishes are still in the sink. I thought we had agreed that each of us would take care of our own dishes promptly. After I've spent a long day at the office, I'd like to come home to a neat kitchen. What do you think we could do to make this situation work better? It

would sure make my day nicer if the kitchen was neater, and I think we'd get along better, too."

Notice that in the assertive "I" statement, the first thing the speaker does is to describe the situation objectively, including the speaker's understanding of the "dishes" agreement. (If there is no agreement about the dishes, then the first step is to negotiate one.) Be careful that your tone of voice does not convey anger or annoyance with the situation. Next the speaker describes his or her desires and suggests that both parties participate in finding a solution. Finally, the speaker spells out the benefits of addressing the problem constructively. The use of assertive "I" statements is less likely to result in conflict—though of course there are times when even assertive communication does lead to interpersonal conflict.

The above is called the DISC approach to communicating assertively. *Describe* the situation objectively. Use *"I" statements* in explaining your feelings. *Specify* what you want to happen. Explain the *Consequences* if things are different.

MANAGING INTERPERSONAL CONFLICT

An important part of assertiveness is being able to respond appropriately to another's anger or criticism. Conflict arises for a variety of reasons—values differ, assumptions are made, expectations don't match, someone takes offense. Actions that are perceived as unfair, wrong, or insensitive can produce conflict. A difference of opinion or perspective is at the bottom of virtually all situations that engender conflict or bad feelings. Even the best relationships can encounter situations that bring up conflict.

Communicating assertively may bring you into conflict with others, especially if they have been used to getting their own way and now you seem to be changing the rules. At such times, you may encounter another person's anger. If this happens, there are ways to make confrontation easier and to facilitate a better outcome. Many of these are listed in Table 8.7.

Depression and Weight Problems

The cluster of depression, overeating, and body image distress is frequently seen in those with obesity and disordered eating. One study found that 74 percent of women seeking treatment for bulimia and 48 percent of those seeking help for binge eating disorder had lifetime prevalence rates for major depressive disorder.[8] Another study found that clinical samples of obese binge eaters had prevalence rates of 65 percent for major depressive disorder or chronic, low-level depression.

Overeating is a known feature of atypical depression.[9] This type of depression is marked by overeating and oversleeping. Research shows that obese individuals consume significantly

Table 8.7
GUIDELINES FOR MANAGING CONFLICT

1. **Don't let yourself get hooked into someone else's anger.** Maintain your "cool" by using supportive self-talk (e.g., "I can handle this") and distress tolerance skills (this chapter). Avoid taking things personally. Stay relaxed. Be careful not to let your "hot buttons" get pushed. If you lose your temper as well, the argument is likely to escalate. Stay mindful.

2. **If someone is angry, don't try to reason with him or her**. Let things cool off, and discuss the situation at a later time. Listen attentively and let the person know that you understand his or her concerns. You can acknowledge that you know he or she is feeling upset, but you do not need to agree that anger is justified if it isn't. Suggest that both of you table the discussion until later if emotions are high. Set a time to revisit the problem, and be sure to get back to the issue when tempers have cooled.

3. **Make conciliatory gestures to defuse another's anger**. You may be able to defuse the situation by finding something to agree with—without necessarily agreeing to everything. For example, in response to the accusation that you never put away the dishes, you might say, "You're right—sometimes I do wait to put away the dishes." Or see whether you can agree in principle: "If you feel I don't ever put away the dishes, I can understand why you're upset." Watch for words such as "always" and "never" in arguments. When you hear these words, you can usually find a chance to agree in part or to agree in principle and defuse anger.

4. **Respond to verbal abuse carefully**. Try not to take it personally. Remember that verbal abuse is the angry person's attempt to gain control or to intimidate you. One way to handle verbal abuse is to state assertively, "Please don't talk to me that way." Then raise the level of assertion if you have to: "If you don't stop cursing and yelling, I am going to leave." If this does not stop the verbal abuse, go to another room, take a walk, or just get out of the house. If verbal abuse looks like it might escalate to physical abuse, or if the verbal abuse continues and you are afraid in the situation, don't hesitate to call 911.

5. **Ask for a time-out**. When emotions escalate, or you start to feel you might lose control, ask for a time-out. A time-out is a break to cool down and collect your thoughts. Be careful that you don't use a time-out to ruminate over anger-engendering thoughts. A time-out should provide a chance for emotions to cool down, and for logical thinking to prevail. You need to have an agreement beforehand with your partner that either of you can call a time-out. Be sure to revisit the disagreement later.

6. **Resolve residual stress**. Once a conflict situation passes, remember that you are likely to have residual arousal. Be prepared to take care of yourself by finding a way to let go of tension. Use relaxation techniques, like progressive relaxation and deep breathing. Take a hot shower, or go for a brisk walk around the block. Don't go to the refrigerator.

more calories than people of normal weight.[10] Eating can be a way of medicating away feelings of depression, but it may be that eating certain foods also contributes to depression (see Chapter 4, Eating for Health) in addition to creating negative emotions and more depression following overeating.

OVERCOMING DEPRESSION

Medications are available that can help alleviate both severe and chronic depression. These include the selective seratonin reuptake inhibitors (SSRIs) such as Prozac, Zoloft, and Lexapro. However, antidepressant medication alone does not generally cure depression. Therapy alone or in combination with antidepressant medication has been shown to produce the best results for overcoming moderate to severe depression.

Several therapy approaches have research to support their efficacy in this regard. Cognitive-behavior therapy (CBT) targets hindering self-talk, cognitive distortions, and core beliefs that contribute to depression. The mindfulness- and acceptance-based therapies (such as ACT) promote mindfulness and active acceptance of troubling thoughts and feelings. Together these therapies address problematic thinking that contributes to depression. An important step in coping with depression is to defuse yourself from such depressive thoughts and beliefs, and to see them instead in the same way that an observer on the shore might watch waves wash in and wash out.

HELPING YOURSELF

In addition to learning CBT techniques and an ACT philosophical approach, there are a number of other things you can do to help yourself overcome depression.

 TIP   A good Internet resource for self-help for depression and anxiety is:
http://helpguide.org/mental/stress_management_relief_coping.htm.

Exercise

Exercise has been found to be as good as antidepressant medication for decreasing depressive symptoms. Research has shown that those who become and remain fit are less likely to suffer from clinical depression. Once depression has developed, exercise can help to reverse it. Starting to exercise does not mean becoming a "jock," or engaging only in aerobic exercise. Weight training can work, as well; simply increasing your regular activities of daily living—by walking the dog, gardening, doing chores around the house—by as little as 30 more minutes a day has important therapeutic benefits.

Sleep

Getting eight hours of restful sleep a night is recommended for good physical and mental health. Lack of good sleep is a contributor to depression—and overweight. Staying up late and sleeping in may be fun at times, but it is important to have a regular sleep schedule. It is important for mental health to practice good sleep hygiene. This was discussed in Chapter 1, Understanding the Relationship between Weight and Health.

TIP For more information on sleep hygiene from the University of Maryland, go to: **www.umm.edu/sleep/sleep_hyg.htm**.

Eat a Healthy Diet

Some people with depression don't feel like eating; others overeat. To help with depression, eat regularly throughout the day—three meals and planned snacks as necessary. Avoid or minimize simple sugars. When it comes to grains, follow this simple rule of thumb: if it is white, replace it with a healthier alternative. Replace white potatoes with sweet potatoes, white rice with brown rice, and white bread with whole-grain bread. Avoid products made of refined white flour (cookies, cakes, pastries, pasta, many types of bread), even if it is enriched. Include lots of vegetables in your diet. Try to have some protein at every meal. Also, choose fish over red meat more often than not. Satisfy your sweet tooth with fruit. Most of all, avoid junk food and fast food.

Minimize or Eliminate Alcohol

If you are depressed, alcohol should be minimized, if not eliminated all together. Alcohol is a central nervous system depressant. Although it may seem to help you to relax at first and help you forget about your problems, there is a good possibility of depressive rebound, especially if you have more than one or two drinks a day. Drinking too much interrupts the body's ability to have a good night's sleep, which leads to fatigue, eating simply to feel better, and often more drinking. And of course drinking alcohol is an easy way to take in lots of calories. Even if your alcohol intake does fall within socially acceptable limits and health recommendations, having a mood disorder such as depression makes you even more sensitive to the effects of alcohol. Even a small amount of alcohol in the midst of depression can cause early morning awakenings and disrupted sleep.

Plan Positive Activities

Some theories hold that depression results from the lack of rewarding experiences. It is easy to get bogged down with boring or tedious chores and forget to include fun activities. Such activities can be as simple as setting aside time to read a book, or take a walk, or arrange to have someone watch the kids while you go to lunch with a friend. Consider what activities you used to do that gave you pleasure in the past—or what you would like to do now or in the near future that would be satisfying. Think of ways to replenish yourself emotionally by balancing have-to activities with some fun activities. Develop a plan for taking action. When you get moving in a positive direction, you are less likely to feel depressed, and less likely to eat as a quick way to feel better for a moment.

Seek Social Support

Social support is helpful in coping with depression. The tendency of many depressed people is to withdraw from social activities. They may sleep too much or watch television (and eat) to distract themselves from feeling down, rather than reaching out to other people. Some depressed people are becoming more dependent on the Internet as a means of distraction—or a substitute for "real" relationships. The comfort of family and friends is a great antidote to depression.

Find a Support Group

Consider group therapy that provides a CBT or mindfulness- or acceptance-based approach for overcoming chronic depression. It often helps to know that others are struggling with similar problems, and the opportunity exists for making new friends for mutual support. Some churches offer self-help groups for depression. Online support for depression can be found by doing a search on "support groups for depression," but be careful of the people who masquerade as "therapists" online. Check credentials before you take the advice of an online therapist, and make absolutely sure he or she is legitimate. There are plenty of people giving therapeutic advice with no training to do so. Ask for their license number and what state they are licensed in. What are they licensed to do? Beware of using psychics; you can pay a lot of money for pseudo-information.

TIP For more help with mood disorders, check the website for the Depression and Bipolar Support Alliance: **www.dbsalliance.org**.

Fight Back against Your "Inner Bully"

Stop blaming, criticizing, and attacking yourself. Don't compare yourself to others or to excessively high standards you (or someone else) impose on yourself, only to find yourself wanting. Be more compassionate with yourself. What you say to yourself matters.

 Two Internet resources expand on the idea of stopping self-criticism. Self-talk and stress is the subject of discussion at **www.lifematters.com/self_talk.asp**. Regarding the subject of stress management and improving your life with positive self-talk, check out **http://stress.about.com/od/optimismspirituality/a/positiveselftak.htm?p=1**.

CHAPTER NINE

Stopping the Binge Cycle

RACHEL CONFESSED THAT SHE WAS A SECRET BINGE EATER. *When she left work in the evenings, she would stop and have a complete dinner at a restaurant, then go home and dine again with her family. Rachel also picked her face; afterward she got upset with herself, just like she did when she binged. Rachel felt completely helpless to stop either the binge eating or the skin picking. Finally she found an app for her smartphone called* **Daytime Affirmations** *that provided support for her effort to stop binge eating. She also found information on overcoming skin picking at* **www.brainphysics.com/skin-picking.php**.

Binge Eating

When most people think of binge eating, they think of bulimia nervosa, an eating disorder that involves binge eating followed by attempts to compensate for the calories consumed in the binge by vomiting, misusing laxatives or diuretics, restricting calories, or exercising to excess. Those with bulimia typically are within the normal weight range, although some may be slightly overweight. Bulimics have concerns about weight and shape that cause great distress. Bulimia is uncommon among those who are obese.

TIP

For information on binge eating disorder and binge eating as it occurs with bulimia, go to: **www.medicinenet.com/binge_eating_disorder/article.htm**. Another good article on eating disorders can be found at: **www.something-fishy.org/whatarethey/be.php**.

BINGE EATING DISORDER

Binge eating is also the central feature in a more recently recognized eating disorder—binge eating disorder (BED). The person with BED also engages in binge eating but does not regularly use the compensatory behaviors that the person with bulimia uses. Those with BED may diet periodically, or even vomit once in a while after an eating binge, but these behaviors do not occur on a regular or frequent basis. Individuals with BED are usually overweight or obese. Those with BED who also overvalue shape and weight tend to suffer more psychological distress—depression, anxiety, eating pathology—than do BED sufferers without significant concern about weight or shape.[1,2] And this is true regardless of what they actually weigh.[3] That is, some large people who binge are not troubled by their size, though they may want to curtail binge eating. Thus they suffer less distress.

Binge eating is often the paradoxical consequence of attempts to restrict calories to lose weight or maintain weight loss. Unable to cope with feelings of hunger or deprivation or other unpleasant feelings, the binge eater eventually succumbs to a seemingly overwhelming urge to eat. Those with BED gain weight because their bouts of excessive eating provide more calories than they expend, whereas those with bulimia or anorexia compensate for excess calories consumed. Between 25 to 50 percent of obese people suffer from BED.[4] The more severely overweight a person is, the more likely it is that binge eating is a problem.

TIP

For comprehensive information on binge eating disorder, go to:
www.helpguide.org/mental/binge_eating_disorder.htm.
The Mayo Clinic also provides information on BED at:
www.mayoclinic.com/health/binge-eating-disorder/DS00608.

Understanding Binge Eating

Some binges are triggered by hunger precipitated by strict dieting. Those who skip meals in an attempt to cut back on calories are particularly susceptible to hunger-induced overeating. Stress and tension can build up to a tipping point and trigger a binge. Feeling bad is another trigger for eating binges. Self-criticism or criticism from others about weight or shape results in low self-esteem and can contribute to a binge. Habit and simple pleasure-seeking can also cause binge eating. In some cases, obsessing or ruminating about desired food can trigger a binge.

Emotional reasons—the desire to be comforted, to avoid upsetting situations, to numb painful emotions, or to be distracted from boredom or loneliness—are frequently triggers for binge eating. In such cases, the binge serves as a way to escape unpleasantness or forget difficulties. Some people are unable to identify specific triggers for binges but report feelings of persistent tension and anxiety that are relieved by binge eating.

TIP Take a test about emotional eating and join a blog conversation at: **http://normaleating.com/blog/2009/11/are-you-an-emotional -eater-take-the-test/**.

WHY DO PEOPLE KEEP BINGEING?

Most people continue to binge because it "works." The binge is often an effective means of escaping from upsetting thoughts and painful emotions, such as anxiety, anger, depression, loneliness, and boredom, or from pain or fatigue. A binge can temporarily shut out self-criticism and negative or hindering self-talk. In some cases a binge provides a certain amount of satisfaction, because it is a way to express anger or to rebel against rules or limitations imposed by dieting or by other people. In other cases it affords a much-needed relief from self-imposed limitations.

The events that follow a binge serve to reinforce it. Escaping thoughts and painful emotions with a binge is reinforcing, because the binge helps avoid pain. Because binge eating "works," it continues to happen, despite later regrets or self-denigration. For example, eating a cookie that tastes good makes you want to have another cookie. The good flavor in your mouth leads to wanting, and probably eating, more cookies. If the cookie didn't taste good to you, you might not have another one unless you are just eating mindlessly. The immediate consequences that follow a behavior make it more or less likely to happen again.

Immediate consequences carry more influence on behavior than do distant ones. The good taste of a cookie *now* is more important than worries about gaining weight later. The desire to escape stress by binge eating is compelling, especially if the binge eater has no other way to cope. Getting something good now, or escaping pain in the present, usually wins out over future consequences—good or bad.

Of course, a binge has its downside. Eating excess calories eventually produces weight gain. After a binge, most binge eaters feel disgusted, guilty, and ashamed of their behavior. Yet these consequences often do not stop the binge behavior from happening again and again. The fact that a binge provides immediate relief from stress or hunger outweighs most of the negative consequences, such as weight gain or bad feelings about weight or size.

IDENTIFYING THE BINGE PATTERN

If you are a person who binges, to stop the binge cycle, you must identify the behavior pattern—the cues or triggers that elicit the binge, the thoughts and beliefs that accompany it, and the reinforcers that perpetuate binge eating behavior. Deconstructing the behavior pattern using the ABC model introduced in Chapter 3, Changing Behavior, helps you decide how to understand and intervene in the behavior pattern in the future. (Recall from Chapter 3 that the antecedents, or As, are events that precede and elicit or cue behaviors and thinking. The Bs—which are often the beliefs we hold and the thoughts we have about an A event—are our behaviors or actions. Consequences, the Cs, follow and reinforce the behavior and influence whether it happens again in the same context.) Once you identify the antecedents or cues, the thinking or behaviors, and the consequences or rewards that reinforce a binge, you are better able to influence the behavior pattern.

Revisit Chapter 3 and review the information on self-monitoring of behavior patterns. Then begin monitoring your binge patterns. Record the date and time, what you ate (not necessarily the calories), what kind of binge it was (more about types of binges on page 236), and what you thought and felt before, during, and afterwards. Consider each binge pattern and write out a plan for coping with the different components of such a binge in the future.

Characteristics of the BED Binge

According to the American Psychiatric Association, a *binge* is characterized by a perceived lack of control over eating (e.g., feeling that one cannot stop or control what or how much one is eating) and eating within a discrete period of time, typically two hours, an amount of food that is definitely larger than most people would eat in a similar period of time under similar circumstances. This description of a binge better fits the type of binge experienced by those who are bulimic or anorexic, rather than the binge that those with binge eating disorder experience.

For most people, a binge means losing control, whether eating or drinking too much or spending too much money. A loss or suspension of control or inability to stop the behavior once it has begun is the hallmark of all eating binges. The amount or kind of food eaten and the number of calories consumed can vary for those with binge eating disorder. Some BED binges may involve eating large amounts of food in one sitting; in other cases, it can have a stop and start pattern. A BED binge may last for days at a time, rather than a couple of hours. Some binges may involve continuous snacking throughout the day that blends into mealtimes. This type of eating is called *grazing*.

A BED binge eater may keep large stores of candy bars or chips in his or her desk drawer to snack on throughout the day. Sometimes grazing begins in the late afternoon and continues until bedtime. Such binges are often associated with watching television or using the computer. Most binges end when a person goes to sleep, but some people arise at night to eat again.[5]

A binge may involve eating a meal before arriving home to eat the meal that was prepared by a spouse (like Rachel did in the chapter-opening vignette). Or a binge may begin by eating just one tasty item and then going to the store to purchase a larger quantity, and then consuming all of it. Binge eating is often followed by self-criticism, which not only is painful but also can lead to more binge eating later to escape the self-inflicted pain.

When a binge involves large quantities taken in more or less all at once, it usually involves eating rapidly, eating when not physically hungry, eating until uncomfortably full, and eating in secret. It is usually accompanied or followed by feelings of disgust with oneself, depression, shame, anger, or guilt. Low self-esteem and dissatisfaction with appearance often accompany binge eating disorder.

The type of food eaten during a binge varies, but it typically includes sweet, high-calorie foods, such as ice cream, cookies, cake, pastries, or candy. Starches and foods made from refined carbohydrates are also preferred binge foods for some—especially bread, cereal, bagels, and the like. For others, chips, nuts, and other salty snacks are preferred. Still others prefer the creamy texture and taste of butter and fatty foods. If an eating episode violates a self-imposed rule about "good" eating, it can trigger a binge.

BED binges are often triggered by negative emotions. Eating serves to block out thoughts and feelings, at least temporarily. Binge eaters are usually distressed about their inability to control their eating and about their weight and shape. In some cases, the person with BED was once anorexic or bulimic. Most have a long history of dieting. Some continue to try diets, whereas others have given up all efforts because of repeated failures. Increasingly, bariatric surgery (surgery that reduces the size of the stomach or alters the gastrointestinal tract to reduce the number of calories consumed or absorbed) for the more severely obese is considered necessary when dieting and exercise efforts fail, though even surgery may not eliminate binge eating.

The BED person does not generally seek to be thin—he or she would be happy to just be average weight or even somewhat above average weight. Binge eaters are often sedentary and may have obesity-related physical problems that interfere with exercising, such as foot or knee problems. Because of their considerable dissatisfaction and shame about their bodies, they may avoid sexual relations. Many obese binge eaters are in marriages that have been asexual for many years. They may believe that looking at them disgusts their spouses; in fact, their own body dissatisfaction is a contributing factor in the lack of sex in their relationships.

TIP

For a good article from the American Psychological Association on the best treatment for BED, go to: **www.apa.org/monitor/mar02/binge.aspx**.

Types of Binges

Depending on the cause or triggers, binges come in a variety of forms. These include the hunger binge, the deprivation binge, the stress (or emotional) binge, the opportunity binge, the vengeful binge, the pleasure binge, and the habit binge.

THE HUNGER BINGE

The hunger binge is triggered by physical deprivation. To most people, dieting means limiting calories. Dieting can also involve eliminating certain foods or food groups, eating fewer times per day, or following an extensive set of rules about what, when, and how much to eat. Studies on starvation show us that fasting and severe caloric restriction produce changes in the body and the brain. Hunger that persists leads to symptoms similar to those of starvation. These include preoccupation with food and eating, and thinking excessively about food or meals one has had or hopes to have. Mood swings are common with starvation and hunger. Dips in blood sugar can trigger dizziness, hand tremors, and headaches. Irritability is also common with hunger-inducing, restrictive dieting.

To thwart the hunger binge, it is important to eat regularly and adequately throughout the day. This means eating at least three regular meals with planned snacks as necessary or eating more frequent but smaller meals. Those who think they are saving calories by skipping a meal—usually breakfast or lunch—are setting themselves up for a hunger binge.

Some people claim that they can't eat three regular meals. They don't eat breakfast because they aren't hungry and can't "face" food that early in the day. Sometimes this is because they have eaten so late the night before that they still feel full. Others don't leave time to eat breakfast as they hurry off to work, preferring to grab a doughnut or muffin on the way or get something from the vending machine at work. Still others, fearing that once they start eating, they won't be able to stop, delay eating for as long as possible. When they do allow themselves to eat, usually sometime late in the afternoon, they are too hungry to stay in control, or they feel that they "deserve" to eat what they want after having not eaten all day. That's when the hunger binge evolves into a deprivation binge.

THE DEPRIVATION BINGE

The deprivation binge results from psychological restriction. Making foods forbidden or off-limits ultimately leads to feelings of deprivation. Add the irritability that often follows attempts to resist desired foods and eat low-calorie foods that are unappetizing, and a deprivation binge is usually not far behind. Foods that are forbidden become all the more irresistible and compelling, especially if you continually think about eating them. Dieters reach a tipping point that often involves having "just one" or committing a small indiscretion, and the binge begins.

One way to curtail deprivation binges is to eat all foods in moderation. However, sometimes it is necessary to stay away from certain problem or "danger" foods (i.e., foods that trigger binges) until you feel more confident about maintaining healthier eating habits. (Such foods are discussed in detail in Chapter 3, Changing Behavior.) Then you can try reintroducing such foods in moderation. If you still cannot eat certain trouble foods without triggering an eating binge, you may need to change your thinking about the foods you choose to include in your way of eating.

Consider the approach taken by Alcoholics Anonymous (AA), the organization that has helped more people overcome alcoholism than any other. They promote a policy of total abstinence from alcohol. One of their sayings is "one drink—a drunk." If you experience "one —bite (of a certain food)—a binge," you may have to decide whether you can learn to live without the particular food that triggers binge eating for you. Just as it is possible to live without drinking alcohol, it is possible to live without a particular problem food—like peanut butter. This requires a change in self-concept—that is, how you think of yourself. Rather than saying, "*I can't* eat sweets," you need to focus on saying, "*I don't* eat doughnuts [or whatever your specific danger food is]." Be careful, however, not to make large categories of food forbidden.

The author's former binge food was Almond Roca. She could eat other candies without caving into overeating, but with Almond Roca she could not eat *just one.* For many years she was okay not eating Almond Roca (and she didn't binge); in fact she had long ago decided she had no need to eat it. She could live without Almond Roca. One holiday a gift appeared at her door; it was a tin of Almond Roca. "After all these years, I can surely eat just one," she thought. To her dismay, she polished off the whole tin in one episode, standing in her kitchen. As a result, she concluded she still could not manage eating Almond Roca moderately. But doesn't this constitute making Almond Roca a forbidden food—and isn't that a bad idea? Banning highly desirable *categories* of foods can lead to feelings of deprivation and is generally not advised. But in the author's case, for undetermined reasons, the taste of Almond Roca was more compelling than simply desired. Thus, deciding it wasn't part of her way of eating did not lead to feelings of deprivation. She decided that she didn't need to eat Almond Roca. She redefined herself as someone who just doesn't eat this one particular food.

To change your self-concept means to revise your beliefs and assumptions about yourself. Take the example of the person who achieves sobriety through AA. He changes one of his beliefs about himself from "I'm trying not to drink" to "I'm in recovery; I don't drink." Notice that the latter statement is focused on the present moment, not a hope for the future. A future-focused statement would be "I'll never drink again." While never drinking again may be his goal, in the words of AA it is necessary to take it "one day at a time." The person in recovery doesn't necessarily have to change all his beliefs in order not to drink. For example, he might say, "I wish I could drink. I liked getting high. I miss drinking." But the bottom line is, "I don't drink." Fortunately, the author, who had Almond Roca binges, didn't wish she could eat that candy; rather, she redefined her eating style such that it did not include Almond Roca.

Carrying this analogy to other self-definitions related to eating, some people define themselves as vegetarians; others say they just don't eat meat. As vegetarians or as non–meat-eaters, they don't pine for meat. Their values—how they think of themselves—guide their eating. Perhaps they chose these values for health reasons, moral reasons, or other convictions. They may reveal that in the past they were not vegetarians or did eat meat, but at this time, they think of themselves differently. Having once defined some aspect of self-concept, whether it is related to drinking alcohol, eating meat, or eating certain types of sweets, this becomes the guide for current behavior. (Of course, it is possible to change again, as some do, and start drinking again or eating meat again, but this is less likely if you are clear about your values.)

THE STRESS BINGE

As stated in Chapter 8, Addressing Stress, a person experiences stress when resources for coping are taxed or exceeded in the face of perceived threat and well-being is endangered. Inability to be appropriately assertive, to manage interpersonal conflict, to have realistic expectations, or to experience losses, failures, unsatisfactory relationships, and disappointments in life are some common sources of stress. Likewise, sadness or depression are themselves stressors, as well as often being the result of stress. Even some occasions that are normally associated with happiness or celebration, such as weddings, retirement, vacations, or the birth of a child, often bring stress as well as joy. Anxiety, anger, depression, boredom, loneliness—these emotions and others—can result from stressors and thoughts about stressful situations. These are at the heart of the stress binge.

When stress or emotional conflicts become too intense or overwhelming, a state that is similar to dissociation can occur. Dissociation involves the breakdown of the usual ability to integrate cognition and behavior. Consciousness, memory, perceptions, and behavior become compartmentalized, or split off from one another. Those experiencing dissociation may feel detached from their bodies or from their mental processes, even though they are still in touch with reality. Dissociation can occur when a person is subjected to traumatic circumstances, including severe physical, sexual, or emotional abuse. Bingeing can incur a kind of dissociation, because it can temporarily numb feelings and provide a feeling of distance from difficulties or troubling thoughts. During a binge, some report they aren't thinking at all—as if they were in some sort of trance or dissociated state.

When a person is under chronic stress, eating often serves as a coping mechanism and a means of day-to-day survival. If eating is limited due to being on a diet, anxiety and tension are likely to increase. The increased stress from not having the coping mechanism of eating at hand eventually brings a return to eating as a means of coping and may initiate a binge. The stress binge is an attempt to escape painful self-awareness and to avoid feeling bad.

To overcome stress eating, it can be helpful to identify your problem thinking, challenge your assumptions and underlying beliefs, use more helping self-talk, and learn new coping skills for managing stress and emotions. Cognition and problem thinking were addressed in Chapter 6, Managing Thinking and Self-Talk, which discussed cognitive distortions, self-talk, and core beliefs. Remember that thoughts and feelings arise and disappear, like waves washing up and out on a beach. You do not have to believe them or act on them. Chapter 8, Addressing Stress, covers both problem-focused coping and emotion-focused coping. Refer back to these chapters for suggestions in managing stress eating.

THE OPPORTUNITY BINGE

The opportunity binge most often occurs when there is easy access to tempting food and high access to privacy. In some cases, the opportunity binge occurs as a result of the combination of boredom and unstructured time. The likelihood of such a binge happening is increased if the person dwells on thoughts of eating highly preferred high-calorie foods. An added factor is the awareness of being able to get away with something. Simply realizing that there will be an opportunity to be alone and binge can trigger thoughts about what to eat. This is followed by going out and buying the desired items.

Another type of opportunity binge involves socially sanctioned eating situations such as vacations, holidays, and celebrations. Any celebration can provide an opportunity to overeat. Even just feeling good or wanting to celebrate might lead to overeating. Some people in weight loss programs who lose some weight between sessions sometimes leave their meeting and get something to eat—to celebrate. Even happy feelings can bring on a binge or unhealthy eating.

Of course, overeating on occasion is not the basic problem for weight management. Most people overdo now and then. It is when overeating—usually occasioned by using some excuse or rationale to permit it—occurs frequently that weight is impacted. Rachel from the chapter-opening vignette admitted that she found lots of excuses to eat at any opportunity: "When I'm out with my friends I want to eat like they do." "Why should I have to set limits on myself?" "It's been a tough day; I need something to feel better." "I might never get to try this again."

Transitions from one task to another provide opportunities to eat. Getting home from work and transitioning to family time can prompt getting something to eat. This is often the "glass or two of wine plus some cheese and crackers" beginning of an opportunity binge. Any change in routine—for example, wrapping up a project, finishing painting the living room, driving home after a meeting—can incite an impulse to get something to eat or drink. Completing a task is often associated with good feelings. Eating serves as a tension reliever and signals it is time to relax. Such transition times can pose a problem if getting something to eat turns into overeating. When eating results in the thought "Well, I've blown it now, so why not go all the way?" a small incident of overeating can trigger a full-blown binge.

The best remedy for the opportunity binge is to bring to bear all the cognitive and behavioral tools you have learned in the preceding chapters. These include managing the environment and planning ahead how to cope. For example, decide in advance how to minimize or cope with unstructured time, holidays, and special occasions, and plan to use self-rewards to encourage better behavior. Normalizing eating (which involves eating three meals a day plus planned snacks as needed), discussed in more detail later in this chapter, as well as allowing yourself to eat most foods in moderation, are core principles for overcoming all binges. Learning to redirect thinking away from the immediate rewards of eating and focusing on your long-term goals and values are also important.

THE VENGEFUL BINGE

Fueled by anger, the vengeful binge is a way of venting hostility. The target is sometimes the binge eater, sometimes another person, and sometimes the situation. Your body may become a target: "I hate my body." Perceived failure can invite self-punishment. A nagging or overbearing parent can be the source of vengeful eating. Having a tough time at work could trigger a vengeful binge. Overeating is just one way of venting frustration and anger when a situation seems out of control.

Vengeful binge eaters are sometimes people who have been injured emotionally. In such a case, the vengeful binge eater perceives himself or herself as wronged, slighted, or in some way hurt by another. She usually doesn't see how her own actions may have contributed. Or perhaps she was indeed hurt through no fault of her own and feels she has no way to alleviate her anger. Binge eating is one outlet. A binge can be a way to suppress the angry feelings. Unfortunately, the vengeful binge eater must bear a double burden—the original injury along with the hurt, anger, and disillusionment, plus unneeded calories from the binge.

Sometimes the vengeful binge is instigated by an inner "Rebel" voice or subpersonality, which resents and rejects authority and takes delight in flaunting poor food choices. The Rebel eschews self-discipline and undermines dieting attempts. The Rebel is often angry about being "different"—having to eat differently from others or having to cope with obesity. Obsession with this unfairness, along with a wish for revenge, prompts the vengeful binge—a symbolic "No!"—when there appears to be no other resolution available. Review Chapter 7, Challenging Your "Inner Voices," for more on dealing with the voice of your inner Rebel.

Overcoming Vengeful Binge Eating

To overcome vengeful binge eating, the underlying anger must be addressed so that forgiveness can proceed. In his book *Forgive for Good*,[6] Dr. Frederic Luskin states that forgiveness involves transforming a grievance against an offending party to a state of acceptance. Another way of thinking about forgiveness is "giving up the wish that the past was different from what it was" and learning to accept and move on. According to Dr. Luskin, forgiving someone for what they have done does not necessarily mean that you condone it, justify it, or forget it, or even that you understand it, or that the person is reconciled with you. Of course, in some cases forgiveness may lead to reconciliation, but this is not a necessary outcome. It may well be advisable not to allow the offending person back in your life. Forgiveness allows you to move on with your life, finding happiness by staying in touch with your values and overarching principles and acting in accordance with them.

Dr. Robert Enright and Dr. Richard Fitzgibbons, in their book *Helping Clients Forgive*,[7] add that attaining retribution for, compensation for, or acknowledgement of the wrong done by the perpetrator is not a part of forgiveness. Neither is forgiveness achieved by passively letting time heal the wound, nor by simply saying, "I forgive you." Some people want to know whether they should confront the person who hurt them. Be warned, however, that doing so may generate new hurt and more anger when the other party sees things differently or is defensive about his or her actions. In situations in which it is best not to confront the other person, writing a letter to the offender expressing what you feel, but not actually sending the letter, can be cathartic. When you write this letter, be sure to explore the deeper meaning to you of the situation, not just what happened. Doing so allows you to work through the experience by expressing your feelings and opinions, even if only on paper. If after writing and, if necessary, rewriting such a letter you can communicate your opinion and feelings assertively and respectfully, then do so. But remember that the other person may still dispute your experience.

Dr. Luskin describes preconditions for forgiving. It is important to look closely at the facts about what happened. In what way did your actions, or inaction, play a part in the outcome of the situation? That is, how are you accountable for the outcome? How did each person involved contribute to the problem? What assumptions did you jump to about the situation? Did you check out your judgments? This may help you see the situation differently as you look back on it and try to understand what took place. Ask yourself what was taken from you, what you lost. Other relationships you valued may have been damaged, or your view of your own self-worth may have suffered. You need to assess the damage, and the consequences to you, caused by the hurt that was perpetrated. How did the hurt alter your view of the world? Perhaps it is now harder for you to trust in the goodwill or honesty of others. Understand your feelings—don't deny them. What was your emotional response then? What is it now? Don't rationalize away how you feel. Most of all, don't stay in denial about the facts, or about your emotional response. This may involve admitting shame, when appropriate, and confronting your anger or other feelings. It also means bearing and accepting the pain of the hurt, especially when there is no other course of action available. The bottom line of forgiveness is acceptance, without resentment, of what was or is.

To help yourself heal, Dr. Luskin advises telling your story to a couple of trusted people, without practicing a victim or grievance story. Remind yourself that clinging to a victim story only reinforces an attitude of "poor me," and thus keeps you stuck in the past. After acknowledging what has happened and recognizing your feelings, it is better to put your energy into looking for a way to get your needs and goals met in the present, rather than rehashing past experiences that have hurt you. Instead of mentally replaying your hurt, seek out new ways to get what you're looking for. When you do, you will no longer need the vengeful binge. Table 9.1, How to Forgive, summarizes the steps for reaching forgiveness.

THE PLEASURE BINGE

The pleasure binge is triggered by the desire for stimulation and entertainment. Obese binge eaters are vulnerable to this type of binge when they have few other sources of pleasure or satisfaction in their lives beyond food. Eating provides a reliable source of reward. Those who succumb to the pleasure binge describe feeling excited by the idea of eating and sometimes spend much time thinking and fantasizing about what they will eat next. They can enjoy food, but later may regret their obesity and its health implications.

Table 9.1
HOW TO FORGIVE

1. Acknowledge to yourself what happened, your grievance, and your anger about it.

2. Write out a description of what happened, including how it made you feel at the time—without changing the facts to reflect how you think you should have felt. Don't turn your description into a guilt trip or an apology for what you felt.

3. Consider what role you played (whether through your actions or your inaction) that contributed to the event. How are you accountable?

4. Tell your story simply to a few trusted people, without clinging to a victim story.

5. Do not expect that the person will be reconciled with you, even if you seek it. And remember that sometimes, even attempting to seek reconciliation can be unwise.

6. Acknowledge the pain or hurt that the incident or situation caused.

7. Put aside resentment, and instead put your energy into looking for ways to meet your needs and goals now and in the future.

8. Focus on getting on with your life by staying true to your values.

For all people, eating should be a pleasure that does not induce guilt or harm health. In every culture, eating and sharing food with others is a central focus of social celebrations and social interchange. For example, the ceremony of "breaking bread" (eating) with another is an acknowledgement of friendship. Although in certain times and places earlier in history, overindulging, even gorging, during a feast was an accepted practice, Christian teaching has labeled the excessive pursuit of pleasure, including by overeating, as the sin of gluttony. In modern Westernized society, eating healthy food in moderation is recommended by health experts. This contrasts with our environment, which invites unhealthy eating and overindulging.

One way to avoid excessive eating for pleasure is to exercise portion control. It is also helpful to eat slowly. Eating should not be the only, or even the main, source of pleasure or satisfaction in a day. Redefining self-concept so that healthy eating and regular exercise become parts of self-identity is also necessary for overcoming pleasure binge eating. Think of yourself as someone who makes healthy food choices and engages in regular exercise. It's a matter of self-perception.

THE HABIT BINGE

The habit binge is the binge that is on automatic pilot—no one seems to be at the controls. This sort of eating involves a basic stimulus–response pattern and is usually mindless eating. The stimulus is readily available food, and the response is eating without much thinking—and often not much pleasure. Unlike the pleasure binger, the habit binger does not especially focus on the taste or pleasantness of food. Another name for the habit binge might be the grazing binge—it's nothing more than continuous, more or less nonstop eating with little conscious effort to control it or any immediate inclination to feel upset about it. Only later, when body weight increases or obesity is obvious, do negative reactions set in.

The habit binge eater is likely to benefit from self-monitoring. Self-monitoring involves keeping daily records of food eaten and the circumstances of the eating (including external events and thoughts and feelings related to these events). Keeping a record of eating behavior makes the behavior more available to conscious control, and therefore more readily changed. Limiting food consumption to prescheduled meals and snacks is important for overcoming all binge eating.

TIP

The smartphone app **Thought Diary Pro (http://appshopper.com/medical/ thought-diary-pro)** takes a cognitive–behavioral approach to self-monitoring and lets you record your thoughts and the circumstances related to the behavior in question. In addition, it helps you identify "thinking errors," (also known as cognitive distortions). You can even use the **Thought Diary Pro** app to e-mail your thought diary to your therapist.

Interrupting the Binge Eating Cycle

Binges commonly have six stages that repeat over and over. The first stage is the tension-building phase, during which threat is perceived and stress is taxing your ability to cope. During this phase, thoughts and how you interpret a situation contribute to stress. At some point, you enter the second stage: stress and tension become so seemingly intolerable that you reach a tipping point, and the binge starts. The third stage is the binge itself, when often there is little thinking going on. At some point, the binge terminates, ushering in the fourth stage, in which self-recrimination and guilt occur. If it was a sugar binge, there may also be a period of fatigue and exhaustion—the fifth stage. This is followed eventually by the final stage: the point at which you resolve not to let this happen again. And then the cycle repeats with the first stage, the tension-building stage, beginning again. Figure 9.1, The Binge Cycle, is a schematic of what a binge looks like in all its phases.

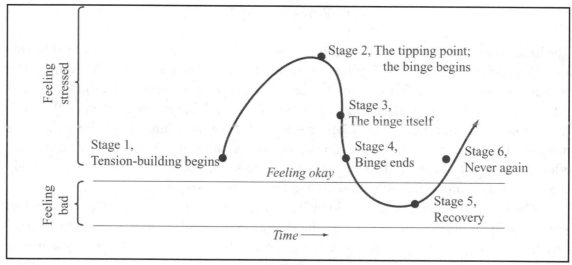

Figure 9.1
THE BINGE CYCLE

The best stage of the binge eating cycle during which to intervene is the first, when tension is building but before you reach your tipping point. Sources of stress and tension—including stress-inducing thinking—need to be identified and reduced before tension becomes overwhelming. Although it is possible to avert a binge just before it begins, it is more difficult to do so if tension has built to a high level. This is especially true if a thought occurs such as, "Well, I've blown it; who cares?" Once the binge has begun, it can be very difficult to stop it from proceeding, mainly because there is an abdication of conscious control.

Success in overcoming a binge is more likely in the future if you identify the prior binge pattern, including the thoughts and beliefs that occurred during the tension-building phase, the triggers that elicited the binge, and the reinforcers that immediately followed the binge (e.g., temporary relief from feelings). More effective stress management will reduce tension buildup and decrease the likelihood of a binge. Avoiding the triggers that set off a binge reduces the likelihood of the binge occurring. Likewise, learning what function the binge serves—how it is a reinforcer of behavior—provides you with information so you can meet your needs better in the future.

TIP To join in a blog conversation about various topics related to binge eating, go to: **www.overcome-binge-eating.com/overcoming-binge-eating-blog.html**.

TRIGGERS

The occurrence of one or more events can serve to trigger or elicit a binge. Thinking and how you understand external events are triggers. It is very important to determine which triggers are most likely to set off a binge for you. An event can be something external that happens—perhaps an argument or a painful remark you hear. An event can also be a thought, a feeling, a disturbing memory, a physical state such as fatigue or hunger, a decision, or a reaction to an external circumstance (such as the opportunity to overeat). A particularly potent trigger involves obsessing about food.

Self-test 9.1, Rate Your Triggers for Binge Eating, lists some events that typically trigger binges. After you take the test, think about how you can use the coping skills covered in Chapter 8, Addressing Stress, to reduce the impact of the triggers that you rate as a 4 or 5. Identify the thinking or self-talk that is likely to trigger a binge for you. Consider pleasurable or satisfying activities you can use to reduce the likelihood of having a binge because of negative emotions.

Obsessing about Food

Some people are troubled by intrusive and persistent thoughts of food and eating. As they ruminate more and more about eating a particular food, they reach a point where they can no longer resist eating. Their focus of attention has become so narrow that they can think of nothing else except *eating that food*. Eating serves to reduce the tension built up by obsessing about eating. In some cases, thoughts that turn to eating follow thoughts about a troubling situation. "Wishing it wasn't so" or worrying about the future both prompt feelings of anxiety, even anger. Both anxiety and anger are emotions that push the thinker to "do something." Boredom

SELF-TEST 9.1
Rate Your Triggers for Binge Eating

Instructions: Rate each of the following from "1," not at all likely, to "5," highly likely to trigger a binge for you. Those you rate a "4" or "5" need your special attention.

Rank   Binge Triggers

_____   1. Experiencing hunger from restrictive eating.

_____   2. Experiencing anxiety or tension.

_____   3. Experiencing cravings.

_____   4. Obsessing about food or eating.

_____   5. Eating anything.

_____   6. Eating something sweet.

_____   7. Breaking a dietary rule or breaking your diet.

_____   8. Experiencing interpersonal conflict.

_____   9. Feeling judged, criticized, blamed, rejected, unappreciated, taken advantage of, or unacknowledged.

_____ 10. Engaging in irrational thinking, cognitive distortions, self-critical thinking, or negative self-talk.

_____ 11. Failing to perform up to your own expectations.

_____ 12. Having unstructured time.

_____ 13. Having access to privacy and food.

_____ 14. Participating in social situations.

_____ 15. Needing to or feeling like rebelling.

_____ 16. Worrying about money, sex, family, etc.

_____ 17. Feeling overwhelmed.

_____ 18. Suffering work-related distress.

_____ 19. Having marital problems.

_____ 20. Thinking about sex.

_____ 21. Suffering pain, fatigue, illness, or debilitating physical symptoms.

_____ 22. Suffering from premenstrual tension.

_____ 23. Drinking alcohol or using certain drugs.

_____ 24. Other: _____

can also prompt ruminations about eating something that tastes good. A vulnerable person's thoughts may turn to eating when it appears there is nothing that can be done about a troubling situation or there is unstructured time in the day. The more the attention is focused on eating and thoughts about food, the more compelling the idea of eating becomes. Finally the binge occurs, and it provides temporary relief from worries, troubles, and boredom—only to be followed by self-recrimination and guilt.

One way to avoid the binges triggered by obsessive thinking about food and eating is to use the problem-focused and emotion-focused coping skills detailed in Chapter 8, Addressing Stress. If thoughts continue to intrude, try thinking to yourself, "That's just my binge thought"; simply notice and acknowledge it. Don't struggle with the thought—that is, don't try to get rid of it. Rather, just let it pass through your mind as you think to yourself, "It's just a thought, and I don't have to attach to it or act on it." If you continue to find yourself obsessing about eating, use distraction: shift your attention to doing something else. Take a walk. Brush your teeth. Drink a few big glasses of water. Call a friend. You may need to try different things, but most of all, don't buy into your thoughts and feelings. (However, if you have intrusive and unsettling thoughts about a number of things and must do something to reduce the anxiety of these thoughts, such as washing your hands or checking the stove, you may have obsessive-compulsive disorder; in such a case, consult a qualified and experienced therapist.)

COPING WITH CRAVINGS

About 50 percent of obese binge eaters report having cravings for certain foods, especially sweet and sugary foods. Both hunger and unpleasant emotions—such as boredom—can set off food cravings. We crave something because we focus on it too much—we fuse with the thought—and often we are seeking to escape pain. The best thing to do is to recognize that you are having a craving, and remind yourself that you don't have to follow through with it. Instead, enlist the Five Ds:

◎   *Delay* at least 10 minutes before deciding when to act on the craving.

◎   *Distract* yourself by doing something else that requires your attention.

◎   *Distance* yourself from the food or temptation.

◎   *Determine* whether giving into the craving is in alignment with your lifestyle values.

◎   *Decide* whether to eat or to do something else in the moment that serves you better. If you do decide to eat, do so without guilt.

To read an article entitled "Coping with and Managing Food Cravings," originally published by *Food Insight*, a publication of the International Food Information Council, go to: **www.fitwoman.com/updates/update_coping_ fall91.shtml**.

Using Rewards

In Chapter 3, Changing Behavior, you learned how to use rewards to change behavior patterns. You can use the calendar-and-stickers method introduced in Chapter 3 and give yourself a re-warding sticker for each day you don't binge. By using a month-at-a-glance calendar or book-let, you will track your progress and see your improvements. Be sure to give yourself a mental pat on the back as well for each day without a binge.

Normalizing Eating Patterns

To break the binge eating cycle, you must normalize your eating pattern. In order to succeed, it is necessary to learn to eat in a way that is naturally healthy. Natural and healthy eating is reg-ulated by feelings of hunger and satiety. However, those with an eating disorder such as BED may no longer tune in to these signals, or else confuse them with other feelings—for example, anxiety may be misinterpreted as hunger. Those who are grazers never let themselves feel hunger, and those who skip meals become overly hungry.

Eating regularly—having three meals and optional, planned snacks each day—is the basis for long-term weight management and prevention of binge eating. If you want to cut calories, eating on a regular basis throughout the day initially may seem counterintuitive. But binge eating will become less likely if you learn to eat regularly. When you eat regular meals, you are not stressing your body or your psyche, you are less susceptible to negative moods, and you are less likely to overeat or binge. Regular eating is also a far more satisfying, healthy, and effective way to manage weight over the long haul. You won't lose weight quickly, but over time your weight will reflect your behavior.

CHANGING YOUR EATING PATTERNS

Normalizing your eating patterns must be done in small, incremental steps. The first step is to decide on the times each day that you will eat your three meals and two or three planned snacks. You can decide each day what your times will be—the times may vary from day to day. Or you can plan several days or a week in advance. You can adjust your eating times as you like to ac-commodate your commitments as long as *no more than three to four hours elapse between eat-ing times.* Once you establish your eating times, eat *only* during those times. Allow yourself only enough time in your schedule to eat your meal or snack. Breakfast or lunch should take no more than 15 to 20 minutes to eat. Supper ordinarily should take no longer than 30 minutes to eat, and a snack no more than 10 or 15 minutes. Focus on eating slowly; remember that binge eaters tend to gulp their food. Eat at the planned times, even if you don't feel hungry, and use portion control. Don't skip meals or planned snacks; and don't eat between times. If you do slip and eat at an unplanned time, or even if you binge, just get back on track as soon as possible.

If you have been on many diets in the past, usually with poor results, the thought of imposing self-discipline, even just restricting meals and snacks to certain times of the day, may feel overwhelming to you. If you have never had much success with setting limits on your eating in the past, you may even doubt that you can. By normalizing your eating with planned eating, you demonstrate to yourself that you *can* exercise control, even if only by limiting eating to certain times of the day. Once you find that you have more control than you may have thought, the next step is to make gradual changes in what you eat, thus moving yourself closer to a healthy diet and a healthier weight. Table 9.2, Steps to Normalizing Your Eating Patterns, sets out a plan for making positive changes to your eating habits.

Once you are eating on a regular schedule, begin to make changes to what you eat. Start with small changes that you feel you can readily accomplish. For example, you might change from whole milk to low-fat milk, and eventually to nonfat milk. Try eliminating butter on bread; then reduce the amount of bread, or change to a whole-wheat bread. Switch from sug-

---

Table 9.2

STEPS TO NORMALIZING YOUR EATING PATTERNS

1. Establish set times for eating three meals a day.

2. Eat planned, healthy snacks, as appropriate.

3. Allow three to four hours between eating episodes.

4. Don't skip meals.

5. Don't eat between planned times.

6. If you have an eating slip, get right back on track.

7. Initially focus on when you eat, more than on what you eat. Once you get the times down, *then* begin to make healthier choices.

8. Focus on overcoming binge eating before worrying about losing weight.

9. Avoid restrictive eating.

10. Focus on changing behavior, not losing weight. Weight follows behavior.

ary soft drinks to water or tea. Reduce the size of your portions. Remove tempting foods from your refrigerator and kitchen—if you don't have something in the house, you are less likely to eat it. Implement some of the changes suggested in Chapter 3, Changing Behavior.

Succeeding with Planned Eating

Success is achieved little by little when it comes to normalizing your eating habits. It is not necessary—even possible—to go from never setting limits on eating to being perfect at doing so. Take it one day at a time, one meal at a time. Just tell yourself you'll do the best you can. Each time you succeed at some small goal—for example, limiting one evening's snacking to a predefined time—count that as a success, and pat yourself on the back. Analyze what helped that allowed you to succeed one time, and do more of what works. Keep your eye on the big picture, and don't get distracted by small slips. Remember that the road to success is always under construction.

Steps for Preventing a Binge

The best strategy for stopping binge eating is, of course, to prevent a binge from occurring in the first place. Normalizing your eating patterns, as we discussed in the last section, as well as implementing the following steps, will decrease the likelihood of a binge:

1. **Start with a healthy breakfast—and *don't skip meals.*** Choose foods that are rich in fiber, such as whole-grain cereal or old-fashioned oatmeal. Fruit or whole-grain breads can give you loads of fiber. Forget "white bread" breakfasts that cause a blood sugar spike and then a premature blood sugar drop. Include a healthy, high-protein food, especially those from plant sources, such as tofu or veggie sausage, at breakfast and other meals. Eat an orange, rather than having just juice, so you can get fiber.

2. **When you eat, eat enough.** That doesn't mean stuff yourself—but also don't skimp on meals or eat tiny diet-sized portions and expect to keep hunger at bay for hours upon hours. Include unrefined carbohydrates such as beans, vegetables, fruits, and grains, all of which are high in fiber.

3. **Know your minimum number of calories per day.** Multiply your desired, healthy body weight by 10 to determine an approximate target minimum number of calories per day. Remember, this minimum doesn't take into account intentional exercise or other activity.

4. **Get exercise, and also get enough rest.** Even if you don't go to a gym, you will benefit from incorporating more movement into your usual daily activity—like taking the stairs or parking in a far corner of the lot. Regular physical activity helps you sleep better. To

ensure better sleep, beware of caffeine and alcohol, both of which can disrupt sleep. Drink a glass of milk, or have some other food that promotes serotonin, such as a piece of whole-grain toast, before bed.

5. **Improve your coping skills for managing stress.** Use problem-focused and emotion-focused coping. Remember that upsetting thoughts are just thoughts—they don't need to be acted on. And the same is true for emotions. Learn to change what can be changed, and learn to accept what cannot. See Chapter 8, Addressing Stress, for more stress management tools.

6. **Live by your values and guiding principles.** Remember that your health and your weight are your reasons for preventing or intervening in the binge cycle. What matters are the benefits you have identified for engaging in an effort to develop a healthy lifestyle that is in alignment with your values. See Chapter 2, Getting and Staying Motivated, for more information about motivation and values.

MORE TIPS FOR PREVENTING BINGES

The best way to prevent a binge is to prevent or reduce the buildup of the tension that initiates a binge. One way we have already discussed of avoiding tension buildup is to normalize your eating patterns and to eat regularly throughout the day so that you don't become overly hungry. Additional strategies include "binge-proofing" your home and rethinking your "forbidden foods" categorization.

"Binge-proof" your home as much as possible. Stock up on healthy foods, and don't buy binge foods. For the obese binge eater, having lots of good food around may provide a sense of security and comfort. The idea of keeping tempting foods out of the house may cause anxiety. When food and eating have functioned as your primary, perhaps only, way of coping, not having food available to eat can make you feel vulnerable. This is where emotion-focused coping is needed. Chapter Eight, Addressing Stress, discusses emotion-focused coping. Find other ways to deal with anxiety. Tell yourself, "Not having my comfort food readily available may be difficult, but feelings are like waves: they build, crest, and pass. I just need to accept my feelings and allow them to pass, and in the meantime, focus on doing something useful."

At the same time, try not to make any foods forbidden or completely off-limits if possible. Instead, categorize foods as "Frequently Chosen," "Sometimes Chosen," and "Rarely Chosen." As mentioned in Chapter 3, Changing Behavior, you may need to add a special category for one or two items that are your binge foods. This last category would be your "danger" foods—those you must treat with care. You may need to avoid them for a while, but eventually you may be able to reintroduce them into your diet. If you find that certain foods are always trouble for you, consider that you can probably live without them if they are something that is proven to set off a binge.

TIP For more information on treatment and medications for BED, go to:
http://psychcentral.com/lib/2006/treatment-for-binge-eating-disorder/.

Medications for BED

Several medications have been found to be helpful in reducing the symptoms of binge eating disorder. It appears that such medications can reduce the frequency of episodes and hopefully help with weight loss. However, drug research for BED is still in its early stages and more studies are needed. The primary medications that have been used to date are discussed here.

Antidepressants known as selective serotonin reuptake inhibitors (SSRIs) appear to help reduce binge eating by increasing the availability of the neurotransmitter serotonin in the brain, which in turn helps improve mood. (Recall that neurotransmitters are the chemicals in the brain that control communication among brain cells.) Examples of brand-name SSRIs include fluoxetine (Prozac) and sertraline (Zoloft). However, once these medications are discontinued, binge eating can reappear. Worse, some people experience weight gain with some of these medications.

The appetite-suppressing antidepressant sibutramine, known by the brand name Meridia, until recently has been used in the treatment of long-term obesity and binge eating. Meridia belongs to the group of antidepressants known as serotonin–norepinephrine reuptake inhibitor (SNRIs) because they target two neurotransmitters—serotonin and norepinephrine. Meridia had been found to suppress hunger and increase feelings of fullness, thus helping to reduce binge episodes. However, it was taken off the market in 2010 because increased health risks were identified in association with its use.

Topiramate, or Topamax, developed for controlling seizures, is used off-label for treating binge eating. (It is approved for treating seizures.) However, it can cause serious side effects, including fatigue, dizziness, problems in focusing, and burning or tingling sensations. For now, the best treatment for BED is psychotherapy.

CHAPTER TEN

Dealing With Backsliding

ETHAN WOULD MAKE GOOD PROGRESS ON HIS WEIGHT MANAGEMENT EFFORT until he went out with his friends for the evening. He told himself he'd just have one beer and no snacks. After the second beer and some peanuts, Ethan forgot about his weight management progress and threw caution to the winds. "Who really cares?" he would think to himself. "After all, I've already blown it—and besides, I deserve a little fun once in a while." Then he would have a cheeseburger with fries, and together with more beers, the calories really added up. In short, Ethan started backsliding when he went drinking with friends. Eventually he had to face a difficult question: Could he keep his drinking (and eating) buddies and maintain healthy habits? Ethan had to recognize that going out with his buddies was a "high-risk situation," and that he needed better coping skills for managing it, lest he have to give up his boys' night out. Ethan also had to decide whether alcohol was a problem for him. He went on the Internet to get more information about relapse prevention for weight management and also to investigate whether or not he had a problem with alcohol. After reading all he could find, he made a plan to eat before joining his buddies and then follow one beer with soda water. If that didn't work, he resolved, he would have to take a hard look at his situation with alcohol and decide if he had to stop drinking and stay away from his drinking buddies.

Understanding Backsliding

Backsliding is a process that can lead to a return to old habits. It is a significant problem for weight management. People may begin to backslide after a period of doing well. Then there is a single small lapse, which may be followed by more lapses. If lapses multiply and continue, backsliding has begun, and this can lead to complete relapse.

Of course, occasional lapses are common in any behavior change effort and are to be expected. When you slip, the important thing is to recover from the slip and recommit to value-driven behavior and the lifestyle change you say you want. Treating a slip as a learning experience, rather than as a prediction of imminent failure, is important. It will help you to understand what causes lapses.

CAUSES OF LAPSES

One of the biggest hazards in terms of succumbing to a lapse is telling yourself that you will have "just one." Such thoughts usually occur in the context of a high-risk situation—one fraught with temptation. When a single lapse leads to more lapses in short order, motivation can begin to wane. A series of lapses, intended or unplanned, accompanied by increasing ambivalence about your ability to maintain success, can result in a precipitous return to old habits. Research on quitting smoking found that total relapse tended to occur within the first ninety days after stopping. However, relapse in any behavior change effort can result at any time if adverse circumstances and hindering thoughts prevail.

A single lapse in a weight management effort usually results from the desire for some short-term gratification—wanting something to eat *now*—and losing sight of your overarching values and guiding principles. For some people, an imaginary line is crossed with a single lapse—eating something deemed to be too much—and when that line is crossed it often leads to backsliding and perhaps a full-blown relapse. This is usually because the person slips into all-or-nothing thinking: "*Now* I've blown it—I may as well give up." If you see the infraction as evidence of your inability to succeed, or if you decide it is just too much trouble to keep going, you may decide to quit trying.

In order to justify having committed one small infraction, you may continue the unhealthy behavior, because you decide you just don't want limits set on your behavior. This weakens your motivation and increases the chances of having more slips. Having more slips sets in motion backsliding and can lead to eventual relapse into old habits. If, on the other hand, you view deviations from your commitment as opportunities from which to learn, you can regain your commitment to change. A single lapse need not lead to total relapse. Developing awareness of the process of backsliding, and learning how to prevent or recover from a lapse and backsliding, are keys to preventing total relapse.

TIP　Psychotherapist Marcia Garceau explains more about slipups, the early warning signs of backsliding, and what constitutes total relapse. To learn more, go to: **www.selfconnect.org/Assets/Web%20Pages/Article_Backsliding.htm**. The site provides a model of the core characteristics of each of the terms (lapse, backsliding, and relapse) and also refers to the stages of change discussed in Chapter 2, Getting and Staying Motivated.

Lapses and backsliding start in the context of an event or situation that involves temptation—a *high-risk situation*. Such situations may catch you unaware, though sometimes you can anticipate a circumstance that will strain your ability to cope. Whether or not you are prepared to cope, and how you mentally react to a triggering situation, can determine whether you will have a lapse and perhaps begin to backslide. The real problem is not the high-risk situation per se; it is the failure to have a way to cope. We will discuss dealing with high-risk situations later in this chapter.

TIP To hear Dr. Kelly Brownell discuss how to approach relapse associated with weight loss, go to: **http://abcnews.go.com/video/playerIndex?id=6760304**.

EXTRINSIC VERSUS INTRINSIC MOTIVATION

When we make a behavior change or any other motivated effort, we do so either because it is more or less demanded by outside sources (external factors) or because we simply choose to do so (internal factors). Effort motivated by external factors is called *extrinsic motivation*, whereas effort motivated by internal factors is called *intrinsic motivation*.

Doing things because of intrinsic motivation leads to better commitment and follow-through. This is because our actions are in line with who we believe ourselves to be, and what we want to be. In other words, our behavior aligns with our chosen values.

When someone else or some outside directive (for example, a diet or a parent) tells you what you can and can't do, you are likely to rebel sooner or later. Because it is coming from an external source and you have not adopted it as your own—you don't "own" it—it is harder to feel motivated and harder to persevere. Lapses and backsliding can be initiated by rejection of behavior change that is not owned. Not only does backsliding portend ultimate failure, but it also hurts emotionally.

EMOTIONAL HAZARDS OF LAPSES

Deciding that a single slip is terrible or that you are bad or incapable of succeeding because you broke the rules moves you closer to slipping into backsliding, and eventually total relapse. Backsliding, and even small lapses, often produces emotional upset and lowered self-esteem. How upset you get depends on several things. If you feel that the lapse wasn't your fault, or that you really didn't try too hard, you might not feel too bad. On the other hand, if you engage in self-criticism and blame, rather than problem-solving, you will feel worse. The more effort you have put into changing, or the more you feel pressured to succeed, the more upsetting lapses are likely to be. Backsliding after you have maintained the new behavior pattern for a long time is likely to be very upsetting. Likewise, regaining a significant amount of weight can be emotionally devastating. If someone you care about is angry or disapproving because of your backsliding, you will probably be upset, too. Feeling that you are losing, or have lost, control produces more negative emotions and may result in abandoning further effort. The more important the thwarted goal is to you, the more upset you will feel.

Backsliding affects not only how you feel, but how you think. You may start to wonder if the goal you are striving for is really worth the effort. (You may begin to focus on the items in the demotivation boxes [2 and 3] of the cost–benefit analysis; see Chapter 2, Getting and Staying Motivated.) You may try to rationalize the actions that led to backsliding so that you can stop feeling guilty about violating your commitment to change. To find a good excuse, you may distort or deny the facts. If you blame someone else for your backsliding (your mother-in-law insisted you eat something), you may resent them for their behavior. If you place all the blame on the situation, failing to acknowledge your own accountability—how you played a role in the outcome—you are less likely to learn from the experience and to reverse the backsliding.

Or, conversely, you may unreasonably blame yourself entirely for the lapse, without also considering the circumstances that surrounded the lapse, with the result that your self-esteem declines and your self-image suffers from excessive self-criticism. Your confidence in your ability to cope takes a nosedive, and you develop an expectation for future failure. To understand that occasional slips are inevitable and can even be valuable in your change efforts (if you use them as learning opportunities), you need to learn more about the factors that can cause lapses and backsliding and the steps you can take to cope more effectively in turning around potential failure. Many things can contribute to backsliding, including high-risk situations, errors in thinking, an unsupportive context, lack of self-management skills, and an unbalanced lifestyle.

TIP

An article by Stanley J. Gross, Ed.D., adapted from his book *Growing Ourselves Up: A Guide to Recovery and Self-esteem*, provides information on relapse prevention and can be found at: **http://psychcentral.com/lib/2006/ relapse-prevention/**.

Determinants of High-Risk Situations

Backsliding almost always begins when a person encounters a high-risk situation and does not have a way to cope with it. G. Alan Marlatt,[1] the psychologist who first identified the role that high-risk situations play in the relapse of alcoholics, broadly defines a *high-risk situation* as "any situation that poses a threat to the individual's sense of control and increases the risk of potential relapse." From his work, he has described two general groups of high-risk situations that influence behavioral addictions: those that occur as a result of intrapersonal/environmental determinants (your reactions to private events or external events) and those that are brought about by interpersonal determinants (your reactions to social events).

INTRAPERSONAL/ENVIRONMENTAL DETERMINANTS

Intrapersonal or environmental determinants are the thoughts you have and emotions you feel in response to environmental factors. They include:

◎ *Negative emotions, moods, or feelings:* Frustration, anger, fear, anxiety, tension, depression, loneliness, sadness, boredom, worry, apprehension, grief, as well as stressful feelings related to such situations as examinations, promotions, public speaking, employment and financial difficulties, personal misfortune or accident, traumatic memories.

◎ *Negative physical states:* Unpleasant or painful physical experiences, such as pain, illness, injury, excessive hunger, or fatigue; bad reactions associated with drugs or from withdrawal from an addictive substance; hormonal or chemical imbalances such as those associated with diabetes, hypoglycemia, or premenstrual syndrome (PMS).

◎ *Private positive emotions:* Satisfaction, pleasure, relaxation, joy, and pride, as well as feeling secure, loved, accepted, or nurtured.

◎ *Tests of personal control:* Deciding to have "just one," pushing the limits of willpower or ability to control, overconfidence in one's capacity for moderate use.

◎ *Urges or temptations:* Wanting, craving, longing for, feeling desire for, strongly attracted to, sudden inclination for.

INTERPERSONAL DETERMINANTS

Interpersonal determinants are influenced by your relationships with other people, and include:

◎ *Interpersonal conflict situations:* Conflict or disagreements you experience in marriage, friendship, family, sales/consumer situations, employer/employee situations, or any other situations involving people that produce frustration, annoyance, anger, arguments, disagreements, fights, jealousy, discord, hassles, anxiety, fear, tension, hurt, apprehension, or guilt.

◎   *Social influences:* Situations in which either an individual or a group pressures, coerces, tempts, coaxes, prepares, condones, or makes a gift that influences a return to old habits, or situations in which such a return to old habits is prompted merely by observation of an individual or group engaging in the unhealthy behaviors.

◎   *Interpersonal positive emotions:* Social situations that generate feelings of pleasure, celebration, sexual excitement, freedom, and the like.

Typical Triggers for Backsliding

According to Marlatt, nearly 75 percent of all backsliding related to behavioral addictions is triggered by just three determinants: negative emotions, interpersonal conflict, and social influences.[2]

Similarly, other research has identified three clusters of typical high-risk situations for weight management. The first of these, social mealtime situations, usually involving friends or family, was the most common. At these times, spirits were often high, and negative emotions tended to be absent. A second cluster of high-risk situations consisted of situations that involved some kind of emotional upset—especially anger, but also anxiety, loneliness, sadness, or depressed mood.

The third cluster of high-risk situations, termed "low arousal," was characterized by eating when alone. Dieters generally reported feeling no particular emotions at such times, though some reported being tired or bored. In addition, low-arousal, high-risk situations involved relaxing, waiting, or being between other activities. The latter, also called "transition times"—when one task has been put aside or finished and another has yet to begin—are often times when dieters find themselves getting something to eat. In these situations, food is present or readily available.

Still other research that investigated high-risk situations for dieters confirmed that high-risk situations involving positive social interactions or negative emotions led to relapse for those trying to lose weight, and additionally that physiological cravings disposed dieters to eating.[3]

Clearly there are a number of high-risk situations that can lead to relapse in weight management. You need to determine your own, and the best way to do that is to use self-monitoring. Another way is to *deconstruct* a lapse, and determine what led up to and triggered the lapse. What were the circumstances? What stressors were involved? What beliefs or self-talk did you use? Did you try to cope and if so, how? In hindsight, what could you have done to prevent the lapse? From this analysis, you should be able to identify the high-risk situation that led to your lapse and the circumstances and thoughts and feelings that played a role.

Recognizing and Coping with High-Risk Situations

Sometimes people don't recognize that they have just encountered, or that they are about to encounter, a high-risk situation. We can all easily recognize that attractive and available foods present a temptation, but other high-risk situations are not so obvious. For example, many people find that feeling good is a high-risk situation—that they not only indulge in food, but also use it to prolong positive emotions. Perhaps they go home and eat more despite having had a nice dinner with friends. Getting bored with a weight loss program is also a high-risk situation. At first there is excitement about embarking on a diet, but over time, diets are wearing. Other high-risk situations can arise from having to tolerate a slow rate of weight loss, having to eat "diet" foods, falling sick, or getting injured (and, as a result, being unable to exercise).

In order to substantially reduce the risk of lapses and backsliding, it is important to learn to identify and cope with high-risk or crisis situations that can prompt overeating. Success is ensured by developing skills for coping with emotions and low-arousal times, dealing effectively with interpersonal conflict, and managing social influences and situations. You need to know how to recover from a small lapse and to not let repeated slips lead to full-blown relapse.

HOW TO COPE WITH HIGH-RISK SITUATIONS

To overcome repeated lapses and backsliding that are triggered by high-risk situations, you can do several things:

1. **Learn to identify the high-risk situations that may cause you difficulty.** Make a list of those situations that you know are hard for you to handle. Once you have identified your personal high-risk scenarios, take steps to avoid those that can be avoided. For those that cannot be avoided, plan ahead how to cope more effectively. Write down the high-risk situations you can anticipate encountering and then plan for handling them.

2. **Be prepared with a coping response.** Know what to do. Mentally remind yourself of your values and of your commitment, and why you made it. Review the motivation boxes (1 and 4) in the cost–benefit analysis you completed in Chapter 2, Getting and Staying Motivated. Tell yourself what to do to cope—and then take positive action. A coping response should involve both thoughts and actions. If you start to slip into excuses and rationalizations, bring in helping thoughts. Remember that you don't have to act on your hindering self-talk. Be willing to take drastic action if necessary—such as tossing candy or chips in the disposal (instead of rationalizing that you'll save it for the kids or for company).

3. **Mentally rehearse.** If you know in advance that you will have to deal with a high-risk situation, mentally rehearse ahead of time how you will handle it. Never let yourself encounter a high-risk situation that you have anticipated without mentally preparing for it. To mentally rehearse, imagine yourself in the situation beforehand. Then imagine handling the situation effectively and feeling good about it. Plan ahead. Determine in advance what you will order in a restaurant, at a wedding, or at a party. Plan how you will say "no" nicely, but firmly. Decide ahead of time what action you will take to avoid lapses or backsliding.

4. **Employ specific skills or techniques for coping.** To avoid backsliding, be prepared to use helping self-talk, exercise, meditation, relaxation, assertive communication, and any other skills or techniques that will help you cope more effectively. Review earlier chapters that discuss how to implement such strategies. Helpful advice and specific strategies are also provided later in this chapter, in the section on Implementation Intervention Plans (IIPs).

5. **Avoid "tunnel vision."** Tunnel vision occurs when your awareness narrows and you focus only on the temptation—eating, drinking—to the exclusion of other factors, such as impairing your health, gaining weight, or sticking to your commitment. You lose sight of your values and guiding principles. Tunnel vision often leads to rationalizations about why you should give up your efforts. Tunnel vision is a precursor to falling into a trance-like state in the bottom of the Funnel of Awareness (see Chapter 6, Managing Thinking and Self-talk).

One trick for avoiding tunnel vision is to keep on hand your cost–benefit analysis from Chapter 2, Getting and Staying Motivated, and refer to it when you expect to encounter a high-risk situation or when motivation starts to wane. Be careful not to get caught up in your hindering self-talk. Talk back to your rationalizations and excuses. Think about your life values and guiding principles. Talk yourself out of giving up; reread the motivation boxes (1 and 4) of your cost–benefit analysis. You need to remind yourself of your reasons for making the commitment and the hard work you have put in to achieve progress with a change effort.

6. **Learn to recover from a first slip**. If at all possible, it is good to avoid a first slip, but if it happens, learning to recover is a crucial coping strategy. Most people do not stop at "just one," and recovering from a small slip like this can be problematic. If you do manage to handle "just one" the first time, you may become overconfident and think you can always handle "just one"—but a succession of "just ones" contributes to backsliding and can lead to full-blown relapse.

Succumbing to a first slip, however, does not have to signal a slide into backsliding. Instead of getting down on yourself, focus on what you can learn from the experience so that it is less likely to happen again. Usually this means becoming aware of what situations present temptation and making sure that you have a way to cope with similar situations if they occur in the future, and then using your coping strategies to avoid or minimize harm.

7. **Use reminder cards**. Another helpful tool for preventing or recovering from a first slip is carrying a reminder card. Like the seat-pocket card the airlines use to tell you what to do in an emergency, a reminder card tells you what to do in case of a threatened or actual first slip. On an index card write a brief reminder of why you made the commitment to change and what your values related to health are. Also note what actions you should take to either avoid a first slip or recover from a first slip if it happens. It's a good idea to include the name and phone number of a friend or weight loss buddy you can call for support and advice. Carry the card with you, and when you need it, use it!

IMPLEMENTATION INTERVENTION PLANS

Planning how to translate intention into action in a specific context promotes goal achievement and weight loss.[4] Planning when, where, and what to eat will help you translate your intentions into actions and reduces the risk of backsliding. Likewise, planning when, where, and how you will exercise helps motivation. Specific Implementation Intervention Plans (IIPs) that spell out a location and a time that a particular behavior will be enacted are more likely to be carried out than vague intentions. Similarly, planning ahead how you will cope with risky or tempting situations increases your likelihood of success. Use IIPs for anticipated high-risk situations. Research has shown that planning behavior helps people lose weight and exercise more.[5]

IIPs promote goal achievement by translating intentions into specific, context-linked plans. In other words, by writing out what you plan to do with regard to a specific category of food—for example, sweets—you are more likely to carry out your intention. For instance, an IIP might list when and where you plan to eat a problematic food. Thus, if you plan to allow yourself to choose a pastry on Sunday when you go out for coffee, write this down on your menu planning form. (For an example, see Figure 10.1). On the other days of the week, you might not choose a sweet. In such cases, you would write down your plan to order only coffee, or to order coffee and some fruit—an alternative strategy for handling sweets.

These eight particular food categories (plus one for exercise and physical activity) are listed on the menu planning form because the behavior-change targets in this sample form are reducing consumption of sweets, fast foods, and processed foods; increasing vegetables and fruit intake; and choosing wisely when it comes to bread, meats and protein, and whole-grain foods.

MENU PLANNING: Week of _____ to _____

Planning when, where, and what to eat as well as when, where, and how to exercise has been found to help people translate their intentions into action. Using this form, make an exact plan of when, where, and what you will eat and when, where, and how you will exercise during the next seven days.

Describe:	Monday	Tuesday	Wednesday	Thursday	Friday	Saturday	Sunday
Sweets, Fats, Alcohol *Time, where, what*							
Bread *Time, where, what*							
Fast foods, Snacks *Time, where, what*							
Processed foods *Time, where, what*							
Vegetables *Time, where, what*							
Fruits *Time, where, what*							
Meat/protein *Time, where, what*							
Whole-grain Products, Cereal, Rice, Pasta *Time, where, what*							
Exercise, Physical activity *Time, where, what*							

Figure 10.1
MENU PLANNING FORM

In addition to completing a menu planning form for each week, you need an IIP to help you anticipate possible difficult situations you could encounter with regard to eating or exercise. Figure 10.2 is a completed IIP plan for coping with difficult situations (used with the permission of an actual person engaged in a change effort). Figure 10. 3 is a ready-to-use blank. After reviewing the sample, complete the blank form, giving as many answers to complete each statement as you can think of. Be specific: What thoughts or actions would you take in each situation? Once you have completed the sentence statements given for difficult situations, make a list of situations that are specific to your particular situation. Write out what the situation is and what you plan to do to cope. For example, what would you do if someone offered you a favorite unhealthy food? How would you manage that situation? How do you plan to maintain a healthy diet? What if family or friends are coming over for dinner? What if you are tempted to forego your exercise session? How do you plan to expend calories in your ordinary, day-to-day activities?

Cognitive Distortions and Backsliding

Cognitive distortions, or misinterpretation biases, were discussed in Chapter 6, Managing Thinking and Self-Talk. You may want to go back and review these now. Cognitive distortions are almost always a factor when backsliding happens, and they contribute to ineffective coping in high-risk situations and can lead to faulty decision-making. Everyone misinterprets now and then, and doing so is not cause for self-condemnation. Rather, learning to recognize when you make such errors in thinking, and taking steps to rectify them, is what is important.

FAULTY DECISION-MAKING

Part of the thinking process involves making decisions about what something means, or about what to do. Sometimes the quality of decision-making is poor, further compounding a problem.

A faulty decision-making strategy known as *defensive avoidance* involves ignoring or denying the existence of a problem. A person who is using defensive avoidance may procrastinate, delaying appropriate action. A defensive avoider may blame others for the problem, constructing wishful rationalizations that make it acceptable to choose a less objectionable alternative and minimizing the probable consequences. Excuses characterize the defensive avoider. An example is the person who rationalizes having "just one" with the thought "I might never have this again." Buying into such a thought leads directly to making poor choices.

Defensive avoidance often allows the problem to get worse until it can no longer be ignored, at which point panic may lead to yet another faulty decision-making strategy, that of

1. **When I am hungry, instead of eating something unhealthy, I plan to:**

   Remember my guiding principles; know that although hunger is uncomfortable, I can take time to make a healthy choice; make a healthy choice that also tastes good; plan in advance to have healthy choices available.

2. **If I have a slip, instead of giving up, I plan to:**

   Think about what led up to the slip; make healthy choices at my next meal, because each moment is a new moment in which to make a healthy choice.

3. **When I go out to eat, I plan to:**

   Think beforehand about what choices will be healthiest; imagine myself taking none or only one piece of bread before dinner; review the menu for healthy choices; stop eating when I am full; eat slowly to enjoy my food and realize when I am full enough (not overly full or stuffed).

4. **When I'm out socializing and having a good time with friends, instead of giving myself permission to eat just anything, I plan to:**

   Remember my guiding principles; know that the only person I have to answer to regarding my eating is me; be prepared for possible hunger before going out; make healthy choices just as I would try to do if I wasn't out.

5. **When someone brings food into work or a meeting, I plan to:**

   Remember my guiding principles so I can make good choices; have my own healthy snacks available so I don't feel deprived.

6. **When I'm feeling mad about having to cut calories or exercise, I plan to:**

   Allow myself to feel my emotions, but know that I don't have to let them take over; be aware of eating out of resentment or anger or rebellion; take a walk or do something interesting to take care of myself at that moment.

7. **When I'm tempted to do something else besides exercise, I plan to:**

   Think about how good exercise feels afterward; consider doing a different type of exercise (e.g., doing a class instead of the elliptical machine); when I start thinking of other things to do, remember that those are just thoughts, and that I don't have to act on them—I just need to exercise.

8. **When I am tired and don't feel like exercising, I plan to:**

   See comments in #7; remember that when I exercise I sleep better; give myself permission to exercise for less time but still enough to get my heart rate up.

9. **When I am feeling overwhelmed and stressed out, I plan to:**

   Talk to my spouse; go for a walk; meditate; schedule a massage; remind myself that stress will pass, and I'll be okay.

(continued on next page)

Figure 10.2

PLAN FOR COPING WITH DIFFICULT SITUATIONS: COMPLETED SAMPLE

10. When I start getting down on myself, I plan to:

Think about my guiding principles and goals; think about the great things I have, like my friends and family, spouse, and job; find something else to do, like read a book, go for a walk, or plan meals.

11. When I am bored, I plan to:

Stay away from the fridge; find something to do, like go to a movie, read, go for a walk, plan a fun, healthy meal to cook, buy a magazine, go to the library, clean up around the house, or go to the storage area.

12. What are my difficult situations? How will I cope?

My difficult situations are boredom, losing motivation, giving up, resentment, rebellion. When these occur, I plan to cope by using all the ways I mentioned above. I have to remember that I am the adult; I am in control of my actions. I have to answer to myself for my heart health, my waistline, and my emotions. My actions are all under my control. I'll remember the support systems I have in my spouse and friends, and I'll talk to them when needed. I'll stay in touch with the values and guiding principles that give direction to my life.

Figure 10.2
PLAN FOR COPING WITH DIFFICULT SITUATIONS: COMPLETED SAMPLE
(CONTINUED)

hypervigilance. This strategy is characterized by searching frantically for a way out of the dilemma and impulsively seizing whatever solution seems to promise immediate relief. An example of hypervigilance would be seeking a quick weight loss program or diet when weight gain has become alarming or there is a special occasion impending.

A better approach to making decisions is to be sure you are in touch with what's really happening. Be on your guard against any tendency to deny or distort feedback information. Armed with a realistic view of things, you can decide first whether there is a problem, and then decide what to do about it. A *vigilant* decision-maker takes care to obtain relevant and accurate information needed to make the decision, is careful not to distort the facts, and considers various alternatives before making a choice. The vigilant decision-maker avoids procrastination and addresses a problem before it gets out of hand.

TIP You might find it helpful to blog about your struggles with backsliding. This will allow you to express your feelings, sharing them with like-minded people on the Internet. First, sign up with **www.lifegevity.com**. Then go to **www.lifegevity.com/blog/?p=102** and blog about your experiences. It helps to know that you are not alone.

Instructions: On a sheet of paper, complete the following sentences by writing down as many ways to cope as you can conceive for each situation. Use additional paper as necessary. Be specific: What **thoughts** or **actions** will you take in each situation?

1.   When I am hungry, instead of eating something unhealthy, I plan to:

      _____

2.   If I have a slip, instead of giving up, I plan to:

      _____

3.   When I go out to eat, I plan to:

      _____

4.   When I'm out socializing and having a good time with friends, instead of giving myself permission to eat anything, I plan to: _____

5.   When someone brings food into work or a meeting, I plan to:

      _____

6.   When I'm feeling mad about having to cut calories or exercise, I plan to:

      _____

7.   When I'm tempted to do something else besides exercise, I plan to:

      _____

8.   When I am tired and don't feel like exercising, I plan to:

      _____

9.   When I am feeling overwhelmed and stressed out, I plan to:

      _____

10.   When I start getting down on myself, I plan to:

      _____

11.   When I am bored, I plan to:

      _____

12.   If I have a binge, I plan to:

      _____

13.   What are my difficult situations? How will I cope?

      _____

Figure 10.3
PLAN FOR COPING WITH DIFFICULT SITUATIONS

Changing What Can Be Changed

Acceptance means changing, or trying to influence, the things you can change, and accepting and working with the things you cannot. If you can't put it (or some subset of the situation) on a "to do" list, you probably can't do anything effective to change a situation. If you are having worried thoughts ("what if . . ."), this is a substitute for taking action. If you can't take effective action, you can't change or influence anything.

Consider the example of one woman who had lost 60 pounds the previous year, but who was now having trouble maintaining her weight loss. She and her husband had started a new business, and money was tight. He was often upset, and he took out his irritation on his wife, blaming her for a variety of problems and criticizing her excessively. And as if this weren't enough stress, their teenage son was involved with drugs and was having problems at school.

The constant stress of this woman's life was making it difficult for her to maintain her new eating behaviors. She was keeping up her exercise, which helped her relieve her own tension and gave her a good excuse to get away from the tension at home, but at home she would fall back into her old strategy for coping with stress—snacking. The *context* of her life was not supporting the maintenance of healthy eating habits, and indeed was actively contributing to a return to old habits. An unsupportive context is a special kind of high-risk situation, because it is ongoing.

What this woman *could* do was continue to exercise and accept that right now, life was stressful. She needed to stop fighting her feelings (and avoid fighting with her husband). She didn't have to snack just because she felt stressed; she could accept that things were tough, and that she needed to stay focused on her values for health.

THE CONTEXT OF YOUR LIFE

A variety of things contribute to the context in which change and the maintenance of change take place. Other people make up an important part of the context. The nature and quality of your interactions with them will influence your thinking, your emotions, and your behavior. The economic situation is another part of the context that influences your ability to maintain change, as is the degree to which you must cope with personal or physical limitations, including addiction, biochemical dependence, genetics, physical handicaps, or the necessity of taking certain medications. Finally, your ability to produce the results you want and to avoid results you don't want is integral to the context of your life.

The context can either contribute to backsliding or help ensure success. When the people in your life are supportive, when your relationships are nurturing (or at least not destructive), when you enjoy an adequate level of economic security, when you are not constrained by outside forces, and when you have abilities commensurate with your needs and goals, you are likely to have a context that supports change and the maintenance of change. Conversely, when the context of your life is not helping to maintain your new behavior patterns, you need to take whatever steps you can to create a context that works to support and encourage the maintenance of change.

CREATING A CONTEXT THAT WORKS

Influencing the context of your life and creating a context that works may seem like a monumental task. The woman mentioned previously was barely holding herself and her family together in order to cope day to day. Yet even in this apparently dire situation, there were things she did that over time influenced and changed the context of her life. Following are some strategies that can help change a difficult context.

1. **Learn to be more interpersonally effective.** One important aspect of becoming more effective in interpersonal relationships is to learn how to communicate assertively. Another is to learn how not to take things personally, especially other people's barbs and nastiness. For some people it is helpful to enroll in programs specifically aimed at helping you become more assertive or better able to manage conflict. Another good option is to seek therapy, either individually or as a couple.

TIP   A resource for managing interpersonal conflict that provides access to a chat room for help with conflict is: **www.abacon.com/commstudies/ interpersonal/inconflict.html**.

2. **Take action to change your environment.** One way to handle a difficult situation is to get out of it. When this is not a realistic option, it is important to identify the resources available to make the situation less noxious. One possibility is to seek the help of a therapist, or to call a local crisis center and ask for suggestions. Often, churches can provide pastoral counseling that may be of assistance. Having a sympathetic friend willing to listen can help a lot. Once you begin asking for help, you are likely to find sources of assistance you didn't know existed.

TIP   A short but useful article on leaving an abusive relationship (you'll have to ignore the ads) can be found at: **www.essortment.com/all/ leavinganabusi_rjjh.htm**.

3. **Don't automatically buy into your limitations.** While it is important to take into account your actual limitations, it is also important not to sell yourself short. You may be able to do more than you think. It is unrealistic to think you will one day compete in the Olympics if you are older or severely overweight, but don't use being over 35 and severely overweight as an excuse for never being able to do something special, such as running a marathon. Challenge your preconceived limitations. They may not be as limiting as you thought, or they may be completely imaginary.

    Real limitations are part of the context; the limitations in your head come from thinking errors. Richard Bach wrote in his book *Illusions*,[6] "Argue for your limitations, and sure enough they're yours." Often limitations are imagined. Take real limitations into account in your planning, but don't let them (or imagined limitations) keep you stuck in a problem.

4. **Use a problem-solving approach.** Sometimes you may make a valiant effort and still not get the results you want. Perhaps you get no results at all, or get results you hadn't expected. You might undertake a particular weight reduction method, following it as recommended, only to discover that you are not losing weight—or, worse, that you are gaining. When something like this happens, don't automatically blame yourself. It may be that the weight reduction method is poorly conceived. Or perhaps you just weren't ready for the effort.

    Instead of throwing up your hands and giving up all efforts to manage your weight, take a problem-solving approach. (Refer to Chapter 8, Addressing Stress, for a discussion of problem-solving.) Ask yourself, "What is the real problem here? Is it a failure on my part, or a failure on the part of the method, or both?" Try to determine how your context may be working against you, instead of assuming that the problem lies entirely with you. If necessary, get professional advice. Use a vigilant decision-making strategy to decide what to do next.

5. **When necessary, make the best of a bad situation.** Some situations are bad and not amenable to much change. One woman with three children and no job skills was married to a man who was an alcoholic. With no family support, she did her best to protect the children from his drunken moods and give them as safe an environment as possible. She was able to get support by going to Alanon and enlisting the help of her pastor.

TIP

For an article on how to build a healthy relationship, go to:
www.helpguide.org/mental/improve_relationships.htm#top.

6. **Seek spiritual support.** Many people find support for coping with a difficult situation through a spiritual path. Depending on your religion, this may involve going to a church, synagogue, or mosque for spiritual support, or it may mean using meditation on a regular basis. Prayer is known to help people cope.[7] Some people derive spiritual connection from hiking in the wilderness or helping others. Whatever your path, spiritual support can help.

For a short article on using prayer for coping with stress, go to:
www.relaxationexpert.co.uk/using-prayer-coping-stress.html.

Restoring Balance to Your Lifestyle

Your lifestyle may be contributing to backsliding. A healthy lifestyle is one that has a relative degree of balance between the things you must do (and that are potential sources of stress) and the things you want to do (and that make life pleasant). An unbalanced lifestyle is characterized by too many "have to" tasks and not enough "want to" activities. There is more work than play, and there are more obligations than rewards. Energy is directed outward, with little time or energy left for activities that give personal pleasure, satisfaction, or an inner sense of self-fulfillment.

If you have an unbalanced lifestyle, you may be attempting to cope with the attendant stress by engaging in one or more negative addictions—abusing alcohol, smoking cigarettes, drinking excessive amounts of caffeine, surfing the Internet, or overeating. Engaging in such behaviors is an attempt to restore some balance and to nurture yourself as well as an attempt to reduce the physical overstimulation that accompanies stress. When your lifestyle is unbalanced, you are likely to feel deprived, possibly with a periodic need for self-indulgence. The probability of backsliding is very high unless you bring more balance into your lifestyle by reducing obligations or increasing opportunities for reward and nurturing.

Stress in life can come either from major life events, such as divorce, illness, loss of employment, or the death of a loved one, or from ongoing daily hassles. Although traumatic life events can be the source of considerable stress, in terms of health—and long-term success in weight management—the ability to handle day-to-day stress is more important.

REPLACING NEGATIVE ADDICTIONS WITH POSITIVE BEHAVIORS

To restore balance to an unbalanced lifestyle, begin with an assessment of your current ways of coping. What strategies do you use to cope with the stress and hassles of daily life? Examine negative addictions listed in Table 10.1 and identify which of these inappropriate ways of coping with stress apply to you.

Having identified your negative coping styles, decide how you will tackle and change them. Where will you begin? What kind of assistance will you need? What positive coping styles do you need to integrate into your life? A balanced lifestyle is characterized by certain positive behaviors, such as those listed in Table 10.2, and by appropriate coping strategies.

Table 10.1
NEGATIVE ADDICTIONS

◎ Eating inappropriately—snacking, skipping meals, eating the wrong foods, overeating.

◎ Obsessing about food.

◎ Smoking tobacco.

◎ Using alcohol to excess to cope with stress, tension, or unpleasant emotions.

◎ Using nonprescription drugs or abusing prescribed drugs to deal with stress.

◎ Sleeping too much—sleeping to escape difficult situations.

◎ Sleeping too little—staying up late and not getting enough sleep.

◎ Overcharging with credit cards or spending beyond your means.

◎ Gambling, betting, playing cards, or playing games such as solitaire or bingo to excess.

◎ Watching television to excess.

◎ Playing video games or surfing the Internet to the near exclusion of social interaction.

◎ Spending too much time on the computer at the cost of other activities.

TIP

www.centersite.net provides an online self-help book of psychological tools for changing behavior and thinking, as well as important other issues relating to mental health. The page "Dealing with Reward-Motivated Behavior: Relapse Prevention" gives useful information for understanding and overcoming backsliding. Read it at: **www.centersite.net/poc/view_doc.php?type=doc&id=9741&cn=353**. Be sure to check out the other "chapters" of the online book at **www.centersite.net**.

Table 10.2
POSITIVE BEHAVIORS

- ◎ Eating a healthier diet.

- ◎ Regularly engaging in a well-rounded program of exercise.

- ◎ Getting enough sleep—about eight hours a night.

- ◎ Getting adequate relaxation and personal satisfaction by engaging in sufficient "want to" activities.

- ◎ Having satisfying social contacts and engaging in interpersonal activities that provide a sense of acceptance and connectedness.

- ◎ Getting adequate satisfaction from your job or career.

- ◎ Having a life philosophy or spiritual grounding that provides guidance for life decisions.

CHAPTER ELEVEN

Overcoming Challenges to Change

MARIA HAD BEEN OVERWEIGHT SINCE ADOLESCENCE. *She worked as a receptionist at a construction company. Until she lost 40 pounds, Maria had always been ignored by the contractors and construction workers who came to the office. Then some of the guys became so friendly they would stop, sit on the edge of her desk, and just chat. Maria didn't know what to make of this. Before, she had felt invisible; now, it was as if a spotlight were shining over her head. She didn't know how to play this game. The rules had changed—and she didn't know what they were. Maria joined the 3 Fat Chicks on a Diet weight loss community (**www.3fatchicks.com/forum/**) and started a blog topic about adjusting to the expectations others seemed to have for her and for others who had lost a lot of weight.*

Changes and Challenges

Common wisdom says that losing weight is only half the battle; making the initial lifestyle changes is just the beginning. The other half is keeping it off—that is, maintaining weight loss and healthier habits. People attempting weight management frequently report losing the same pounds over and over again. Regaining lost weight causes some people to give up and try to live with being overweight or obese rather than continue the frustrating yo-yo cycle of dieting, losing, regaining, and dieting again. Why, after all the effort involved in losing weight, does success slip out of so many people's hands? One important reason is that they don't permanently change their habits and lifestyles. Often, this is because they have not defined the values they want to live by. In the absence of defined values and guiding principles, they gradually resume overeating and under-exercising, and along with these old bad habits comes weight gain. Another important reason for regaining weight is that even many of those who are successful at losing weight are not prepared to meet the other challenges of changing.

TIP For good information on yo-yo dieting and weight cycling, go to: **www.freedieting.com/yoyo_dieting.htm**. Another good site (though you'll have to ignore the ads) is **www.weight-loss-for-busy-people.com/ yo-yo-dieting.html**.

In addition to making permanent lifestyle changes, those who succeed in losing weight and maintaining good habits must be able to cope with factors that can undermine success. As Maria discovered, sudden "visibility" is one challenge that must be faced. Having to cope with compliments on appearance during and after weight loss is another challenge. Coping with new demands placed upon those who lose weight, both by other people and by themselves, is still another. Spouses, family, and friends can begin to treat people who lose weight differently—and not always supportively. Shopping for normal-size clothes and dressing attractively during the weight loss process can be anxiety-producing. The fear of regaining weight haunts some of those who succeed in losing weight. Others become overconfident and think they no longer need to maintain their healthy eating and exercise habits. For people whose relationships have become asexual, the possibility of engaging in sex again can be quite a challenge. Relationship problems once kept in the background by weight issues may now surface. A body image that has not quite caught up to reality can wreak emotional havoc. A number of sometimes surprising pitfalls await the newly-at-a-lower-weight individual. Thankfully, many of the skills you developed to help you lose weight in the first place can be applied to helping you live successfully at a lower weight.

TIP An interesting app, **Weight Loss Now**, that employs hypnosis to help you lose weight is available for a fee at **www.maxkirsten.com/iphone/ weightlossnow/index.asp**. The app includes audio and video sessions along with an explanation of hypnotherapy. The developer of this app, Max Kirsten, is a clinical hypnotherapist and NLP practitioner.

CHALLENGES FOR WEIGHT LOSS SURGERY PATIENTS

Severely obese people who undergo weight loss surgery (e.g., with procedures such as the Roux-en-Y or gastric banding) face all the problems just listed, as well as still other problems. How can they avoid cheating? How do they socialize when food is often a central part of social events? How do they deal with the fact that there is no going back once this very serious step of surgery has been taken—at least in the cases of the more invasive surgeries? Even though they chose the surgery, the changes it forces on them can cause initial resentment. Will they be able to adopt new eating behavior habits, or will disordered eating become reinstated? What if they become preoccupied with food again, as they were before the surgery? Will sex with their partner improve? Will they need cosmetic or reconstructive surgery after losing weight in order to deal with sagging skin? The challenges involved in dealing with a thinner body and maintaining weight loss are significant for all who manage to lose weight, and most people aren't aware of them.

> **TIP** The Weight Loss Surgery Channel is the world's first television network devoted exclusively to the weight loss surgery community. It provides information, encouragement, and support to people considering bariatric surgery, as well as to post-operative weight-loss surgery patients and their family, friends, and caregivers. For more information, email them at **info@wlschannel.com**, or check them out on the web at: **www.weightlosssurgerychannel.com/about/**.

Eating Successfully

Perhaps you did just fine managing food and eating while you were losing weight. You were a "good dieter" and felt in control while dieting. Or perhaps you didn't have to manage food, because you were on a program so tightly prescribed that it took the choice out of eating. If you had weight loss surgery, you were initially prevented from eating too much, but gradually you have become able to eat more normally. The problem for many dieters begins when it is time to transition to a weight maintenance phase. If you gradually changed your eating and exercise habits during the weight loss phase, this problem may not be as serious for you, especially if you did so with your life values firmly in mind. Likewise, if you stay connected to others who are engaged in maintaining weight loss, your odds of keeping it off are increased. The pitfall that leads to regaining weight is going back to old eating habits and not meeting the challenges of maintaining success. Obesity is acknowledged to be a chronic problem, and ongoing effort is required to maintain a healthy lifestyle.

One of the most difficult challenges for the person who is approaching the weight at which he or she wants to be is integrating more food and calories back into the diet without regaining weight. Often people don't know how to do this. They go back to eating the way they did before undertaking a weight reduction effort, and they let exercise slide. This results in weight gain. Binge eaters can fall back into the pattern of eating to cope with emotions. Those who have undergone weight loss surgery and are constrained initially by the size of their stomachs may soon learn they can cheat by consuming liquids or eating small amounts of food more or less continually throughout their day.

SHIFTING TO THE MAINTENANCE PHASE

If you have created a new way of eating for yourself that is guided by your values related to health, you will naturally come to a weight that is right for you. Weight follows behavior, and as your new eating pattern settles into a routine, your weight will stabilize where it should be for your body. The challenge then is to continue your no-longer-new behavior and meet the challenges of maintenance with mindfulness and values-guided behavior. If, however, you have reached a new weight by dieting and restricting calories, you will need another strategy for stabilizing your weight.[1]

There are several strategies for introducing more foods and calories at the weight maintenance level. One is systematically to add back calories—for example, 100 per day for a week—and observe the effect on your weight. Then add back another 100 per day the next week, and continue so until your weight holds steady where you want it. Or you can gradually add back certain foods one at a time and in moderation, allowing your weight to be a guide to what you eat. It will still be necessary to consume problem foods carefully. An old Weight Watchers strategy is to "stay on program" on weekdays and allow yourself moderate treats on the weekend. Your ultimate goal is to eat a varied diet of moderate calorie intake appropriate to your age, gender, and level of exercise.

TIP A good blog for advice on weight maintenance is **www.diet-blog.com**. For more information on weight maintenance, go to: **www.cheaphealthygood.blogspot.com**. In addition to its blog, this website has lots of recipes and information on food as well.

The best strategy is to maintain the way of eating, or style of eating, that you have developed over the time you have been losing weight. Your eating "style" is an internal set of guidelines you define that may sound something like the following:

I eat X or Y foods for breakfast though occasionally I eat something special. I usually choose from among certain foods (A, B, or C) for lunch, but sometimes I choose a food from the Sometimes Chosen Foods list. Dinner involves eating lean protein (chicken, fish, or lean meat) with vegetables and some fruit. I try to make two or three main meals a week vegetarian or meatless. On special occasions, or when I just want to, I might choose from my "Rarely Chosen Foods" list. I eat healthy planned snacks as appropriate.

No matter what strategy you use, eating in moderation and using food only to provide nourishment and non-guilty pleasure is the key to eating successfully during maintenance, as well as for the rest of life. This is best accomplished by being guided by the overarching values about health that you want to guide your life, and referring to these regularly.

Making Movement a Permanent Part of Your Life

The evidence is overwhelming: to maintain weight loss, you must make regular exercise and physical activity an integral part of your lifestyle.[2] In one study of men and women who used a variety of methods to lose at least 20 percent of their body weight and kept it off for at least two years, the common denominator for all of them was sticking to an exercise program after reaching goal weight.

Chapter 5, Getting Started with Exercise, contains the information you need to start an exercise routine and maintain it. The idea of making exercise a permanent part of your daily routine may seem overwhelming, especially if you have never exercised. If you are older, you may worry that it is too late to get started. However, there are many people who do. The news periodically includes human-interest stories such as that of an 84-year-old man who water-skis barefoot or a 91-year-old woman who completes a marathon, despite never having run until age 89. And although they are not as newsworthy, plenty of Americans walk, hike, bike, play golf or tennis, or engage in other physical activities well into their senior years.

Unfortunately, most Americans of all ages tend to be sedentary. To become active requires a shift in self-concept from "I have to" (or even "I don't want to") to "This is who I am, and this is what I do," because I value my health.

Accepting the Loss of Invisibility

Many people who are seriously overweight say that they feel invisible to the world much of the time. Feeling invisible—and perhaps wanting to be invisible—is something that many who struggle with weight know. If you are obese you may find that few people on the street look you in the eye, and that many people tend to "look past" you. Conversely, if you are obese and are shopping for food, you may be the target of disapproving looks or stares. You may dress to minimize your shape and to avoid calling attention to yourself.

Once you lose weight, you are likely to lose your social invisibility. People passing you on the street may look at you, and may even say hello or stop to talk. In stores, clerks may seem to offer help more readily. You may be offered a seat on the bus, or be provided with other new courtesies. Instead of living in the shadows, once you lose weight, it can seem as if you are on stage. It seems as if the rules of social behavior have changed and you no longer know what they are.

Maria's story began this chapter. After she lost 40 pounds, she found that men in her office paid attention to her in a new way. Before she lost weight, they had just walked by, often without so much as a hello. Once she lost weight, they stopped, chatted, and even lingered. She wasn't sure what to make of it. She was flattered by this attention, but at the same time she felt uncomfortable. She was used to doing her work more or less unnoticed. She had grown used to being "invisible," and it felt comfortable. Now she didn't know how to respond.

 To read about the experiences of others who lost their invisibility after weight loss, go to: **www.enotalone.com/article/18619.html**.

COPING WITH INCREASED VISIBILITY

Being prepared for your increased visibility helps ensure weight loss success. Realize that unfortunately the rules governing social behavior change when you lose weight. Before, people didn't engage you much because of your size. Thinner, you become more noticeable. Other people check you out. You may feel uncomfortable at first when you receive new attention; give yourself time to sort out the meaning of changed behavior on the part of others. You no longer have to acquiesce to the needs of others to gain their acceptance. During your period of adjustment, tell yourself, "This may be uncomfortable now, and I can handle it. I'm learning how to adapt." You may need to learn to engage in small talk. And you'll need to learn how to handle compliments. You may find it helpful to join a support group or online community to interact with others who are having the same adjustment problems.

TIP   Social networking can help you lose weight and maintain weight loss. Select an app such as **SparkPeople** or **LoseIt**, or an Internet program like **Weight Watchers Online**, or one of many others that include online communities, and register for the site. Use the online social network tools such as blogs and forums to link with others who are managing weight. Blog to pose questions, express your feelings, get and give tips, and create new friendships. For more information on how to use social networking for weight management, go to: **www.ehow.com/how_2331036_use-social-networking-lose-weight.html**.

HANDLING COMPLIMENTS

Learning how to handle compliments is another challenge. Being complimented on your appearance is likely to be unfamiliar, and it can be confusing and uncomfortable. You may be unsure whether the compliment is being offered sincerely or as a joke. Nayeli, who lost 25 pounds, was confused when a stranger referred to her as "tiny." She had certainly not ever thought of herself as "tiny," and she didn't know what to say in response. Miguel got upset as more women started noticing and complimenting his appearance. He already had a girlfriend, and this new attention was disconcerting.

When someone keeps complimenting you on your weight loss, you may begin to feel increasingly uncomfortable. You may worry: "What if I regain weight? How could I face them if I fail?" A compliment about your weight loss may make you wonder whether your eating is under surveillance. For example, at first, Grace was pleased with the compliments she got about her weight loss, but eventually they became tiresome. Questions such as "How did you do it?" and "How much have you lost?" became increasingly irritating. She just wanted to be seen as a "regular" person, not always singled out because of her weight loss and her appearance.

Receiving compliments and not knowing what they mean or how to respond can be exhausting. The first step is to take a compliment at face value: assume it is sincere. Say simply, "Thank you." Don't discount it in your mind, or verbally to the other person. For example, don't say, "Oh, it was just because I got sick," or "It wasn't such a big deal."

If you find yourself worrying that all this attention puts a demand on you to maintain weight loss and you aren't sure you can, tell yourself, "Just take it one day at a time and do the best you can. What *they* think is not in my control." Then turn your attention to something else, and don't get fused with the idea of failing. Learn to accept compliments as rightfully deserved, and use them to affirm your self-worth. If worried thoughts keep occurring, just notice *that* you are worrying, then choose not to buy into the fear. Stay focused on one day at a time.

When compliments no longer have a positive effect, or are making you too self-conscious, you might try saying something assertive like, "You are so wonderful to notice my weight loss, and I know it may sound odd, but I'm starting to feel uncomfortable about all the attention I'm getting. What I'd most like right now is just to be treated like anyone else. I'm fine with getting compliments on my appearance, but please don't focus exclusively on my weight loss. Thanks so much for understanding."

 To read one man's success story in losing weight and keeping it off, go to: **www.secondhelpingonline.com/?p=925**. *Second Helping Online* is an online magazine that provides success stories for weight loss.

Coping with Others' Expectations

The expectations other people have for you can present another hazard. At your previous higher weight, you knew what to expect of others, and what they expected of you. At a lower weight, it may not be so clear. A spouse may want you to dress in a sexier fashion. Your boss may give you more responsibility. You may not want to do what is requested, or you may feel uncomfortable doing so. You may find that all of a sudden friends or strangers seem to want something more from you.

Miguel lost weight and discovered that women were now looking at him and flirting with him. Some slipped him cards with their contact information. He already had a girlfriend, and he was unsure how to respond in this new situation. He felt guilty about enjoying the flirtations of other women, but he didn't want to lose his girlfriend. Eventually, he was able to adjust to the new situation by blogging about it with his online weight loss support group.

Although you will always be influenced to some degree by others' expectations for you, you need to sort out what you want for yourself and what others want from you. Just because another has some expectation of you or indicates in some way that he or she wants something from you does not mean you must comply. On the other hand, don't retreat to safe behaviors just because you are uncomfortable with new expectations. Consider what you want, and if it's appropriate, have the courage to try something new.

Dealing with Social Challenges

Sometimes others feel threatened by your success. A spouse may not want you to be slimmer—even if he claims he does. He may even try to sabotage you by bringing you candy or insisting on going out to fast-food restaurants. Or he may simply be insensitive to your current needs. Likewise, friends may drift away or have no time for you once you have lost weight, especially if they see you as a threat. They may be envious of your accomplishments or fear that you might steal their spouses. Samantha discovered after losing weight that her next-door neighbor didn't visit for coffee any more. Lily's overweight coworkers urged her to gain weight by repeatedly telling her, "You are too thin; you look awful." (She didn't look "awful," but she took their comments as an excuse to go back to old habits, and she regained the weight and more.)

You may be able to reassure a fearful spouse or significant other by talking honestly and openly about your commitment to the relationship and to a healthy weight. To pacify a friend who feels uncomfortable about your weight loss success, make extra efforts to reach out; invite him or her to socialize with you. But be prepared for some of your relationships to change.

The rules that governed your relationships before you lost weight may now be up for renegotiation. A spouse who criticized your weight as a means of controlling you no longer has that power. Toby used his wife's weight as an excuse to do what he pleased—stay out late, spend money on nonessentials that they could not afford, watch endless football games on television, and generally indulge himself. Whenever she complained about these things, he brought up the subject of her weight. When she said nothing in the face of his indulgences, he ignored her weight. Once she started losing weight, his license to do anything he wanted was threatened. His loss of control over her and her newfound strength eventually led them to go into couple's counseling to deal with the power struggle that threatened their marriage.

Similarly, a friend or spouse may not embrace your weight loss if it means that your changed eating habits affect him or her. For example, both Carl and Connie loved to eat, and both were overweight. When Connie started losing weight, Carl became angry. He liked cooking gourmet meals and going out to nice restaurants. He didn't want to have to change his habits because of her newly found value of healthy eating. Their arguments became more frequent as he tried to pressure her to go along with his eating habits. They eventually divorced.

Unfortunately, some relationships break up when one partner succeeds in losing weight and the other is unable to adapt. Usually such relationships were relatively unhealthy to begin with, and weight loss merely brought pre-existing problems into the open. If your weight loss is bringing problems in the relationship into the open, it is time to seek the help of a therapist who is trained to work with couples. Control is often a major issue underlying relationship problems, and therapy may help the partners face the issues in their marriage and save or improve the relationship.

For an insightful article on how weight loss can change relationships, go to: **www.thats-fit.com/2009/03/27/weight-loss-will-it-change-your -relationships/**. To learn the five signs that weight loss is affecting your relationship, go to: **www.sparkpeople.com/resource/motivation_ articles.asp?id=1187**.

Shopping and Dressing

Although shopping and dressing in smaller sizes is thrilling for many who have successfully lost weight, others find that initially shopping after weight loss, especially if they have been very obese, can cause a lot of difficulty. As a heavier person, you were used to shopping in stores or departments that carried your size, and choosing clothes to disguise your weight. Going to a clothes rack with smaller-size clothes is often disorienting and distressing because you are no longer sure what your size is. Jasmine, who was used to shopping for a size 22, moved down to an 18, and then to a 16. When the size 16 was too big, she left the plus-size clothing store, unsure where to continue shopping. Hailey, who had lost over 100 pounds, was taken gently by the arm by a clerk she knew well from the plus-size clothing store. The clerk said kindly, "Honey, you don't belong here any more." That, too, was distressing. The now-thinner customer lost not only a familiar place to shop but a clerk who was friendly to her. Yet another woman, Evelyn, sent her sister into the regular-size women's section of a department store to bring home possible choices in various sizes for her to try. Evelyn feared that if she showed up in that store, she would be told to leave because they didn't have sizes that would fit her.

Some people solve the shopping difficulty by shopping online. Some may even make their own clothes or have them made. Others keep wearing ill-fitting clothes too long. Most just keep trying until they can tolerate the stress of finding the right dress or pant size. The good news is that eventually this anxiety passes, and dressing as the thinner person provides much satisfaction.

Despite the anxiety that shopping can produce, dressing well *while losing weight*, even if your desired final weight has not yet been achieved, is important. Many people say they don't want to invest the money in new clothes only to be unable to wear them when they lose more weight. Even so, feeling good because you know you look good as you are losing weight is part of the adjustment to becoming thinner and building self-esteem. Discount or consignment clothing stores offer one option. Another is to buy separates or clothing that can be taken in. Some people save their larger-size clothes because they reason that they might need them if they regain weight. (And, too often, this has been their experience before when they have lost weight.) While this may be a prudent financial strategy, psychologically it gives you permission to let weight return—your grasp of your guiding principles and values may be shaky. If you can't bear to get rid of your larger-sized clothes, at least pack them up into boxes and put them in storage. Get back in touch with your values and guiding principles.

Regaining Some Weight

Some people who reach goal weight live in fear of regaining weight. They repeatedly think catastrophizing thoughts: "what if" thoughts about how awful it would be to regain weight. The more they worry, the more anxious they become, until finally some of them can't stand it any longer, and they abandon the good habits and values that ensure maintaining a lower weight. These people have become "fused" with their fear. Instead of realizing that it is simply a fear and allowing it to pass in its own time, they become hostage to the thought or idea of regaining weight.

Worrying excessively about regaining weight is like holding a grenade with the pin pulled; it is just a matter of time before it blows up. One woman awoke each morning fearing "this will be the day I start gaining weight." Eventually she did. Rather than focusing on "what if," keep your attention on what you need to do this day, at this moment. Remind yourself that a thought or a feeling does not have to be acted on or acted out. Live one day at a time. Eat regularly, and have planned snacks as needed. Take care to eat moderately and be physically active. Increase your activities of daily living whenever you can. Participate in some kind of regular exercise. Get exercise on your calendar; try exercising early in the day so that exercise won't be displaced by other urgent needs that arise later in the day. Your healthy weight will settle to the right place for you if you live a healthy lifestyle. If you slip, just pick yourself up and get back on track. Focus on living a healthy life that includes fun and satisfaction.

If you do regain some weight, you need to do problem-solving: Where are you getting the extra calories, and why? Is your exercise adequate, or have you let it slide? Refer back to the cost–benefit analysis from Chapter 2, Getting and Staying Motivated, to boost your motivation. Review your reasons for wanting to maintain a lower weight. Are your actions being guided by your life values? What do you need to learn from regaining this weight? What do you need to do to get your lifestyle back in balance? Remember, the road to permanent change is not straight; it has twists and turns, and the important thing is to keep going in the right direction.

AVOIDING OVERCONFIDENCE

On the opposite end of the spectrum of the fear of regaining weight is overconfidence. The essence of overconfidence is thinking: "I've got this knocked. I don't have to worry any more." Exercise slides, good eating habits erode, and eventually weight comes back. It is easy to be drawn into feeling overconfident if you test the limits and get away with it a few times. You might indulge yourself and find that you don't immediately gain weight. As a result, you decide you don't have to worry about eating or weight any more—that somehow, magically, you have become a naturally normal-weight person, adopting the wrong-headed notion that normal-weight people don't monitor their food and eating. Before long, a series of excesses leads to some weight regain, and then some more. You discover too late that you now have a weight problem again.

Don't allow yourself to become overconfident, but also don't obsess about every little thing you eat. Eat moderately in all things. Be guided by the eating style you have adopted while losing weight. Don't let a couple of slips turn into a major relapse. Be sure to get exercise and be active. Live a healthy lifestyle, and your healthy weight will be a natural outcome of how you lead your life. Stay in touch with your values and avoid fusing with your thoughts and feelings. Stay mindful.

Facing Sex Again

Some people find that weight loss incites their partner to have an increased or renewed interest in sex. This is not always a welcome turn of events. The slimmed-down person may feel resentful or angry that he or she is only desirable now that he or she is slimmer. Whatever else he or she may have contributed to the relationship seems to count for little. For example, Dayanna managed the household and the children while her husband traveled on business, but he rejected her sexually because of her weight. He even refused to engage in gestures of caring such as holding hands or hugging. The only way he would have sex with her she found belittling and distancing and she did not enjoy just indulging him. He badgered her to lose weight, saying that he was turned off by her size. When she finally did lose weight, she was so angry about the way he had treated her that she wanted nothing more to do with him.

Others who have lost weight and had assumed that their sex life would become revitalized as a result of the weight loss discover that their weight was not really the reason their relationship had become asexual. For instance, even though Valerie lost weight and even had some cosmetic surgery, her husband still seemed not to be interested in her or her activities.

LOW SEXUAL DESIRE

A satisfactory sex life is one of the hallmarks of a happy marriage. The desire to participate in sexual activity is a normal part of life. Many overweight or obese people are in sexually satisfying relationships. But some people (overweight and normal weight) are in marriages or long-term relationships in which sexual relations have been absent for years. This can be the result of one or both parties' having low sexual desire. One-third of sexual problems in relationships are the result of low sexual desire. Excess weight is often the excuse given for this situation, and usually overweight people blame themselves for their partner's lack of sexual desire. Often after weight loss, the excuse needs to be reexamined. Or low sexual desire may be a problem for the one who has lost weight. There are many reasons, including low sexual desire, for sexual relations to change in a partnership.

Both physiological and psychological factors influence sexual motivation. Sometimes these factors are linked to issues about weight, but sometimes they are not. It is helpful to understand what may be contributing to low sexual desire and to seek professional help if this is a problem in your relationship.

For more information on inhibited (low) sexual desire and its causes and treatment, go to: **www.nlm.nih.gov/medlineplus/ency/article/001952.htm**.

Physiological Factors

Physiological factors affect sexual desire. Hormone disorders can be a factor in low sexual desire for both men and women. Sufficient levels of testosterone are necessary for desire, particularly in men. A man who has a "low libido" should see his physician to have his level of this hormone checked out. After menopause the level of testosterone in women also falls, and a decrease in estrogen makes it harder for the vagina to lubricate. This can cause pain with intercourse, which reduces desire. A variety of drugs, including antidepressant medications, can also suppress desire, as well as the ability to maintain an erection (for men) or reach orgasm (for both men and women). Other physiological factors that can reduce sexual motivation include depression, pain, fatigue, the use of certain street drugs, and alcohol abuse. Conversely, physical stimulation through massage, stroking, and touching increases sexual excitement. Try setting aside a time for lovemaking when you know you won't be rushed or stressed. Obtain a good lubricant and try lighting some candles and putting on music—which helps psychologically, too.

Psychological Factors

Psychological factors are also involved in sexual desire. One psychological suppressor of sexual desire is perceiving your partner to be unattractive. Of course, what is considered "attractive" or "unattractive" is subjective and completely up to each individual. Studies show that men are naturally more tuned in to visual stimuli, which may be one reason they like women to wear lingerie. Finding a woman physically appealing may be enough, at least initially, for a man to become aroused. A woman is usually more accepting of physical shortcomings in a partner, though a good-looking person can excite her, too (especially if she is a young girl or woman). As a relationship develops, a "beautiful" body is not all there is to sexual desire. Factors other than physical appearance become important in the relationship. Having similar values and interests contribute to the long-term viability of a relationship. Attributes such as the other person's sense of humor or warmth become important. With time, the couple's history together increasingly is a binding factor.

The longer partners are in a relationship, the more history they build together. This history may include major life experiences such as having children and also includes good memories and the experience of having withstood together the crises that life presents. The age-related changes that occur naturally in both partners' bodies are more acceptable, because a relationship is not just about sex. Family becomes an important binding factor. (Of course, some people throw away family for another partner.) It is true that some people do find excess weight to be a sexual turn-off. And it may not be the normal-weight person who is turned off. Some overweight people are so self-conscious about their weight or shape that they avoid sex, even if their partners are interested.

Some people find themselves in relationships with partners who may have been attractive at one time but have eventually become unappealing to them. Many factors other than weight can make a sexual partner unattractive. Bad breath or poor hygiene can actually lead to sexual aversion—extreme repugnance or disgust that causes avoidance of sexual behavior. Likewise, intolerance of the idiosyncrasies of a lover can cause sexual distaste. Paige, for example, eventually became so irritated by her boyfriend's habit of taking the pillowcase in his teeth and growling as he approached orgasm that she finally broke off the relationship.

Other psychological inhibitors of sexual desire include emotions such as anger, anxiety, and sadness. Anger is especially likely to inhibit sexual desire. Some couples claim that their best lovemaking is right after having had a fight. This is probably because anger is an emotion with a lot of energy behind it, and arguments are tension-producing. Making up and having sex reduces that tension. Even so, anger, especially unresolved anger, is usually an emotion that impedes the desire for sex. Long-harbored resentments are likely to bring avoidance of sex, and a partner who is prone to anger is often a turn-off.

Cultural or personal attitudes about sex can also contribute to low sexual desire or other sexual problems. For example, in some cultures women who are having their menstrual period are considered to be unclean; as a result, men would not consider having sex at such times. Some religious beliefs deem certain sexual behaviors as wrong, inappropriate, or unclean. If parents convey to a child that sex is dirty or disgusting, this message is likely to affect the child's comfort being sexual as an adult. Discomfort with touching of genitalia or having one's own genitalia touched may lead to avoidance of sexual behavior and low desire. The longer the avoidance persists, the more difficult the situation becomes. Disgust with bodily fluids and products may also depress sexual desire. In these cases, the help of a qualified therapist is appropriate.

PROMISCUOUS BEHAVIOR

Being at a lower weight may make you feel good about your body for the first time. But feeling as if you have become a swan after being an ugly duckling can loosen your constraints around sexual behavior. In some cases, a newly thinner person may take advantage of newfound confidence by engaging in promiscuous behavior. This can ultimately produce shame and guilt for some people, and it should be regarded as another potential pitfall of losing weight. You need to be alert to this phenomenon so that you can avoid behaviors that might make you feel bad later.

Addressing Relationship Problems

Weight loss can unmask underlying marital or relationship problems in addition to sexual ones. A spouse who is emotionally unavailable to you or to the family, or who is angry much of the time, or who is critical and controlling, can be at the root of some marital problems. Of course, these characteristics can all be present; they are not mutually exclusive. Such issues can make having sex unsatisfactory, or may even lead to avoidance.

THE EMOTIONALLY UNAVAILABLE SPOUSE

Women, more than men, complain about spouses who are "emotionally unavailable." Often this means that the spouse works a great deal and is not home much of the time; their participation in family life is minimal. Parenting is left primarily to the other parent, while the emotionally unavailable partner justifies long hours as necessary for the family's finances. The other parent and the children are left to emotionally fend for themselves. Eventually, the emotionally unavailable spouse may find it difficult to be a part of their interactions and dynamics.

Sometimes a partner is emotionally unavailable because of alcohol. Wilson started drinking at cocktail hour—5 o'clock for him—and didn't stop until he fell asleep on the sofa in the evening. His wife felt lonely and abandoned. She muted her dissatisfaction with eating. Once she undertook a weight reduction effort and could no longer blame her dissatisfaction on her own weight issues, she had to come to grips with the fact that her marriage had problems and her husband was likely an alcoholic. Richard had another problem: he liked to go out and party at the bar with his friends. After 8 or 10 drinks, he came home late to his wife and children. He often lied and made up stories—*it was a friend's birthday or I had to take out a client*—to excuse his being out and drinking.

In some cases, the partner is not a workaholic and does not abuse alcohol; he or she just isn't "present" in the marriage. Watching television, surfing the Internet, playing computer games, or engaging in sports activities or other hobbies to excess can take up a lot of time and energy. Adam, for example, obsessively collected, sorted, and read through his comic book collection, neglecting interaction with the rest of the family; Katelyn, on the other hand, spent so much time tending to her horses that her husband and children had to fend for themselves at mealtimes. They ended up eating frequently at fast-food restaurants.

When a spouse is emotionally unavailable in the relationship, the partner may turn to food and eating to fill up the emptiness he or she often feels. As a result, the neglected partner gains weight, and then his or her attention becomes focused on the weight problem, rather than the underlying problem in the relationship. Once weight is lost, a person with an emotionally unavailable spouse must face the possibility that the loneliness and dissatisfaction in the marriage may not have been simply related to his or her being overweight. The help of a therapist may be needed to help your spouse become more emotionally available to you and the family. When all else fails, it may be necessary to create a separate life—one with your own interests, activities, and friends—within the relationship if you are not willing to leave it.

THE ANGRY SPOUSE

Many overweight people are conflict avoidant and tend to be people-pleasers. This type of person often ends up in a relationship with a partner who openly and frequently expresses anger. One angry woman felt she had the right to tell everyone, especially her husband, when she thought they were wrong, and she did so frequently. Overeating was his way of rebelling against her as she complained about his weight and his eating, as well as about other things that annoyed her. Another man angrily expressed to his wife resentments about her, his work, his coworkers, her family, and his family. He was unable to see that he had an anger problem and left a couple's therapy session complaining about the ineptness of the therapist. Finally, his wife divorced him.

If you are in a marriage with an angry person, you may have thought he or she was angry with you for being overweight. When you lose weight and the anger is still there, you may have to face the fact that your spouse's anger is a problem that your being slimmer cannot solve. Bringing the anger problem to his or her attention may help—and you should urge your spouse to seek professional help if he or she cannot overcome it alone. Of course, your doing this may trigger more anger. Review Chapter 8, Addressing Stress, and in particular the section toward the end entitled, "Managing Interpersonal Conflict." Most importantly, don't blame yourself or your weight for your spouse's anger.

On the other hand, you may be the angry one. If so, you may be using food to express your anger. Kara was always irritated or annoyed about something—usually something that interrupted her usual routine or that surprised her in an unpleasant way. She could easily go from annoyed to all-out angry. She made critical comments to her partner that usually resulted in defensive rebuttals on his part. Getting nowhere with her attempts to feel in control, she often resorted to eating something sweet to sooth herself.

THE CRITICAL AND CONTROLLING SPOUSE

The desire to be in control is the central characteristic of critical and controlling people. They believe that their way is the "right" way and are not open to differing opinions. In their view, they are right and everyone else is wrong. They often zero in on some minor detail and can't seem to focus on anything else. They argue about small points and lose sight of bigger issues. Such people often demand perfection of themselves and of everyone else around them. When they encounter opposition, they become irritable or angry. Little things tick them off. They live by rigid rules and expect everyone else to do the same.

Critical and controlling people don't generally think they are critical or controlling. Their point of view is: "If only others would see things my way and do things the way they are *supposed* to be done, everything would be fine." But everything needs to be done "their way." Sometimes such people explain that they are not criticizing, but just "helping." When partners or family members withdraw or turn angrily on the person doing the criticizing, the criticizer feels attacked and unappreciated. Gil, for example, repeatedly criticized his wife for her eating habits, her weight, and her lack of fitness. He also criticized his children for not being fit and for eating poorly. When one of his daughters developed anorexia and another child became disruptive in school, he couldn't understand why they were behaving so badly.

Eating is one way some people cope with critical and controlling spouses. Eating functions to suppress the pain, as well as their own anger at constantly being criticized, and can be used to rebel against the controlling behavior of others. And, of course, people other than spouses can be controlling and critical. Parents and bosses often fall into this category. It can be difficult to lose weight if eating is your only means of coping with such people in your life. Once you have lost weight, coping more successfully with critical and controlling people is essential to maintaining weight loss success.

To cope more successfully, you first need to take a good look at yourself and your behavior in the relationship. Too often, both people in a relationship insist that the other one always wants to be in control. Before you label your partner a "control freak," pause and consider how you may be contributing to or be part of the situation. Next, you need to bring this problem out into the open. Talk to your spouse about your perceptions and feelings. Negotiate a new way to relate to each other. Decide who is best at certain tasks, and who will be in charge of them. For example, if you are the one who cooks and cleans up afterward, your spouse needs to give up his or her attempts to control how you load the dishwasher. Once you delegate roles and decide who is responsible for what, your life with a controller may be easier. That way, when he or she starts criticizing how you load the dishwasher, you just say, "We agreed this is my domain, and I get to decide how to do it." And, by the way, your eating and your weight are your responsibility. If someone starts criticizing you, stand your ground and emphasize that you are responsible for handling your eating and your weight.

GETTING PROFESSIONAL HELP

Weight loss can reveal underlying relationship problems that are often too complex or touchy for the partners to work through alone. Sometimes one or both partners are verbally and perhaps even physically abusive. The help of a therapist experienced in working with such issues is usually required to help the couple overcome problems.

When choosing a therapist, interview several on the phone. Give each a brief summary of the problem and ask how they would work with you to resolve the situation. If you don't get a good feeling on the phone when talking with the potential therapist, don't make an appointment. Once you do make an appointment with a therapist who seems to be caring and competent on the phone, give your partner and yourself a session or two to decide whether this therapist seems like a good choice for both of you. Don't hesitate to change if you feel you aren't understood and aren't making progress. Credentials are important, of course, but the therapist's ability to connect with you is equally important. Contact one of the national organizations on the Internet for a referral to a therapist in your area. The Association of Behavior and Cognitive Therapy (**www.abct.org**) is one such organization. Another possibility is to contact your local county psychological association, listed in the phone book under "Psychologists." Many therapists and professional organizations also have websites; the latter provides information via their referral service on the names of therapists in your area. If you need to use insurance, contact your insurance company for a list of therapists in its network.

Changing Your Body Image

A poor body image is another problem that comes with overweight and obesity, especially when a weight problem is accompanied by binge eating behavior. Some experts define body image as the mental representation or perception a person has of his or her body at any given moment in time. Another way of putting this is that body image is your picture of your body as seen in your mind's eye. In reality, body image is more than just an image in the mind. It is made up of all the perceptions, thoughts, attitudes, emotions, and concepts you have about your body. Body image encompasses the emotional significance of the body.

Those who lose a lot of weight often find that initially they still have a "fat" mental picture of themselves. (And sometimes people who have always been slim are surprised to discover they have a weight problem.) It takes a while for body image to catch up with the reality of a changed body. Some people have difficulty accomplishing this transformation and continue to think of themselves as fat (or slim when they aren't).

Problems with body image arise when unhappiness reaches such a level that a person cannot accept his or her appearance and this dissatisfaction interferes with relationships or personal development. When a person focuses primarily on being unhappy with some aspect of physical appearance, there is a problem with body image. Losing weight does not automatically cure a poor body image. Fortunately, a poor body image and dissatisfaction about weight or shape can be overcome. It helps to understand how body image develops and changes as you mature.

 Emelina, a layperson, writes about her struggle for many years with a poor body image and body dissatisfaction. To find out what she learned and how she changed, go to: **www.emelina.com/building.html**.

HOW BODY IMAGE DEVELOPS AND CHANGES

Influenced by temporal, environmental, and interpersonal factors, your body image begins to emerge in infancy and continues to develop and change throughout your life. Each person organizes and constructs his or her body image through the integration of many perceptions and experiences over the course of a lifetime. In society today, the emphasis on a thin body as the cultural ideal negatively impacts many people's perception of their bodies. When a person is teased or criticized by others about weight or appearance (or praised for it), body image is affected. Parents who worry out loud about a child's weight can plant the seeds of a negative body image. Media images of fashion models who are dangerously underweight or whose technically enhanced images are on magazine covers contribute to body dissatisfaction for many people. The person who comes to believe that appearance determines self-worth is vulnerable to developing an eating disorder—and a disturbed body image.

Body image is complex and dynamic. The body changes with age, and thus body image gradually changes over time. But small fluctuations and changes can and do occur over short periods of time. Even during a single day, body image can vary. After strenuous exercise, a person may feel "thin and fit" for a while, but a few hours later after eating something filling, that same person may "feel fat." But "feeling fat" is not really a feeling; it is a perception arising from the interpretation of physical sensations. In such cases, the person has fused with the thought "I feel fat" and it feels like the truth, even though it may not be. A good idea is to be more objective about your body and choose to see it and accept it as it is, without wishing away perceived flaws or inventing ones that aren't really there.

IDENTIFYING THE SOURCES OF A NEGATIVE BODY IMAGE

The first step in overcoming destructive body dissatisfaction is to identify the sources of self-consciousness. What cultural, developmental, interpersonal, or emotional influences have contributed to your concern about appearance? Teasing from peers or parental criticism contribute to body weight and shape concerns. Parents with body image issues of their own may demand that the child diet with them or may even enroll their child in a weight loss program. Fueled by images in the media of unrealistic bodies, self-criticism picks up where external factors leave off. Eventually, many people start to ruminate about their appearance and what they deem is "wrong" with how they look.

In addition to identifying the source of your body image, two other important steps in creating a more positive body image are identifying the expectations others may have placed on you and relinquishing self-criticism. You need to understand and reconcile the discrepancy between the ideal self (what you wish you were) and the actual self (what you actually are). The reasonableness of the "ideal body" as portrayed by media, culture, family, or friends should be examined and challenged. It is important that you reevaluate and accept your perceived actual self. Emphasize your positive qualities in a way that goes beyond appearance. Replace critical and disparaging internal dialogues with more helpful thinking, and replace hindering self-talk and self-critical thinking with self-accepting and supportive, helping self-talk (see Chapter 6, Managing Thinking and Self-Talk, for more on how to do this). Remember that hindering thoughts are, after all, just thoughts. They are ideas that come into your mind and may or may not reflect reality. In either case, get some distance between you and your hindering thoughts. You do not have to act on them or get drawn into the pain they probably produce.

To change the thinking that contributes to a poor body image and identify the influences that contributed to the development of your body image and what conclusions you made about yourself as a result of these influences, create a body image history for each of the following periods of your life: early childhood (up to 8 years old), later childhood (8 to 12), early adolescence (12 to 16), later adolescence (16 to 21), early adulthood (21 to 29), middle adulthood (29 to 40), later adulthood (40 and up), and during the past year. Depending on your age, you may not be able to complete a history for all these periods, but be sure to at least answer as far as you can, including for the past year.

For each period, *describe your body* in terms of whether you were underweight, overweight, or normal for your age. Also describe other aspects of your shape and appearance: Were you taller or shorter than most others your age? Did you wear glasses? Did you have braces or acne? Did you develop earlier or later than others? Indicate if there were other characteristics that made you self-conscious. What do pictures from that time period tell you about your weight and body?

Then answer the following questions at each period: *How did others treat you?* Were you teased, criticized, or rejected because of your weight, shape, or appearance? Were you called names? If so, by whom? Or did your appearance attract positive attention that made you uncomfortable? Did participation in a sport or activity play a role in your feelings about yourself and your body? *What messages did you get about your body and your appearance at that time?* And finally, *What conclusions did you reach about yourself at each period?* Indicate whether you continue to hold these convictions today. For example, did schoolyard teasing convince you that you were unattractive when you were in elementary school? Did a parent's criticism make you feel ugly or uncomfortable as a teen?

For 10 tips from Loyola University on improving your body image, go to: **www.loyola.edu/campuslife/healthservices/counselingcenter/weight.html**.

COUNTERING HINDERING BODY TALK AND AVOIDANCE BEHAVIORS

Body talk is how you think and talk to yourself about your body. In Chapter 6, Managing Thinking and Self-Talk, you learned that self-talk is one type of thinking. Certain kinds of self-talk (that is, thoughts) can contribute to or accompany painful emotions. Some self-talk, especially if it focuses on how you don't measure up or what you hate about yourself, promotes body dissatisfaction. Examples of hindering and destructive body talk might be, "My rear end is so huge," "They think I'm ugly," "I hate my looks," "They don't like me because of my size," and "I wish I were thin like her." Believing such thoughts is a problem. To do so is to become fused with these ideas. Remember that thoughts are just thoughts; they do not necessarily represent reality. Or if they do, all you can do is accept what is and do your best to cope effectively.

Thoughts come from your interpretation of events—that is, the meaning you give to them. Hindering body talk may prompt dieting, and it can lead to avoidance behaviors. You may start wearing baggy clothes so that others can't see your body. The thought of having to wear a bathing suit may make beaches off limits. You may avoid social occasions or situations in which you think you might be scrutinized or criticized by others. Perhaps you skip working out in a gym or stop going outside and walking because you don't want to be seen. You may avoid mirrors or large windows that reflect your image. You avoid scales. You engage in these avoidance behaviors in an effort to avoid feeling anxious. But a better approach is to tolerate the anxiety of being in these situations, and to substitute supportive thinking for destructive thinking. For example, when catching a glimpse of your image in a store window, you might choose to say to yourself, "I'm not happy about this, and I'm taking the steps to improve myself." Or, if your weight is decreasing but you still criticize yourself, just notice the thought and remind yourself that thoughts come and go—and that this one is a hindering thought. Try finding something supportive to say after the critical thought happens. Thus, if you automatically think, "My waist is still too big," then follow that thought with one like, "and I've come a long way." Accepting yourself at your present weight and committing yourself to take action for a healthy lifestyle is the best solution.

In a journal, record the anxiety-producing situations that you tend to avoid—like wearing a bathing suit or going to a party. List at least six such situations, ranging from low-anxiety to high-anxiety situations. Rate each one from 1 to 10 according to how anxiety-producing it is, with 1 meaning low or no anxiety and 10 being the worst anxiety possible. Tackle the low-anxiety ones first. Make yourself encounter the situations, rather than avoiding them. For example, go out for a walk even though you worry that someone will call attention to your weight. Or go to the gym wearing regular workout clothes. After you have succeeded with the low-anxiety situations, move on to the medium-anxiety ones, and then finally to the high-anxiety ones. Make notes about how well you did and what you learned each time you tolerated the anxiety, using a journal to record these thoughts and situations as they occur. Be sure to continue exposing yourself to such situations.

Positive or helping body talk calls attention to the positive aspects of your physical appearance and reflects self-acceptance. In your journal, make a list of the hindering body talk you find yourself engaging in. After identifying the criticism you direct toward your body, write down some helping self-talk in response to each criticism. Consider what positive body thoughts you might use to counter destructive thoughts. Some examples of positive body talk might include, "I need to keep my focus on leading a healthy lifestyle," "I am more than my weight or my shape, and my health is what is most important," "I may not be perfect, and I am doing the best I can," and "I need to make friends with my body, nourish it with a healthy diet, and give it lots of exercise and love."

Remember that these examples of helping body talk are not affirmations in the usual sense of the word: They are not simply nice ideas you aspire to. A positive thought affirms a truth and reminds you what to do or provides a supportive message. A helping thought reminds you of your values and guiding principles.

Making Friends with Your Body

Many people who have had a weight problem regard their body as the enemy. They don't trust it. They dislike it. They are afraid of it. They punish it or fight with it. And they reject it. This war between yourself and your body must end. You need to find a way to make friends with your body—not conditionally, as in "when it reaches a certain weight or achieves a certain shape," but now, just the way it is. This can begin by engaging in peace talks with your body.

This is a difficult exercise for many people, but it is worth trying. The idea is to open a dialogue—peace talks, if you will—with your body. In the privacy of your room, face yourself in the mirror, preferably completely undressed. Inspect your body carefully. Talk to it about what you like and what you don't like, what you would like to change and what you know you have to accept. If you can't find anything you truly admire about your body, find something that is at least acceptable. Let go of negativity and really try.

Then thank your body for what it does for you. Apologize to your body for having mistreated it—for having starved it, put it on restrictive diets, denied it good nourishment, fed it too much, exercised it too little, ignored it, criticized it, rejected it, hated it. Ask your body for forgiveness, and ask what it needs from you now. In your imagination, listen to what it says. Write down your body's response so that you can reread it as needed. If you cannot initially do this exercise actually standing in front of a mirror, do it first in your imagination. As you make friends with your body, you will be better able to face it in the mirror and each time experience more self-acceptance. Repeat this exercise often.

Create a Supportive Script

Another way to program helping thoughts is to create a script that acknowledges your body's positive aspects as well as its faults and to be accepting of it while still committing to healthy action. Then record this script in your own voice on an iPod or a tape recorder. Here is an example of such a script:

> *I accept my body in all its aspects, and I commit myself to caring for it with my actions. I acknowledge that I may weigh more than I would like. I apologize for picking my face until it is raw. I don't always take care of my hair or wear the most flattering clothes. I commit myself to making healthy food choices in moderation, starting now, in order to allow my body to reach whatever weight is right for it. I will take my dermatologist's advice, and I will keep the mirror at a distance. I will dress my body to show I am proud of it and care for my hair so that it shows that I care about my body. I apologize to my body for all the indignities it has suffered at my hands. I promise to love it and take care of it, always keeping in mind my value of healthy living.*

Once you have written and recorded your script, listen to it as often as possible—several times a day even. Listen to it until you practically have it memorized. Then repeat it to yourself often.

FIGHTING BACK AGAINST BODY DISSATISFACTION

A certain amount of body dissatisfaction is normal, especially at this image-conscious time and in our culture. It can be painful to feel that you aren't as pretty or as slim or as popular as someone else is. This is especially true for adolescents, but can also be true for adults. However, you have to work with what you have. Beating yourself up with destructive body thoughts about not measuring up to society's or other people's standards—or your own—only makes things worse. Self-acceptance is important, but it does not mean abandoning all restraint, eating whatever you want, and forgetting about your health. Rather, self-acceptance involves developing a healthy self-concept that includes the "good" news and the "bad" news, as you understand it. It means accepting what you can't change about your body shape or weight, and focusing on what you can change—your eating and exercise habits.

To fight back against destructive body talk and body dissatisfaction, you can do several things. Identify hindering thought sequences and challenge the erroneous assumptions and misguided conclusions that underlie your thinking. Next, formulate and use helping positive body talk. Finally, make friends with your body. Table 11.1 summarizes the steps for improving your body image.

TIP

To find a good article on overcoming body dissatisfaction, go to: **http://psychcentral.com/library/id188.html**. To learn more about why we look in the mirror so much and find fault, go to: **www.sirc.org/publik/mirror.html**.

Realistic Expectations for Weight Loss

With all the pictures of young, slender bodies in magazines, on television, and in other media, the person undertaking weight loss may hope that it will also bring a return to youth and a youthful figure. It can be quite a shock when a 43-year-old (or older) body ends up not looking like the 23-year-old (or younger) bodies shown in advertisements. The long-time, seriously overweight person, especially one who has led a mostly sedentary lifestyle, can have sagging skin and stretch marks with an atrophied muscle structure after significant weight loss.

Losing weight is not the modern version of the Fountain of Youth, but there is a lot that can be done to improve appearance during and after weight loss. Adding weight training to an

---

Table 11.1
STEPS TO AN IMPROVED BODY IMAGE

1. Stop criticizing yourself and holding yourself to unrealistic ideals.

2. Learn the difference between what you can change (your behavior) and what you must learn to accept (such as the size and shape determined by your genes).

3. Practice self-acceptance. Every time you look in the mirror, repeat: "It's true that I may not be just the way I want to be, but I need to remember that the one thing under my control is my behavior."

4. Fight back against cultural and socially defined labels and images. Remind yourself that what you see in magazines and on television is computer-enhanced and not true to life.

5. Remind yourself that the positive energy you put out into the world is more important than your physical appearance.

6. Stop judging others on their size and weight.

7. Stop comparing yourself to others.

8 Develop new sources of self-esteem other than shape and weight.

9. Forgive your body for not being perfect.

---

aerobic exercise routine is a good way to build and reshape muscle structure. Ultimately, the important thing is to accept your body with all its perceived shortcomings, instead of rejecting it, striving to make the healthy choices that will keep it in the best shape possible. Make sure your expectations for yourself are reasonable. Life is not about watching your weight; it's about being as healthy as you can be so that you can live a full, meaningful, and satisfying life.

TIP To read about people who have lost weight and kept it off for years, check out the National Weight Control Registry at **www.nwcr.ws**, and click on "Success Stories."

CHAPTER TWELVE

Considering Weight Loss Surgery

LESLIE HAS BEEN OVERWEIGHT ALL OF HER LIFE. Currently she weighs 240 pounds and is only 5 feet, 3 inches tall. She has tried virtually every diet, diet product, and diet program, only to meet with failure time and again. Until recently, she resigned herself to being obese. Then her doctor told her that she was dangerously close to developing diabetes, and that her blood pressure was high. He suggested that she consider bariatric surgery. But the idea frightened her. Nevertheless, she started investigating information on weight loss surgery. She started with the Internet and learned a lot about different surgery options, as well as what to expect before and after surgery. Her next step was to select a program and surgeon to discuss the matter further. Leslie was leaning more toward the least invasive surgeries, but wanted to be sure she would lose enough weight to make it all worthwhile. She also talked to her family members, who at first were against the whole idea. However, gradually they came around to Leslie's argument: her health was in question, and surgery was her last best hope, since she had not succeeded with other approaches to losing weight.

Severe Obesity on the Rise

As has been widely reported in the media, the percentage of Americans—and citizens of other Westernized countries—who are obese has been accelerating rapidly over the last 20 years.[1] According to a 2009 report by the Trust for America's Health and the Robert Wood Johnson Foundation, during 2008 adult obesity (BMI >30) rates increased in 23 states—and did not decrease in a single state. While the percentage of adults in the overweight category (BMI of 25 to 29.9) has remained about the same, the percentages of those in the obese category (BMI between 30 and 39.9) and those who are extremely obese (BMI greater than 40) have increased dramatically. Furthermore, the percentages of obese or overweight children in thirty states are at or above 30 percent—and childhood obesity rates have more than tripled since 1980. Sadly, obese children tend to become obese adults.

To learn more about health risks associated with severe obesity, go to: **www.surgeongeneral.gov/topics/obesity/calltoaction/1_2.htm**.

HEALTH RISKS ASSOCIATED WITH SEVERE OBESITY

Severe (or morbid) obesity (BMI >40) is often accompanied by, or contributes to, various medical concerns.[2] All of the health risks associated with overweight and obesity that were discussed in Chapter 1, Understanding the Relationship between Weight and Health, apply to those with severe obesity. These include coronary heart disease, cancer, type 2 diabetes, and sleep apnea. When one or more of these is present together with obesity, and weight loss attempts have failed, weight loss by means of bariatric surgery—also known as weight loss surgery (WLS)—may have to be considered. And in addition to the aforementioned health risks, additional risks accompany severe obesity. These include polycystic ovary syndrome, increased pulmonary risk, gastrointestinal problems, orthopedic complications, incontinence, gout, skin conditions, and venous stasis. Those who are severely obese often have a poor quality of life as well as additional medical co-morbidity. (In medicine, the term co-morbidity refers to the presence of one or more disorders [or diseases] in conjunction with a primary disease or disorder.)

For an overview of the medical and lifestyle problems associated with severe obesity, go to: **http://emedicine.medscape.com/article/123702-overview**. Scroll down to and click on the second figure, "Co-morbidities of Obesity." For the specific risk numbers for various conditions, published by the Centers for Disease Control, also check out: **www.robertorizzi.com/co-morbidities.htm**.

Polycystic Ovary Syndrome

Polycystic ovary syndrome (PCOS) is characterized by cysts on the ovaries (not all women with such cysts have PCOS), menstrual changes, acne, or excessive hair growth—a sign of hyperandrogenism (excessive male hormones)—which can occur on the face, chest, or back. More than half of women with PCOS are obese, and obesity may be a factor in the development of PCOS in some women. Those with PCOS are at greater risk for hyperlipidemia, hypertension, diabetes, and the metabolic syndrome. The relationship between PCOS and the metabolic syndrome may make it difficult to lose weight, because people with the latter have abnormalities in insulin metabolism that make them resistant to insulin.

Increased Pulmonary Risk

People who are severely obese tend to take smaller and shallower breaths, in what is known as *Pickwickian syndrome.* These small, gasping breaths may not deliver as much oxygen into the blood as needed, leaving the obese person feeling chronically tired.

Many overweight and obese individuals have asthma, and obesity is a factor that can worsen its symptoms. Extra weight makes it harder for the lungs to work right, particularly at night when a person is lying down. This may also cause asthma-like symptoms without actually being asthma. Instead, these symptoms may result from restrictive lung disease, which is best helped by weight loss rather than by inhalers. In severe cases, the restriction that excess weight puts on the lungs can lead to *obesity hypoventilation syndrome*—a condition in which blood oxygen decreases and carbon dioxide increases because the lungs cannot function properly. This condition can lead to daytime sleepiness and eventually to congestive heart failure. It is important to note that shortness of breath can also sometimes indicate undiagnosed heart disease.

Obstructive sleep apnea (OSA) is common among the severely obese and is characterized by loud snoring and interrupted breathing. Although only 1 to 4 percent of all people have sleep apnea, about 24 percent of overweight men and 9 percent of overweight women do. OSA is a link to cardiovascular disease and can be fatal. A sleep study can diagnose OSA; often the patient is subsequently put on a PAP (Positive Airway Pressure) machine at night to help with breathing.

Gastrointestinal Problems

Those who are obese can suffer from a number of gastrointestinal problems, including diarrhea, bloating, abdominal pain, nausea, and vomiting—all symptoms associated with irritable bowel syndrome (IBS). For some obese people, exercise can exacerbate these symptoms, making it difficult to stay motivated to exercise. Other gastrointestinal problems are also associated with obesity.

Obese women have twice the risk of developing gallstones as women of normal weight, and those with BMIs over 45 have seven times the risk. Symptoms of gastroesophageal reflux disease (GERD) are also more common in people who are obese. Obesity is associated with liver problems as well. *Nonalcoholic fatty liver disease* (NAFLD) is currently the most common cause of abnormal liver tests in the United States, and is often seen in association with obesity, diabetes, hypertension, and high triglycerides (another type of blood fat). People with NAFLD often experience no apparent symptoms, with only abnormal laboratory results pointing to it.

In one study of the liver biopsies of the morbidly obese who were preparing to undergo gastric bypass surgery, 65 percent had moderate to severe liver damage, 12 percent had advanced fibrosis, or scarring of the liver, and 33 percent had nonalcoholic hepatitis.

Orthopedic Complications

Extra weight puts more stress on the joints, especially those in the legs, hips, feet, and lower back. For every two-pound increase in weight, the risk of developing arthritis increases 9 to 13 percent. Pain from arthritis can make it difficult to carry out an exercise program; eventually, knee or hip replacement may be necessary.

Incontinence

Many obese women experience stress incontinence, a condition that can cause leakage of urine from the bladder when they laugh, sneeze, or even go for a walk. The condition develops when the abdomen increasingly exerts pressure on the bladder. Medications or surgery to correct the condition can be helpful, but the best solution is to lose weight.

Gout

Gout is caused by a buildup of uric acid to amounts that exceed what the kidneys can filter out. The acid buildup in the joints can cause swelling, inflammation, and pain, most commonly in the big toe or ankle joints. Obesity increases the risk of developing gout, as does alcohol consumption, a diet high in uric acid (found in red meat, red wine, and cream sauces), and kidney failure. There may also be a link between gout and high blood pressure. Although gout is best managed with dietary changes, weight loss will help prevent its recurrence.[3]

Skin Conditions

Obese persons often have areas of hanging skin folds, particularly around the breasts, abdomen, and inner thighs. These can become chafed, irritated, and difficult to keep clean. Superficial fungal or bacterial infections can result, along with bad odor. Deep-tissue infection can also occur. The severely obese, especially those with diabetes, tend to have decreased circulation to their hands and feet and delayed healing of skin infections.

Venous Stasis

Venous stasis is a condition in which there is slowed bloodflow to the leg veins; this can lead to damage to the valves in the leg veins. A sedentary lifestyle further inhibits bloodflow. Obesity can worsen this condition if regular exercise is not undertaken. Venous stasis runs in families and can contribute to superficial varicose veins, which are benign but can be a cosmetic concern. A serious complication of venous stasis is *deep venous thrombosis*—that is, a blood clot in a deep leg vein. Leg swelling and pain can indicate this type of blood clot.[4]

Understanding Weight Loss Surgery

Given that most obesity treatments for severe obesity have only modest effects, bariatric weight loss surgery procedures offer a viable and cost effective alternative. According to 1991 recommendations of the Gastrointestinal Surgery for Severe Obesity: Consensus Development Panel, patients with BMIs greater than 40 and those with BMIs between 35 and 40 with two or more coexisting medical conditions are candidates for surgical weight loss procedures. Even so, weight loss surgery (WLS) should not be undertaken lightly.

TIP To view a video (and read the transcript of the video) of Michael Turnoff, M.D., Tufts University School of Medicine, talking about two procedures for bariatric surgery, go to: **www.insidermedicine.com/archives/If_I_Had_Morbid_Obesity_Dr_Michael_Tarnoff_MD_FACS_Tufts_University_School_of_Medicine_2966.aspx**. Be advised that the video is quite graphic.

Bariatric surgery procedures necessitate a dramatic change in eating behavior and lifestyle. Patients seeking WLS need to be fully informed and must clearly understand the implications of the step they are taking. Those who are ineligible for WLS are those who cannot fully understand and carry out the dietary and lifestyle modifications required. In addition, patients may be denied WLS because of poor surgical risk status, advanced age, untreated endocrine or other medical disorders, or active addiction behaviors. Alcohol abuse or dependency must be overcome before having surgery. If a candidate is severely depressed or has suicidal thoughts, WLS is typically delayed until such conditions abate with the help of therapy, and possibly antidepressant medication.

UNDERSTANDING THE DIGESTIVE PROCESS

In order to understand bariatric procedures, it is important to learn about normal digestive processes. Normally, as food moves along the digestive tract, digestive juices and enzymes digest food and absorb calories and nutrients.[5] Figure 12.1 illustrates the anatomy of the digestive process. After we chew and swallow our food, it moves down the esophagus to the stomach, where strong acid continues the digestive process. The normal stomach can hold about three ounces of food or fluid at one time. The stomach expands and contracts in the process of di-

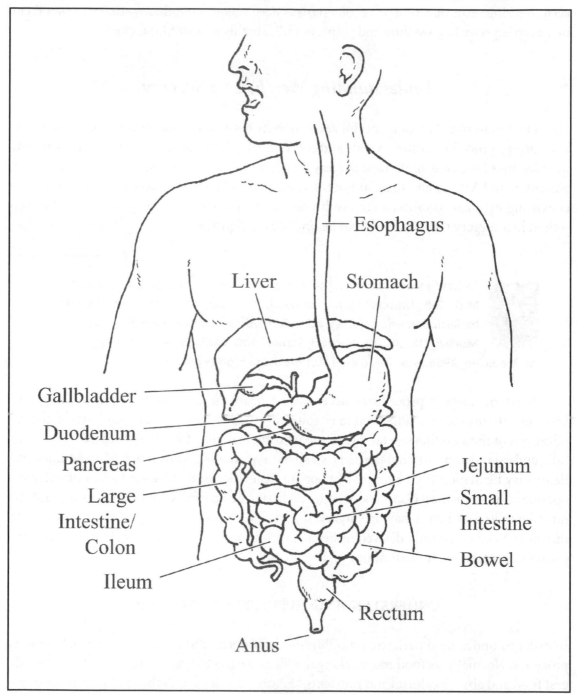

Figure 12.1
THE DIGESTIVE SYSTEM

gesting food. When the stomach contents move to the duodenum, the first segment of the small intestine, bile and pancreatic juices speed up digestion. In the jejunum and ileum, the remaining two segments of the nearly 20 feet of small intestine, the absorption of almost all calories and nutrients is completed. The food particles that cannot be digested in the small intestine move into the large intestine and are eventually eliminated through the rectum. The bowel includes the large and small intestines; it extends from the stomach to the anus.

HOW BARIATRIC SURGERY PROMOTES WEIGHT LOSS

Gastrointestinal surgery for obesity, technically known as *bariatric surgery*, alters the normal digestive process. These operations can be divided into three types: *restrictive*, which limits food intake by creating a narrow passage from the upper part of the stomach into the larger, lower part of the stomach, reducing the amount of food the stomach can hold and slowing the passage of food through the rest of the stomach; *malabsorptive*, which does not limit food intake but instead excludes most of small intestine (the ileum and the jejunum) from the digestive tract so that fewer calories and nutrients are absorbed (malabsorptive procedures can result in severe nutritional deficiencies because of this); and a *combination* of restrictive and malabsorptive procedures, using stomach restriction and a partial bypass of the small intestine.

OPEN OR LAPAROSCOPIC WEIGHT LOSS PROCEDURES

Bariatric surgery may be performed through "open" approaches, involving large incisions in the abdomen, or by laparoscopy ("lap"). In the laparoscopic approach, sophisticated instruments are inserted through half-inch incisions and guided by a small camera that sends images to a television monitor. Most bariatric surgery today is performed laparoscopically because it requires smaller cuts, creates less tissue damage, leads to earlier discharges from the hospital, and has fewer complications, especially postoperative hernias. (A hernia is a protrusion of an organ or part of an organ, such as the intestine, through connective tissue, or through a wall of the cavity such as the abdomen, in which it is normally enclosed.)

Not all patients are suitable for laparoscopy. Those who are extremely obese, who have had previous abdominal surgery, or who have complicating medical problems may require the open approach. However, new procedures are being developed all the time. Surgeons are currently investigating surgery through the vagina, known as "natural orifice translumenal endoscopic surgery."

Sometimes a "lap" procedure must be followed by an "open" procedure because of complications following the laparoscopic procedure. A few people have needed multiple procedures with long hospital stays to achieve a stable outcome.

A number of websites provide information on bariatric surgery. A good website to start with is **www.yourbariatricsurgeryguide.com**.

Surgical Options for Weight Loss

The primary surgical approaches used to treat obesity in the United States include the adjustable gastric band (AGB), Roux-en-Y gastric bypass (RYGB), biliopancreatic diversion with duodenal switch (BPD-DS), and vertical sleeve gastrectomy (VSG).

The AGB and VSG are restriction procedures, while the others both restrict the amount of food that can be consumed and involve malabsorption of nutrients. Each of these procedures can have several variations, and each variation has its own benefits and risks. If you decide to undergo WLS, your surgeon will help you select the option that is best for you, taking into account the operation's benefits and risks, along with many other factors, including your BMI, eating behaviors, obesity-related health conditions, and previous operations. For example, a WLS candidate who has had difficulty mainly with portion control may be directed to the AGB, while another patient with diabetes could be advised to have the gastric bypass.

ADJUSTABLE GASTRIC BAND (AGB)

Adjustable gastric banding is a *restrictive* type of weight loss surgery. It works by placing a small, silicone band with an inflatable inner collar around the upper stomach to produce a small pouch about the size of a thumb. The band narrows the passage to the lower stomach. This smaller passage delays the emptying of food from the pouch and causes a feeling of fullness. The silicone band is connected to a small port that is placed on the outside of the abdominal wall (usually placed under the breast), which allows the band to be tightened by injecting saline through this port. See Figure 12.2 for an illustration of what happens to the stomach with AGB surgery.

It can be helpful for someone who has already had banding surgery to check in with a message board, forum, or blog. The site visited should be specific to bypass surgery or banding surgery, because the problems and issues can be different. The main lap band surgery site is **www.lapbandtalk.com** (it has a lot of ads, but they can be ignored). It has a huge forum with all sorts of subforums organized by patient status (e.g., pre-op, post-op), location, and date of banding. This

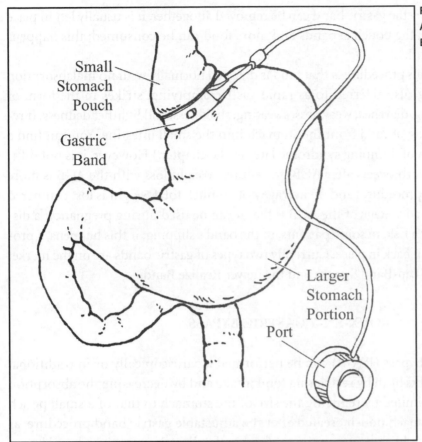

Figure 12.2
ADJUSTABLE GASTRIC
BAND PROCEDURE

Small
Stomach
Pouch

Gastric
Band

Larger
Stomach
Portion

Port

forum involves patients talking to patients and does not include first-hand medical advice from professionals. It can be helpful to know what others are going through or how they have handled a particular problem or issue. Another popular and active blog with worldwide membership is **http://health.groups.yahoo.com/group/DRWBandsters/**. A site specific to those with the Realize band, and more of a personal tracking site than a support site, is **www.realizemysuccess.com**.

The stomach needs to heal from the surgery before the band is adjusted for the first time. This adjustment typically occurs about six weeks after surgery, at which time the band is filled with saline to inflate the band and restrict food from entering the larger stomach. Swelling from the surgery may initially help restrict food intake before the first fill. Gastric bands need to be adjusted (i.e., filled) an average of four to six times in the first year. Adjustments are done to tighten (or sometimes loosen) the band to encourage continued weight loss.

Although technically the gastric band can be removed altogether, it is usually left in place permanently. Over time, the pouch expands and more food can be consumed; this happens after about 18 to 24 months.

The advantage of this procedure is that food is digested normally with no malabsorption or dumping. (Dumping, also referred to as rapid gastric emptying, strikes in the form of cramps, nausea, vomiting, diarrhea, weakness, sweating, shakiness, and lightheadedness. It results from rapid emptying of food from the stomach into the small intestine. You can find a more detailed discussion of dumping syndrome later in the chapter.) However, it is not difficult to consume and absorb sweets after AGB procedures. Weight loss with the AGB is more gradual than with other procedures and on average not as much total weight is lost compared to other procedures. An advantage of the AGB is that it can be used during pregnancy; a disadvantage is that there is a risk, in some patients, of the band's slipping; if this happens, a procedure is required to put it back in place. Currently two types of gastric bands are on the market in the United States: the Lap-Band System and the newer Realize Band.

ROUX-EN-Y GASTRIC BYPASS

The Roux-en-Y gastric bypass (RYGB) can be performed laparoscopically or in traditional open surgery. RYGB works both by restricting food intake and by decreasing the absorption of food. Food intake is limited by reducing the size of the stomach to that of a small pouch similar in size to the stomach pouch created after the adjustable gastric band procedure, as shown in Figure 12.3. In addition, absorption of food in the digestive tract is reduced by excluding most of the rest of stomach, duodenum, and upper intestine from contact with food by routing food directly from the pouch into the small intestine. Since fewer nutrients enter the bloodstream, people who undergo gastric bypass require higher amounts of daily vitamin and mineral supplements to avoid becoming nutrient deficient. The RYGB is currently considered the gold standard bariatric surgical procedure in the United States for those with a BMI between 40 and 55, because it produces quick and substantial weight loss. For those with a BMI over 55, the Biliopancreatic Diversion with Duodenal Switch (BPD-DS) is recommended.

TIP

Roux-en-Y or gastric bypass surgery patients will want to visit **www.obesityhelp.com**. Another helpful blog for bypass candidates is **http://weightlosssurgeryblog.net**.

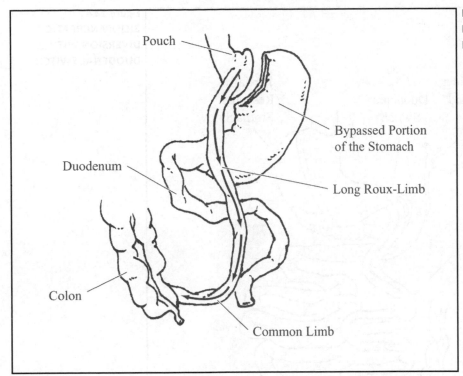

Figure 12.3
ROUX-EN-Y GASTRIC
BYPASS PROCEDURE

Pouch

Bypassed Portion
of the Stomach

Duodenum

Long Roux-Limb

Colon

Common Limb

BILIOPANCREATIC DIVERSION WITH DUODENAL SWITCH (BPD-DS)

BPD-DS, usually referred to as a "duodenal switch," is a complex bariatric operation that actually involves two operations. Figure 12.4 shows the completed duodenal switch after both operations.

The first procedure, shown in Figure 12.5, involves reducing the size of the stomach to create a more tubular "gastric sleeve" stomach by removing about 85 percent of it, thus restricting food intake. This operation is actually a VSG procedure. The gastric sleeve is about the size and shape of a banana; the excised stomach is much larger.

The second operation needed to complete the duodenal switch involves rerouting food away from much of the small intestine to partially prevent absorption of food, and rerouting bile and other digestive juices which impair digestion. The smaller "gastric sleeve" stomach remains connected to a very short segment of the duodenum, which is then directly connected to a lower part of the small intestine. This operation leaves a small portion of the duodenum available for food and absorption of some vitamins and minerals. However, food that is eaten bypasses the majority of the duodenum. The distance between the stomach and colon is made much shorter after the second operation, thus causing malabsorption. BPD-DS produces significant weight loss. However, there is greater risk of long-term complications because of

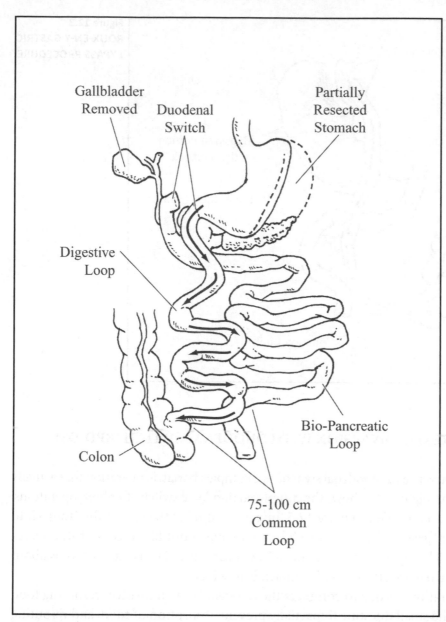

**Figure 12.4
BILIOPANCREATIC
DIVERSION WITH
DUODENAL SWITCH**

decreased absorption of food, vitamins, and minerals. Thus BPD-DS is a combination of a restrictive and a malabsorption procedure.

The BPD-DS procedure is usually reserved for those with a BMI of 55 or higher. The long-term results show the best excess body weight loss with maintenance at 70 to 75 percent in the majority of patients. Patients can eat much larger quantities of food and still achieve and maintain weight loss. Because of the potential complications relating to malabsorption, BPD-DS patients require lifelong vitamin and mineral supplementation and medical follow-up.

VERTICAL SLEEVE GASTRECTOMY (VSG)

Vertical sleeve gastrectomy (VSG), shown in Figure 12.5, historically has been performed only as the first stage of BPD-DS (the creation of the gastric sleeve in the first operation; see previous section) in patients who may be at high risk for complications from other types of surgery. These patients are considered at high risk due to very high body weight or complicating medical conditions. However, more recent information indicates that some patients who undergo a VSG procedure can actually lose significant weight with VSG alone, avoiding the second follow-up BPD-DS procedure involving rerouting. It is not yet known how many patients who undergo VSG alone will need a second-stage BPD-DS procedure. VSG is now being used for patients with lower BMIs and is considered to be an alternative to the AGB and the RYGB. A VSG operation restricts food intake but does not lead to decreased absorption of food. Most of the stomach is removed (about 85 percent), which is believed to decrease production of

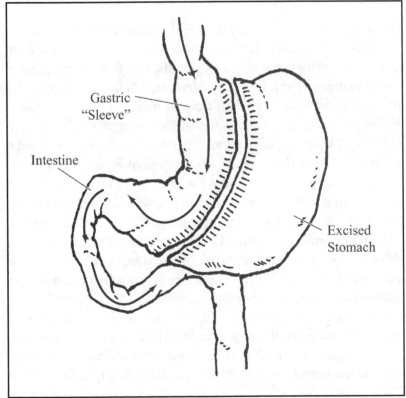

Figure 12.5
VERTICAL SLEEVE GASTRECTOMY

Gastric "Sleeve"

Intestine

Excised Stomach

the hormone ghrelin. A decreased amount of ghrelin may reduce hunger more than other purely restrictive operations, such as gastric banding. VSG is not reversible. (The only procedure that is reversible is the gastric band, but the band is usually left in place.) Once a large portion of the stomach is excised, it cannot be reconnected.

WEIGHT LOSS BEFORE SURGERY

Often surgeons require that a prospective patient lose an amount of weight—10 to 30 pounds—before surgery. The reason surgeons recommend—or require—pre-surgery weight loss is for the patient to demonstrate a commitment to making better food choices. This can give rise to the complaint, "If I could do that, I wouldn't need surgery." Some patients even use the pre-surgery time to indulge themselves and gain even more weight prior to surgery. Consequently they go into surgery with further to go to get to goal weight than had they lost some weight on their own. They have to play "catch-up," which can be demoralizing, and it can increase their risk.

Risks Associated with Weight Loss Surgery

Weight loss surgery entails all the risks that any surgery does and necessitates a period of recuperation with discomfort. Complications can occur, such as bleeding, infection, leaks from the site where the intestines are sewn together, and blood clots in the legs that can progress to the lungs and heart. Post-surgery malnutrition can be a problem, especially for patients who fail to take prescribed vitamins and minerals or to get sufficient protein.

The risk of death is 1 percent, or one in every 100 patients. This compares to a 2 percent risk with heart bypass surgery. About 1 percent of patients experience gastrointestinal leaks, which must be repaired. There is a 2 percent risk of bowel obstruction or a puncture (fistula) of the intestine. Ventral hernia (which occurs when the bowel or intestines protrude through a weakened abdominal wall) happens in about 16 percent of patients, while 24 percent reportedly suffer gallstones (hard, pebble-like deposits that form inside the gallbladder). Because some people start abusing alcohol when they can no longer use food to cope with stress, incidents of death from alcoholic cirrhosis of the liver have been reported. (More about alcohol abuse and surgery follows.) Under no circumstances should surgery in a foreign country be considered. An ill-advised effort to save money could cost you your life.

Other complications may be possible, and these should be discussed with your surgeon. Anyone considering such surgery should carefully weigh the benefits and potential risks before going ahead. They should be prepared for the dramatic changes that will take place—not only physically and psychologically, but socially as well. The patient's family is likely to be concerned about safety, given the risks of surgery. They may be more supportive of surgery if they understand that the person has truly exhausted other weight management options and is likely to face significant health risks if they don't undergo surgery. One should not ignore the risks, or be blinded by the wish for a slimmer and more socially acceptable body.

TIP For a thorough explanation of risks associated with bariatric surgery, go to: **www.bariatricsurgerypittsburgh.com/surgery/risks.html**.

Other Issues to Consider

There are other issues related to weight loss surgery that must be considered very carefully when contemplating the procedures. Clinically severe obesity is a serious and often chronic condition with physical and mental health consequences. Some of these medical concerns were discussed previously, but there are additional concerns as well.

QUALITY OF LIFE

Quality of life refers to a person's perspective on his or her physical, mental, and social functioning.[6] Poor quality of life is often the case for those who are severely obese and who also binge eat—as many as 49 percent of those seeking treatment for obesity with bariatric surgery are binge eaters.[7, 8] In several studies, morbidly obese persons who binge eat were found to be more psychologically impaired than those who did not binge; they reported greater depression and lower self-esteem. The severely obese binge eaters also reported less satisfaction with their sexual lives and greater difficulties with work and career compared to those who did not binge.

There are also logistical problems with severe obesity that contribute to a poor quality of life. The seriously obese can have difficulty walking even short distances, going up and down stairs, traveling on airplanes, and fitting into chairs at restaurants and other places. The obese usually suffer low self-esteem, social stigmatization, depression, difficulty maintaining hygiene, and difficulties in relationships. Research has found that the effect of morbid obesity on quality of life is more severe than the effect of other medical conditions such as cancer or chronic respiratory disease.[9] Fortunately, successful weight loss surgery can help with these conditions. Reversing or significantly reducing these problems is a strong incentive to undertake weight loss surgery.

WEIGHT REGAIN AFTER SURGERY

Before weight stabilizes post-surgery, some small weight regain is normal; this usually occurs 18 to 24 months after surgery. Unfortunately, some patients regain considerable weight; a few even return to pre-surgery weights. This occurs mainly because some people sabotage their own success by cheating and not exercising. They may discover that they can eat high-calorie food in small amounts, and they take up grazing again.

Sometimes, the amount of weight lost from surgery is not as much as the patient expected or hoped for. There is no way to predict how much weight any given patient will lose. On average, those who choose a banding procedure do not lose as much weight as bypass patients, and their weight loss is slower. In addition it takes more time and greater effort on the part of the patient to lose weight after a band procedure. Disappointment with slow progress can lead some people to make the wrong choices—and regain weight.

A new and innovative revision procedure for those who have the RYGB and who have regained weight due to a stretched stomach pouch or enlarged stomach outlet is called StomaphX and is becoming increasingly available at some bariatric surgery centers.

Overall, about 15 percent of patients who undergo bariatric surgery have unsatisfactory weight loss or regain much of the weight that they lost. This is usually due to frequent snacking on high-calorie foods, or to lack of exercise. Sometimes technical problems occur, like a stretched pouch or a pouch that was initially made too big. Continued use of food to cope with emotions is often a culprit in disappointing weight loss or regain.

PHYSICAL ACTIVITY

At a lower post-surgery weight, it is easier for the patient to engage in physical activity. Adding daily exercise to the lifestyle ensures weight maintenance. Gradually, over a year or two, depending on the operation performed, the stomach expands to accommodate more food. In some cases the stomach expands enough that the patient will be eating more or less normal portions. In the meantime, post-surgery patients must develop a new way of eating that will last a lifetime. They cannot use food to cope with stress or take advantage of opportunities to "get away with" inappropriate eating.

The 18 to 24 months post-surgery should be thought of as a sabbatical from your previous lifestyle that gives you time to develop a new, healthier lifestyle and way of eating; it is a time to decide how you will eat—what your personal guidelines for eating are—and how you will incorporate exercise into your lifestyle. Failure to make this transition will result in regaining weight. By the end of two years, you should have established a new lifestyle that supports your lower weight.

EMOTIONAL REACTIONS TO SURGERY

Some people who undergo weight loss surgery may find that initially they are angry about the eating restrictions imposed by the surgery. Fortunately, anger subsides as they begin to see that indeed they do lose weight. Other emotions such as grief over the loss of food or anxiety from not having food to cope can also be present after surgery. Post-surgery patients may not know how to socialize or celebrate holidays without food being central.

Social Support

Some form of social and psychological support is needed for weight loss patients to help them cope with the new demands of life after surgery and to help them develop better coping strategies for stress. Most WLS patients say they want post-surgery support, but only about a quarter of them attend available support groups. Attending such groups normalizes what the person is experiencing at a given stage of recovery and provides suggestions and help from those who have gone before. Some patients find support in website forums and blogs.

TIP A number of blogs provide support to WLS patients. One of them is: **http://livingafterwls.blogspot.com**. For additional blogs, check out: **www.wlslifestyles.com/all-blogs.php**.

Other patients seek psychotherapy before and after surgery. They feel that engaging in therapy helps them sort out the issues that have led to and maintained a weight problem in the past, prepare for surgery, and make the adjustment to being thinner. Therapy before WLS may be necessary for binge eaters because losing weight rarely cures binge eating.

A crucial aspect of success is to have social support, especially from family. The best time to establish this is before surgery. Family and friends need to be informed about what the WLS patient will need from them after surgery. Specifically, the person who is in charge of shopping and cooking needs to be on board with the intention to help and the knowledge of what to do. When such support is not forthcoming, success is jeopardized.

Weight Loss Surgery Results

Before considering research results regarding weight loss surgery, it is necessary to define what is meant by "success." Various definitions are used. Some research defines success as "weight loss down to a BMI of between 20 and 25." Another definition is "maintaining a BMI <35 for five years." Still another is "loss of >50 percent of excess weight." A less precise definition is "weight loss sufficient to meet the patient's expectations and see improvement in general health, life expectation, and quality of life." Finally, some research simply uses arbitrary categories to refer to results, such as "excellent, good, failure," without providing standards for these terms.

Some general conclusions can be drawn from the research evidence. The average patient loses about half of his or her excess weight. The amount of weight lost varies by procedure. Weight loss with gastric banding is slower than with the gastric bypass, and less weight is lost, although more research is needed to verify these conclusions.

The Roux-en-Y (RYGB) procedure shows the best long-term weight loss results for those with a BMI between 40 and 55. With RYGB, the odds of losing a larger percentage of excess weight are much higher than that of the adjustable gastric banding procedure, on which fewer studies of long-term results have been conducted. Of patients who undergo RYGB, on average 75 percent lose 65 to 85 percent of excess weight and keep it off four years or longer. Generally RYGB results in 60 to 80 percent excess weight loss over the course of the first year for most patients, with long-term weight stabilization at 50 to 60 percent loss of excess weight in nearly 80 percent of patients.[10] One study that defined success as "BMI <35 and loss of excess weight >50 percent" found that the Roux-en-Y had a success rate of 58 percent at 33 months after surgery.

A study of 274 patients with long-term follow-up of five years and who had undergone gastric bypass for various levels of severe obesity revealed a success rate (measured by a BMI of <35) of 93 percent for patients in the obese and the morbidly obese categories. In the super-obese patients, 57 percent succeeded.[11]

The vertical sleeve gastrectomy (VSG) procedure alone is still too new to have much data on outcome. However, the existing data suggest that on average about 55 percent of excess weight is lost. In addition 50 percent of patients indicated that they experienced an absence of cravings for sweets. This is probably due to the decrease in the hormone ghrelin, which is produced primarily by the excised (resected) portion of the stomach.

The long-term results of the duodenal switch (BPD-DS) show the best excess body weight loss with maintenance at up to 75 percent in the majority of patients. This is also the most invasive procedure and is usually reserved for the superobese.

TIP For a good overview of what is involved in weight loss surgery, plus some before and after pictures, go to: **www.metrohealth.org/body.cfm?id=1548&oTopID=1548**.

THE "GOOD NEWS"

The good news is that research at three years post-surgery found that, for successful WLS patients, previous disturbed eating patterns were less of a problem. With some procedures there was less hunger, overeating, guilt after eating, and obsessing about food or about eating. In fact, in one study, some WLS patients reported less preoccupation with food than did the normal-weight comparison group.

Overweight and obese men may experience sexual problems that include erectile dysfunction and shortness of breath during intercourse. Women who are overweight or obese are more likely to suffer low sexual desire, mainly because they don't feel sexy. In a study of obese men (average BMI of 46) who had WLS and lost 40 to 100 pounds, weight loss was found to be directly linked to improved testosterone levels, as well as improved levels of the sex hormone estradoil. Those who lost weight reported improvements in the quality of their sex life.

One study of the consequences of weight loss surgery on sexual attitudes and behavior in female WLS patients reported that, before surgery, only 44 percent stated that sex with their partners was satisfying and frequency of intercourse was regular. One year postoperatively, 63 percent said they enjoyed sex more, and 12 percent said they enjoyed it less. Postoperatively, 20 percent said their partnership had changed positively, while 10 percent said it had changed negatively. Depression and social problems that existed before surgery have been shown to improve dramatically after surgery for many patients.

FAILURE OF WLS

Of course, there are those for whom WLS is not as successful as they had hoped it would be. This is usually because they were not well informed before surgery—or were in denial—about what would be required of them after surgery. Even though they met with a dietitian beforehand and were told about food restrictions, they may have secretly decided to do it their way. For example, Careena, who had the band procedure, didn't want to give up steak and red meat, even though she was told it was too fibrous for the pouch. Naturally, she ran into trouble and experienced severe disappointment when she realized that she really couldn't eat the way she wanted. Other people may think they understand what it will be like after surgery, but when they encounter the post-surgery realities, they become angry or depressed. WLS forces changes in fluid and food intake, which affects the ability to eat "normally" on social occasions. Another woman who refused to give up full-calorie Coca-Cola found that her weight loss was disappointing. Effort and commitment to change on the part of the patient are required to achieve WLS success.

Challenges Post-surgery

WLS can be divided into several stages: the first is the decision stage when you are considering whether to proceed. This involves gathering information, finding a surgeon and program, getting insurance lined up (so far, Medicare has made it easier to get this procedure), getting medical tests and clearances, telling family and friends, losing some weight, and setting a date for surgery. The second stage is the actual surgery and immediate post-op period during which any immediate complications that might occur are addressed. The third stage involves coping with the challenges of the later post-surgery period, the first month or so post-op to several years out. The post-surgery stage also involves making the transition to maintenance and living a new, healthy lifestyle. A number of challenges can arise during the post-surgery stage.

THE HONEYMOON PHASE

Those who have gastric bypass surgery often experience a "honeymoon" when weight seems to drop off without effort and expectations are high. None of the challenges that may come later have yet presented themselves. In these heady early times, patients may delude themselves into thinking they won't really have to make the drastic lifestyle changes they have been repeatedly warned about. Following the doctor's orders seems relatively easy. As time goes on, however, it gets harder for some people, and they fail to conform to recommended eating and food choices. Some think they don't really have to exercise after all, and they may forget the warning that they must take vitamin and mineral supplements. They may then lie to the surgeon about their behavior.

CONVERTING TO SOLID FOOD

Initially the WLS patient will be on a liquid or soft diet during the healing phase just after surgery. The duration of the liquid diet depends on the procedure and the program. Usually in about two to three weeks, patients begin the transition to solid, protein-based meals. Eating protein three times a day assists with satiety, because solid food leaves the pouch more slowly. Some patients delay making this transition because liquids and soft foods are easier to consume. In order to avoid hunger—and subsequent wrong food choices—it is necessary to convert to solid foods.

ADDRESSING HUNGER

Hunger typically wanes with surgery, but some procedures, like the adjustable gastric band, do not seem to reduce hunger as much as other procedures do. This makes sticking to the prescribed three meals a day, with no snacking, especially difficult. The hormone ghrelin is produced by the stomach and regulates feelings of hunger. When the stomach is still intact, even though a pouch has been created, ghrelin is still being produced. If the pouch is not made small enough, hunger may persist due to the continued production of ghrelin. If hunger is a problem after surgery, this needs to be discussed with the surgeon. There may be ways to help alleviate this difficulty.

CHANGING EATING HABITS

Weight loss surgery requires permanent lifestyle changes to ensure long-term success. The procedures substantially decrease the size of the stomach, and as a result, the patient cannot eat very much. Initially, the patient is only able to eat about a half-cup of food at a time. At first liquids and soft foods are consumed but gradually the patient needs to transition to solid foods to ensure enough protein is consumed. Solid foods must be chewed very well, and foods that are difficult to digest need to be avoided. This includes red meats, which must be avoided due to their high fat and fibrous tissue content. Foods or beverages high in sugar must also be carefully avoided, because they can cause cramps, nausea, vomiting, diarrhea, weakness, sweating, shakiness, or lightheadedness. This distress is referred to as the *dumping syndrome* (see the section that follows) and results from rapid emptying of food from the stomach into the small intestine. Dumping syndrome is only a problem with bypass patients, but all patients can experience vomiting. Gastric bypass procedure patients specifically may also experience lactose intolerance—the inability to metabolize lactose, a sugar found in dairy products—because of a lack of the required enzyme lactase in the digestive system.

Dumping Syndrome

Dumping—also known as *rapid gastric emptying*—typically starts during, or immediately after, eating in those who are post-WLS. Consuming simple carbohydrates such as those in sugary drinks or ice cream typically triggers the process. Dairy products can also produce dumping. Sugar has a high molecular density, and consuming foods containing a high concentration of sugar attracts a correspondingly large amount of fluid to the small intestine. It then becomes stretched, which causes cramping. In turn these cramps trigger hormonal and nerve responses that cause the heart to race, resulting in heart palpitations. The patient may become clammy and sweaty. Finally, as the small intestine tries to expel the problem, the patient experiences vomiting or diarrhea.

In some cases, dumping occurs later—one to three hours after eating. This is caused by fluctuations in blood glucose levels in patients whose digestive system has been altered by gastric bypass surgery. When sugar is eaten it is rapidly absorbed into the bloodstream, triggering a rapid rise in blood sugar levels. The pancreas responds by secreting a large amount of insulin to soak up the excess blood sugar. However, because the amount of sugar that started this process was small relative to the amount of insulin secreted, there is now too much insulin in the blood, and this triggers common hypoglycemic symptoms such as weakness, dizziness, fatigue, and late dumping.[12] (Hypoglycemia is the medical term for a state produced by a lower than normal level of blood glucose.)

Vomiting

Overeating or drinking too much fluid at one time can cause vomiting in post-WLS patients, regardless of which procedure they opted for. This is because the whole idea behind the surgery is to make it harder for patients to consume food in large enough quantities to make them overweight and obese. To avoid vomiting, some patients, who will not or cannot comply with physician recommendations, graze (eat small bites) more or less all day long. But this is not a good idea, because if they make poor food choices (and often they do) they end up without satisfying the recommendation that patients eat three protein-based meals per day. This is likely to derail weight loss post-surgery. Likewise, consuming sugary soft drinks to satisfy a sugar craving defeats weight loss efforts and invites dumping.

To avoid vomiting, it is necessary to pay attention to physical signals that warn of impending vomiting. When your body signals these warnings, you must stop eating and wait before eating any more. Sometimes an amount you can consume easily one day is not so easy an amount to consume a few days later. Learning to listen to your body and to figure out what to eat, when to eat, and how to eat is a process of trial and error.

CHEATING

It seems foolhardy to undergo a bariatric surgery procedure, with all the pain, discomfort, and expense involved, only to cheat—i.e., make wrong choices—and risk slowing down weight loss or even regaining weight. Yet some people do just that. Some may do so because they suffer hunger pangs, but others do so because they have not really made the commitment to a lifestyle change that involves drastic changes in food choices. They may eat in small bites between meals to satisfy a craving. Or they eat high-calorie, "slippery" foods like ice cream, milkshakes, fruit drinks, and other sugary drinks. At first this may not seem to make a difference, but gradually weight loss will slow down, hunger will return, and because the habit of cheating has developed, weight will be regained.

Some people who cheat are playing out old roles—like rebelling against setting limits on food and eating. Others use food to cope with stress. If you find yourself cheating, review previous chapters on managing stress and self-talk, and then recommit to making permanent lifestyle changes in food and eating. Review Chapter 2, Getting and Staying Motivated, in particular the section on values.

FACING ADDICTIONS, OLD AND NEW

Binge eating is an addictive behavior driven mainly by an inability to cope with emotions and stress. After surgery, the ability to eat for comfort, to soothe sadness or anxiety, to fill the void of loneliness or boredom with food, is no longer viable—at least not in its old form. Instead, it can take on other guises, such as sneaking small bites or eating slippery foods. Cheating can also be an attempt at emotion regulation as discussed in the prior section. Refer to Chapter 8, Addressing Stress, for help with managing stress if cheating becomes a problem. Becoming obsessed with food again is likely to lead to more cheating and weight gain.

A more destructive way used by some people to quiet nerves and achieve relaxation post-WLS is consuming alcohol. Alcohol is metabolized quickly after WLS and leads to a swift high. Because of this, some people fall into alcohol abuse in their ill-advised efforts to manage stress. Indeed, a new addiction to alcohol is a pitfall for a number of people post-surgery, and in extreme cases can lead to alcoholic cirrhosis of the liver. In some cases, a surgery candidate may have been addicted to, or may even have abused, alcohol before surgery, but concealed his or her addiction so as not to be turned down for surgery or have it delayed. This, of course, is self-defeating, as the alcohol addiction is not addressed by WLS. If the patient abuses substances or food after WLS, he or she must seek professional help to overcome the behavioral addiction in order to succeed post-surgery.

DEALING WITH SLOW WEIGHT LOSS

Patients who choose the adjustable gastric band often find that weight loss is slower compared to that of patients who undergo other procedures. This can lead to disappointment, discouragement, and eventually giving up. As a result, such patients may start cheating, which further impairs weight loss efforts. Those with the AGB must work harder to lose weight than those with other procedures. This includes making regular and adequate exercise a part of their lifestyle. Older and more sedentary patients are at special risk for slower weight loss and need to increase the amount and intensity of their exercise.

Yolanda had a band put in, and did 45 to 60 minutes three days a week on the stationary bike she had at home. However, her heart rate rarely went high enough, nor did she break a real sweat. For her, that seemed like a lot of exercise, especially compared to her previous sedentary lifestyle, but to lose weight she needed to be exercising five days a week or more, and hard enough to keep her heart rate up (see Chapter 5, Getting Started with Exercise). She originally chose the band AGB procedure because it was less invasive, but she didn't fully comprehend the necessity of sufficient exercise after surgery to improve success. She also was often hungry and didn't succeed in reducing calories enough to lose a satisfactory amount of weight.

REGAINING WEIGHT

As mentioned earlier in this chapter, regaining some weight after a year or two is expected, but regaining a lot of weight—even going back to baseline—is devastating to the post-surgery patient. Causes include cheating, not exercising enough, and forgetting, or never buying into, the absolute need to convert to a new lifestyle including a changed relationship to food and activity. Other setbacks, such as injury or sickness, can trigger behavior that leads to weight regain. In these cases, the solution is to get back on track with eating and exercise as soon as possible.

Another hazard for regaining weight is pregnancy. The pop star Carnie Wilson lost 150 pounds in 16 months after WLS, but in two subsequent pregnancies she gained 70 pounds and 64 pounds, respectively. Although she was able to lose weight after the first pregnancy, her weight gain after the second one persisted. Her explanation was that she kept making excuses to allow herself to eat whatever she wanted. In fact, she never fully accepted a lifestyle change, as evidenced by the fact that she is producing a line of low-fat cheesecake. Such food, even though it is promoted as low-fat, is not part of a healthy diet for a post-WLS patient. Carnie Wilson now stars in a comedic reality show about her efforts to lose weight.

COPING WITH LOOSE SKIN

Just losing excess weight is the dream of many obese people. But there is a dark side to this dream. Loose skin can hang from the underarms, thighs, abdomen, and back after surgery, especially for older patients. Breasts can become droopy and hang over the chest wall. This "redundant" skin brings similar problems as overlapping skin did before surgery—i.e., fungus infections, odor, chafing, rubbing. Walking can be problematic with excess skin between the thighs. As a result, there is a need to wear compression garments that bind up the skin. Folds of loose skin can be an issue in intimate relations. Many people need reconstructive surgery post-WLS, but insurance will not usually reimburse for this, deeming it cosmetic. Furthermore, more than one surgery is often needed. Possible surgeries include the arm lift, the bra-line back lift, panniculectomy (removal of unwanted hanging fat and skin in the abdomen that often results from massive weight loss), buttock implants or buttock lift to help firm up the buttocks, or a whole body lift (to improve the appearance of the abdomen, thighs, breasts, and buttocks). Taking vitamin and mineral supplements as advised by the surgeon is crucial for healing from reconstructive surgery.

CARETAKING OTHERS

Many people with weight problems, not only the obese, allow themselves to slip into the role of caretaker for others. They put others first and their own needs last. Often there is a hidden bargain: "If I'm nice to you, you won't notice or comment on my weight." The caretaker is the one who stays late at work after others leave on time and does the extra work. When a friend needs something, the caretaker is there, no matter what the cost. If friends or family need something, the caretaker tries to anticipate and provide. Often the caretaker is taken for granted by others. And caretakers do not protest. Instead, they eat. After WLS, the caretaker has to learn to say "no," to be assertive (see Chapter 8, Addressing Stress), and to take time for himself or herself first.

Transitioning to a New Lifestyle

The biggest challenge to success is making a permanent transition to a new lifestyle of healthy choices and adequate exercise. At first, WLS forces changes in eating. But these changes can be sabotaged by cheating or the adoption or resumption of addictive behaviors such as alcohol abuse or emotional eating.

The immediate post-surgery phase is an emotional roller coaster during which moods can swing from happy to sad to content to irritable. Learning to cope with emotions without food is new for a number of patients. Many people come to realize for the first time after WLS that they bear sole responsibility for their choices with food and exercise—and their reactions to circumstances in life.

A lot of unhealthy eating is an attempt to control your experience—to feel better (rather than to *get* better), or to escape something unpleasant. Too often you get caught up in the seeming "importance" of thoughts or feelings instead of simply realizing that they are just passing thoughts and feelings. They are like waves that wash onto the shore and wash out again, to be followed by more thoughts and feelings, washing in and out. It is not necessary to act on thoughts and feelings; better to sit on the shore and watch them come and go. When you can keep in mind what you want out of life—not in the immediate moment, but in the long run—passing thoughts and feeling take on less importance.

Transitioning successfully to a new lifestyle means accepting the loss of unhealthy choices such as sweets, packaged foods, fast foods, and unhealthy snack foods—at least as a regular part of your daily diet. It means giving up on what hasn't worked—i.e., diets and dieting. A key to the transition is mindfulness and the principles of intuitive eating and mindful eating. You need to define for yourself the values that give meaning to your life, to consciously commit to these values, and to take actions in accordance with such values. For the bariatric surgery patient, it means following your surgeon's advice.

Once you realize that it is your *choice* to make healthy decisions or not, to exercise adequately or not, to choose a healthy lifestyle or to put your head in the sand about health risks down the road, you have taken the first step toward lasting success. Of course, the choices you make depend on what you value—immediate gratification or long-term reward. Make no mistake—immediate gratification has a powerful pull for everyone. The only thing that can help overcome that pull is to stay conscious and aware of your values—the overarching, guiding principles that define your life.

Acceptance of the tenets of a healthy lifestyle as emblematic of your life values is necessary for long-term success. Values are not goals; they are the direction you wish your life to take. Actions are chosen with reference to these values. Being willing to make and maintain the changes necessary for a healthy life means giving up immediate gratification and giving up trying to avoid your moment-to-moment experience. When anxiety presents itself, you must acknowledge it and take appropriate action that is in alignment with your values. When sadness comes, you must not try to escape it by eating. When boredom sets in, you must still keep exercising. Part of you may want to escape. But the part of you that has redefined who you are in relation to food, and what you do with your body, is stronger when you have transitioned to success.

Use of the Internet and Smartphones for Weight Management and Physical Activity Improvements: A Brief Review of the Literature

JOYCE D. NASH, PH.D.

Given that more than 60 percent of U.S. adults are overweight or obese, and that weight loss is recommended to reduce the health impact of obesity and type 2 diabetes, finding ways to make weight loss, weight maintenance, and physical activity programs more widely accessible is a national health care priority. Over the past decade the use of the Internet, smartphones, and other new communication technologies (e.g., PDAs, iPods, iPads, podcasts, blogs, chat rooms, interactive video and television, computer-aided instruction) has experienced rapid growth for a variety of health-related problems. Thousands of applications and programs now exist on the Internet or on smartphones, including such options as calorie counters, pedometers, blood pressure monitors, and health and fitness information. Programs with new features such as self-monitoring and feedback capabilities are being added frequently to help people lose weight and increase physical activity levels.

A VALUABLE RESOURCE FOR HEALTH CARE PROFESSIONALS

For health care professionals, the Internet can be a source of information and technology-based therapy, and it can be used as a supplement helping patients to augment the benefits provided during and after office visits.[1] (For example, Kaiser Permanente is a leader in creating such resources for its members.) These resources can benefit integrated weight loss and lifestyle change programs at clinics and hospitals, as well as the smaller practices of dietitians, doctors, health psychologists, and health educators who have limited support. Patients need to be informed of technology resources and need to be guided to choose among them.[2] Some information on the Internet lacks scientific basis or is too academic and beyond the comprehension of many patients. Likewise, not all programs or applications include evidence-based components that enhance outcomes. Web-based programs have only recently been studied as a medium for delivering behavioral programs for weight loss, weight maintenance, and physical activity. However, web-based interventions show promise for lifestyle change. Research is beginning to document this.

McTigue and colleagues studied the feasibility of translating an evidence-based lifestyle curriculum into a clinical setting by adapting it for delivery via the Internet.[3] They adapted the Diabetes Prevention Program's lifestyle curriculum to an online format comprising sixteen weekly and eight monthly lessons, and conducted a before-and-after pilot study of program implementation and feasibility. The program incorporated behavioral tools such as e-mail prompts for online self-monitoring of diet, physical activity, and weight management, and produced automated progress reports. As-needed communication with lifestyle coaches integrated the intervention with clinical care. Fifty patients from a large academic general internal practice participated; 76 percent were female with an average age of 51.94 years ± 10.82 and an average BMI of 36.43 ± 6.78. At 12 months of enrollment, 50 percent of participants had logged in within 30 days. On average, completers ($n = 45$) lost an average of 4.79 kg ± 8.55 kg of weight. Systolic blood pressure dropped 7.33 mm Hg ± 11.36 mm Hg, and diastolic blood pressure changed minimally (+0.44 mm Hg ± 8.55 mm Hg). The researchers concluded that an Internet-based lifestyle intervention may overcome significant barriers to preventive counseling and facilitate the incorporation of evidence-based interventions into primary care.

THE APPEAL OF THE INTERNET, SMARTPHONES, AND TECHNOLOGY

With the explosion of Internet accessibility, online delivery of weight control and physical activity/exercise programs offers potential for significantly greater reach of evidence-based help for adults. These applications and programs reduce barriers to treatment for rural, low-income, and minority individuals. Such programs may also have appeal to working adults who are constrained by lack of time or to those with social anxiety that makes them unwilling to join a group. In addition to being free or low-cost to use, such programs offer convenience and 24/7 availability. They are used in the privacy of one's home, which provides anonymity. In addition, Internet and new technology programs and applications avoid the cost in time and money of traveling to off-site group programs.

INTERNET UTILIZATION

Although research on Internet usage is still sparse, what research exists finds that Internet utilization continues to grow, with a 7 percent increase in utilization between 2005 and 2006 in the United States overall.[4] Over 75 percent of American adults in 2007 reported using the Internet, including 64 percent of individuals living in rural areas, 61 percent of adults in the lowest-income groups, and 56 percent of African Americans. In a large-scale study by Stanford University of 2,514 adults interviewed in households nationwide, nearly 70 percent reported regular Internet use, and nearly 14 percent found it hard to stay away from the Internet for several days at a time.[5] A 2008 study found that 75.9 percent of the U.S. population were Internet users, while 23.9 percent of the world had access to the Internet.[6]

Of Internet users, 79 percent reported obtaining health information online.[7] From 2002 to 2004, there was a 7 percent increase in the use of the Internet for information about diet and a 6 percent increase for exercise and fitness.[8] A large majority of Internet users, 93 percent, reported that it is convenient for them because they can use it at any hour of the day.[9]

Apart from experiencing the Internet on computers, mobile Internet is also becoming more common now. Since the advent of Internet connectivity in Apple iPhones in 2007, mobile Internet search has never been easier. As of October 2008, 10 million iPhones had been sold. In a recent Mobile World Congress, Google revealed that iPhone originates 50 times more searches than any other mobile handset.[10] According to AT&T, the iPhone hosts more Internet usage than other mobiles services. Per user, the Internet usage of iPhone users is almost double that of a person with another standard mobile handset. Google is optimistic that other handset manufacturers will go Apple's way in making web access easy, and that the number of mobile searches will overtake fixed Internet searches in the next few years.

When Apple released the iPad in 2010, first-day sales exceeded 300,000, and some analysts project as many as 7 million units sold by the end of 2010, with triple that number projected by 2012. Analysis indicates that most users are between 30 and 54 years of age. The iPad is especially useful for productivity apps, social networking, and any program that requires a time investment. By contrast, the iPhone and other smartphones are for those on the go who want quick access. The iPad provides apps and access to the Internet the same as a smartphone.

INTERNET USAGE OF WEIGHT LOSS PROGRAMS

A number of factors are relevant to Internet usage of programs for weight loss. Younger people have grown up with computers, but what about senior citizens? How is age a factor in using the Internet for weight loss? How often do people login, and for how long are they logged in? How satisfied are users? Can the Internet provide social support? What about motivation for self-monitoring? Some research has addressed these issues as they relate to weight control programs on the Internet.

Age

Van der Mark and associates in Sweden conducted a study to determine whether older people with less computer training would make use of the new technology for an Internet-based behavioral weight loss program compared to younger people.[11] The researchers examined how members above the age of 65 years performed compared to younger members of a heath consortium. Altogether, 4,440 active weight club members were assessed over a six-month period for their use of the Internet-based program. The number of logins, food intake, and weight records were examined. Participants were divided into age tertiles (thirds) separately for men and women. The oldest tertile was further subdivided into two groups: those above the age of 65 and those below. Results found that participants aged 65 or older were more likely to remain active in the weight club for at least six months compared to younger age groups. This group had the highest amount of weight loss (5.6 kg, 6.8%). Men above 65 years of age had the highest number of logins, on average 161 times during the six-month period. The researchers concluded that older participants are performing equally well, or even better, in an Internet-based behavior weight loss program than younger participants.

Usage and Satisfaction

McConnon, Kirk, and Ransley investigated use of and satisfaction with a website designed for weight control for obese participants.[12] Questionnaire data were collected at 6 and 12 months. In addition, use of the website was automatically recorded when subjects logged in. Subjects ($n = 111$) were part of a larger, community-based, randomized control trial for evaluating the effectiveness of a website. Fifty-nine participants (53%) reported using the website at 6 months, with 32 participants (29%) still using it at 12 months. The average time spent on the website per visit was 21.1 minutes ± 16.6 at 6 months and 13.6 minutes ± 9.3 at 12 months, with an average number of logins of 15.8 ± 15.2 over the trial period. In general, participants reported satisfaction with using the website except for the social support sections. These were used least and received the lowest satisfaction scores.

Social Support

Another study by Kwang and associates investigated social support for weight loss shared by members of a large Internet weight loss community.[13] Interviews and content analysis of discussion forum messages yielded qualitative data relating to social support themes. Survey respondents were primarily white (91.4%) and female (93.8%), with a mean age of 37.3 years and a mean BMI of 30.9. They used the forums frequently, with 56.8 percent reading messages, 36.1 percent replying to messages, and 18.5 percent posting messages to start a discussion. Major social support themes were encouragement and motivation, mentioned at least once by 87.6 percent of survey respondents, followed by information (58.5%) and shared experiences (42.5%). Subthemes included testimonies, recognition for success, accountability, friendly competition, and humor. Members valued convenience, anonymity, and the non-judgmental interactions as unique characteristics of Internet-mediated support. The researchers concluded that the investigated weight loss community played a prominent role in the participants' weight loss efforts. They further suggested that clinicians recommend such communities to patients.

Motivation for Self-monitoring

Webber, Tate, Ward, and Bowling examined changes in motivation and the relationship of motivation to adherence to self-monitoring and weight loss in a 16-week Internet behavioral weight loss intervention.[14] Sixty-six women, aged 22–65, each with a BMI between 25 and 40, received a face-to-face initial session followed by the 16-week Internet program. Adherence to self-monitoring and weight loss were the main outcome measures. Results showed that autonomous motivation increased initially and remained high for those who ultimately achieved a 5 percent weight loss, but declined over time for those who did not achieve a 5 percent weight loss. Autonomous motivation at 4 weeks was a predictor of adherence to self-monitoring and 16-week weight loss. The researchers concluded that targeting motivation for self-monitoring is important in an Internet-based weight loss program.

TRADITIONAL BEHAVIOR THERAPY

Structured, facilitated behavioral therapy is the standard treatment for mildly or moderately overweight individuals. Traditional interventions for weight loss provide written behavior therapy materials to participants and involve weekly face-to-face individual or group contact lasting from 12 to 24 weeks, usually with some follow-up after the active treatment period. These are considered the "gold standard" for the dissemination of lifestyle advice in terms of maximal, long-term effectiveness. They are time intensive and costly. Typically they produce an average of 9–10 kg weight loss in 20–24 weeks, or about a 5–10 percent reduction in baseline weight.[15] Such weight losses are compelling based on substantial evidence that many obesity-related conditions are improved with weight losses of this magnitude.[16] However, potentially due to the cost or inconvenience of current traditional weight loss treatments, few people who could benefit are participating in them.[17]

Traditional Behavioral Therapy vs. Internet Therapy

Traditional behavior therapy consists of certain key features: self-monitoring, supportive tools for behavior change (e.g., stimulus control, response change, use of reward), written guidelines for nutrition and physical activity, social support, check-in accountability, problem solving, and relapse prevention training. These are usually delivered in some combination of bibliotherapy (books, brochures, handouts) and face-to-face contact. The lifestyle intervention materials used in research have been created by organizations such as HealthPartners in Minnesota.

These components were included in the design and implementation of interactive websites for studying Internet delivery of weight control therapy.[18] Researchers either have created their own websites for studies or those created by other researchers, or they have created proprietary online diary interventions or podcasts for their studies. The use of existing programs and smartphone applications has not been well studied.

WEB FEATURES AND SUCCESSFUL WEIGHT CONTROL

Given the proliferation of online weight-control programs, it is important to know which components impact weight loss and weight maintenance. Krukowski and his associates explored the utilization of web-based weight-loss techniques with 123 study participants.[19] The focus of the study was the VTrim website (now available to the public, though at significant cost), which included food and exercise self-monitoring journals, a chat room, and a bulletin board, as well as standard behavior modification strategies for weight loss components (i.e., stimulus control, problem solving, goal setting, social support, and relapse prevention). The first six months were the active weight loss treatment program, followed by six months of monthly maintenance meetings targeting maintaining skills learned during the active treatment phase. During the weight loss phase (first six months), facilitators provided weekly, personalized feedback on self-monitoring journals and homework assignments. Website usage (i.e., number of logins and utilization of various web features) was automatically tracked. Participants logged on to the website on average 190.9 ± 138.5 times during the treatment phase and 94.6 ± 96.1 times during the maintenance phase.

During the active weight loss phase, three factors were identified as important—motivation/support, feedback, and education. Only the first two predicted weight loss. Different and additional factors were identified as important during the maintenance phase. Social support was the most highly related to weight change. Other, less significant features included dietary planning, skill building, calorie information, and calculators such as those for body mass and target heart rate.

The researchers concluded that overall website usage was strongly correlated with weight loss success. Higher login rates were likely a factor in the higher weight losses seen in this study compared to previous research. During the weight loss phase, "feedback" (which included progress charts, physiological calculators, and journals) was the best predictor of weight loss. (It should be noted, however, that other research has identified visual representations of goal progress as also important, along with contact with the facilitator.) The "motivation/support" feature included a bulletin board, contact with other participants via e-mail, and motivational tips.

During the maintenance phase, a different pattern emerged. Participation in the "social support" aspect, which included web chats and e-mailing other participants (forming a support group among participants), was the best predictor of weight loss and avoidance of weight regain. Perception of peer support has been shown to be related to higher login frequency in previous research.

In summary, use of web features that provided participants with visual representations of goal progress, self-monitoring feedback, and social support were predictive of weight loss and maintenance. During the weight loss treatment period, factors most predictive of weight loss were use of progress charts, physiological calculators, and journals. During maintenance, participation in web chats and e-mailing fellow participants was the best predictor. In addition to participants interacting, participant/therapist contact was also important. Despite the inclusion of behavior therapy elements in web-based programs, weight loss with Internet programs was less than that of person-to-person, traditional programs, but better than self-help alone.

e-Counseling

An important feature of recent research studies on lifestyle counseling, behavior therapy, and Internet-based therapy for weight management is that of e-counseling (i.e., distance counseling). This involves lifestyle counseling by phone or e-mail. Previous studies assessing e-counseling for weight management have shown mixed results. Currently e-counseling is a standard component of Internet-based therapy studies. Adding therapist contact via email or phone to online weight-loss programs appears to improve success.[20]

Recently, van Wier and his colleagues studied e-counseling in a work setting of 1,386 overweight employees in the Netherlands.[21] The researchers defined three groups: intervention materials delivered with phone counseling (phone group), web-based intervention with e-mail counseling (Internet group), and usual care getting lifestyle brochures only (control group). The main purpose of the study was to ascertain effects on body weight of a lifestyle program with 10 biweekly counseling sessions by phone as well as by e-mail compared to self-help materials alone, in overweight workers, at six months. Secondary purposes were to determine effects on weight circumference, diet, and physical activity and to compare the effects of e-counseling by phone with the effects of e-counseling by e-mail. Results of the study showed that lifestyle e-counseling by phone and e-mail was effective for reducing body weight and waist circumference and that phone contact was effective for reducing fat intake and increasing physical activity.

EFFECTIVENESS OF INTERNET THERAPY FOR WEIGHT LOSS

Two meta-analysis reviews of the literature were conducted on studies published up to 2008.

Meta-analysis Studies

Wantland and his colleagues conducted a meta-analysis to provide information on patient knowledge and behavioral change outcomes after web-based interventions as compared to outcomes seen after implementation of non-web-based interventions.[22] Twenty-two articles from the years 1996–2003 met criteria for analysis. Data was extracted from a total of 11,754 research participants, split evenly between the sexes. The average age was 41.5 years, and the average dropout rate was 21 percent. Time spent per session per person ranged from 4.5 to 45 minutes. Session logins/person/week ranged from 2.6 logins/person over 32 weeks to 1,008 logins/person over 36 weeks. The effect size comparisons in the use of web-based interventions compared to non-web-based interventions showed an improvement in outcomes for individuals using web-based interventions to achieve the specified knowledge and/or behavior change for the studied outcome variables. These outcomes included increased exercise time, increased knowledge of nutritional status, increased knowledge of asthma treatment, increased participation in health care, slower health decline, improved body shape perception, and 18-month weight loss maintenance.

The authors concluded that the use of web-based interventions improves behavioral change outcomes. Those interventions that directed the participants to relevant, individually tailored materials reported longer website session times per visit and more visits. Additionally, those sites that incorporated the use of a chat room demonstrated increased social support scores.

Neve and associates conducted a systematic review and meta-analysis identifying studies related to web-based interventions for weight management from 1995 to April 2008.[23] Eighteen studies met the inclusion criteria. Of these, 13 aimed to achieve weight loss, and 5 focused on weight maintenance. There was great heterogeneity among studies, and the authors concluded that it was difficult to determine effectiveness.

Pilot Studies

Booth, Nowson, and Matters conducted an evaluation of an interactive, Internet-based weight reduction program in Australia.[24] In their pilot study, the online program including dietary advice plus exercise was more effective than an exercise-only program. Both the intervention and the control group wore pedometers and set weekly goals to increase daily steps through an interactive website. The intervention group received tailored e-mail assistance. Both groups increased their daily steps, but only the intervention group reduced their energy intake. Nevertheless, there was no difference between groups in weight loss.

Randomized Controlled Trials

Morgan and associates conducted a study to evaluate the efficacy of an Internet-based weight loss program for men in Australia.[25] In total, 65 overweight/obese males with an average age of 36.9 years ± 11.1 and an average BMI of 30.6 ± 2.8 were randomly assigned to either an Internet group or an information-only control group. Both groups received one face-to-face information session and a program booklet. The Internet group used the website to self-monitor diet and activity with feedback provided based on participants' online entries on seven occasions over three months. Results showed a significant weight loss of 5.3 kg at six months for the Internet group and 3.5 kg for the control group. Those who complied with the program lost more weight than those who did not. The researchers concluded that simple weight loss interventions can be effective in achieving statistically and clinically significant weight loss in men. However, strategies to improve engagement in online programs need to be explored further.

EFFECTIVENESS OF INTERNET THERAPY FOR WEIGHT MAINTENANCE

Research on using the Internet to facilitate maintenance of weight loss is sparse. Harvey-Berino and her colleagues conducted a study published in 2002 of 122 healthy, overweight adults to investigate the effectiveness of a weight maintenance program conducted over the Internet.[26] Subjects participated first in a 6-month clinical behavioral weight loss trial with in-person behavioral obesity treatment, followed by a 12-month maintenance program conducted with either frequent in-person support or minimal in-person support or Internet support. Subjects' average age was 47.4 ± 9.6 with a mean BMI of 32.2 ± 4.5; 18 males participated. Results showed that weight loss did not differ by condition during treatment. However, during the maintenance phase, the Internet-only group gained significantly more weight and sustained significantly smaller weight loss that either of the in-person groups. Researchers concluded that Internet support does not appear to be as effective as minimal or frequent, intensive, in-person therapist support for facilitating long-term maintenance of weight loss.

Stevens and associates investigated the development, implementation, and usage of a web-based intervention program designed to help those who have recently lost weight sustain their weight loss over one year.[27] The website was developed over the course of a year and was expensive, complex, and time-consuming to develop. Key interactive features of the final website included social support, self-monitoring, written guidelines for diet and physical activity, links to appropriate websites, supportive tools for behavior change, check-in accountability, tailored reinforcement messages, problem solving, and relapse prevention training. The weight loss maintenance program prompted participants to return to the website if they missed their check-in date. If there was no response, a staff person followed up. The mean age of the 348 participants assigned to use the website was 56 years; 63 percent were female, and 38 percent were African American. Weight loss data were not available at the time of this reporting, but results showed that website use remained high during the first year, with over 80 percent of the participants still using the website during month 12. During the first 52 weeks, participants averaged 35 weeks with at least one login. E-mail and telephone prompts were very effective at helping participants sustain ongoing use.

An Encouraging 2008 Large Study

In contrast to other research, a study published in 2008 in the *Journal of the American Medical Association* was more encouraging. Svetkey and colleagues conducted a comparison of strategies for sustaining weight loss in a randomized control trial.[28] This was the largest and longest trial to test different weight maintenance strategies. The study initially enrolled 1,685 overweight or obese adults with high blood pressure or high cholesterol or both. Of the 1,685, 1,032 lost an average of 18.7 pounds during an initial 6-month weight loss intervention involving 20 weekly group-counseling sessions that emphasized a heart-healthy dietary pattern and three hours a week of physical activity. They were then randomly assigned to one of three strategies for weight loss maintenance: monthly personal counseling on diet and physical activity, web-based intervention with the same advice, or self-direction in which participants received minimal further intervention from study staff. Personal counseling sessions were brief and mainly by telephone. At the end of the study, participants who received personal counseling retained an average weight loss of 9.2 pounds, compared to an average of 7.3 pounds for those using the web-based intervention, and an average of 6.4 pounds for the self-directed group. Most people in the study regained at least some of the weight they initially lost. However, both the personal counseling and the web-based program modestly alleviated weight regain for up to two years, with the personal counseling ultimately proving to be the most beneficial by the end of the 2.5-year study.

EFFECTIVENESS OF INTERNET THERAPY FOR PHYSICAL ACTIVITY

Not only do the Internet and smartphones show potential for weight loss and maintenance of weight loss, they also have potential for increasing physical activity—an important part of weight loss, weight maintenance, and health. Regular physical activity is associated with lower morbidity and mortality rates from cardiovascular disease, diabetes, cancer, and osteoporosis. Despite these benefits, the majority of adults in Western nations do not meet the public health recommendations of physical activity. (Physical activity and exercise represent different concepts: physical activity is defined as any bodily movement resulting in energy expenditure; exercise is a subset of physical activity that is planned, structured, repetitive, and aimed at improving or maintaining physical fitness.)

Hurling and his associates investigated a physical activity program based on the Internet and mobile phone technology provided to individuals for nine weeks in the United Kingdom.[29] A total of 77 participants with BMIs of 19–30 took part in the study and were randomly allocated to a test group and a control group. The test group was provided with accelerometers (pedometers) to monitor physical activity and a Bluetooth wrist-worn device for assessing movement. The Internet, e-mail, and mobile phone behavior change system was similar to that used in previous studies. Participants identified their perceived barriers to physical activity, were offered solutions, and wrote out a commitment. In addition to the Internet intervention, participants could choose to receive e-mail and/or mobile phone reminders to exercise.

More than 85 percent of the test participants logged in each week during the first four weeks, decreasing thereafter to a plateau around 75 percent for the last five weeks. The average number of logins per week was 2.9 ± .5 with an average duration of 7.5 minutes ± .9. The most frequently used components of the system were the activity charts (showing the accelerometer feedback data), the weekly exercise planner, and the chat room–style message board. All components of the system were accessed by at least 33 percent of participants during the intervention period. Typically participants formed an idiosyncratic preference for a few components of the system and then repeatedly used these throughout the intervention. More than 70 percent of participants continued to login to the website at least twice a week for all nine weeks of the study. Usage is an important factor in success of any Internet-based program, and it is essential that automated systems engage people in order for the behavior change program to have an impact.

The researchers concluded that the Internet-based behavior change system enabled the test group participants to maintain their elevated level of physical activity. The size of the difference in physical activity between the test and the control group was substantial: an increase of 2 hours, 18 minutes per week represents 92 percent of the recommended physical activity level. Likewise, the test group lost a significantly higher percentage of body fat compared to the control group, indicating that the increased physical activity may have led to greater muscle mass. The researchers concluded that "An Internet-based behavior change system that improved diet as well as increasing physical activity may lead to more substantial losses of body fat and reduced BMI."

Literature Review Studies

Van den Berg and her colleagues conducted a systematic review of the literature on Internet-based physical activity interventions.[30] Ten studies met criteria and were investigated. All found a greater increase in physical activity in the Internet-based intervention compared to a waiting list control. Contact (e-mail or phone) with supervisors or counselors improved results. However, the studies reviewed all had methodological shortcomings.

In another review of the literature by Vandelanotte and colleagues, 15 studies were considered.[31] The focus of the review was to identify relationships of intervention attributes with behavioral outcomes. Of the 15 studies reviewed, 8 showed improvement in physical activity with website–delivered physical activity interventions. Better outcomes were identified when interventions had more than five contacts between participants and counselors and when the time of follow-up was three months or less. There was no clear association of outcomes with other intervention attributes. Furthermore, there was limited evidence that these programs helped maintenance of physical activity changes. The reviewers concluded that much more research is needed in this area.

CONCLUSION

This brief literature review of web-based weight loss therapy and interventions to prevent weight regain suggests that the Internet is a promising modality for promoting weight loss, weight maintenance, and increased physical activity. The more recent studies show that improvements to programs and applications have been increasing over time, and such improvements are likely to continue. Incorporating behavioral therapy principles and therapist contact via phone, e-mail, or possibly other technical means appears to improve success of online behavioral change programs. web-based programs promote peer-to-peer support through chat rooms and bulletin boards, and they facilitate self-monitoring more successfully than in-person programs do.[32] Research shows that web-based programs are more effective than self-help programs for weight loss and weight maintenance.

Suggestions for Using Lose Weight, Live Healthy

Lose Weight, Live Healthy provides evidence-based, behavioral information for those who want to lose weight and adopt a healthier lifestyle. This book can be recommended as a stand alone intervention; it is different from similar weight management books in that it also informs readers about using technology to help them achieve success. Another possible choice for the health professional is to recommend a particular web-based program to an individual patient to be used with this book and then supplement this intervention with e-counseling. Yet another possibility is to form groups which receive a single, face-to-face session about how to use the book and technology for weight loss or weight maintenance, to be followed by e-counseling. An excellent and popular weight loss, web-based program that is available on smartphones, that is free, and that includes social support as well as weight-tracking tools is the **SparkPeople** tool (46 percent of users of such programs voted it best among similar programs). Such a program could be used by professionals in combination with this book and possibly e-counseling. Another possible partner web and iPhone tool is the **LoseIt** app, which includes diet, nutrition, exercise, accountability, and group interaction. Another possibility is to use this book to provide material for face-to-face group programs led by a health professional. The advantage in using *Lose Weight, Live Healthy* is that it not only provides evidence-based behavioral weight loss information and strategies, but it also points the way to using the Internet and smartphones for weight loss and weight maintenance, without professionals having to have access to large-scale, university-based, or research-only web-based programs.

A MESSAGE TO HEALTH CARE PROFESSIONALS

1. Goldstein, D. J. (2004). The Internet and obesity treatment. In Goldstein, D. J. (Ed.), *The Management of Eating Disorders and Obesity* (2nd ed.). Totowa, NJ: Humana Press.

2. Ibid.

3. McTigue, K. M., Conroy, M. B., Hess, R. et al. (2009). Using the Internet to translate an evidence-based lifestyle intervention into practice. *Telemedicine Journal of e-Health 15*(9):851–858.

4. Pew Internet and American Life Project. Demographics of Internet users. (2008). See also http://www.pewInternet.org/trends/User_Demo_2.15.08.htm.

5. See http://med.stanford.edu/news_releases/2006/october/internet.html.

6. See http://www.google.com/publicdata?ds=wb-wdi&met=it_net_user_p2&idim=country:USA&dl=en&hl=en&q=internet+usage#met=it_net_user_p2&idim=country:USA&tdim=true

7. Fox, S., Madden, M., Pew Internet and American Life Project. Generations online. (2005). http://www.pewInternet.org/pdfs/PIP_Generations?Memo.pdf.

8. Fox, S., Madden, M., Pew Internet and American Life Project. Health information online: Eight in ten Internet users have looked for health information online, with increased interest in diet, fitness, drugs, health insurance, experimental treatments, and particular doctors and hospitals. (2005). http://www.pewInternet.org/pdfs/PIP_Healthtopics_Mah05.pdf.

9. Fox, S., Rainie, L., Horrigan, J., Lenhart, A., et al., Pew Internet and American Life Project. The online healthcare revolution: How the web helps Americans take better care of themselves. (2000). http://www.pewInternet.org/pdfs/PIP_Health_Reports.pdf.

10. See http://www.zdnet.com/blog/apple/google-at-t-shocked-by-iphone-usage/1316

11. Van der Mark, M., Jonasson, J. Svensson, M. et al. (2009). Older members perform better in an Internet-based behavioral weight loss program compared to younger members. *Obesity Facts 2*:74–79. Epub 2009 April 9.

12. McConnon, A., Kirk, S. F., Ransley, J. K. (2009). Process evaluation of an Internet-based resource for weight control: Use and views of an obese sample. *Journal of Nutrition Education and Behavior 41*(4):261–271.

13. Kwang, K. O., Ottenbacher, A. J., Green, A. P., et al. (2010). Social support in an Internet weight loss community. *International Journal of Medical Information, 79*(1):5–13.

14. Webber, K. H., Tate, D. F., Ward, D. S., & Bowling, J. M. (2010). Motivation and its relationship to adherence to self-monitoring and weight loss in a 16-week Internet behavioral weight loss intervention. *Journal of Nutrition Education and Behavior*, epub ahead of print.

15. Tate, D. F., Wing, R. R., & Winett, R. A. (2001). Using Internet technology to deliver a behavioral weight loss program. *Journal of the American Medical Association 285*(9):1172–1177.

16. Blackburn, G. L. (1995). Effects of weight loss on weight-related risk factors. In Brownell, K. D., Fairburn, C. G., (Eds.) *Eating Disorders and Obesity: A Comprehensive Handbook* (406–410). New York: Guilford Press.

17. Jeffery, R. W., Sherwood, N. E., Brelje, K., et al. (2003). Mail and phone interventions for weight loss in a managed care setting: Weight-To-Be one-year outcomes. *International Journal of Obesity and Related Metabolic Disorders 27*:1584–1592.

18. Stevens, V. J., Funk, K .L., Brantley, P. J. et al. (2008). Design and implementation of an interactive website to support long-term maintenance of weight loss. *Journal of Medicine and Internet Research 10*(1):31.

19. Krukowski, R. A., Harvey-Berino, J., Ashikaga, T., et al. (2008). Internet-based weight control: The relationship between web features and weight loss. *Telemedicine and e-Health 14*:775–782.

20. Tate, D. J., Jackvony, E. H., Wing, R. R. (2002). Effects of Internet behavioral counseling on weight loss in adults at risk for Type 2 diabetes: A randomized trial. *Journal of the American Medical Association 289*:1833–1836.

21. Van Wier, M. F., Ariens, G. A., Dekkers, J. C., et al. (2009). Phone and e-mail counseling are effective for weight management in an overweight working population: A randomized controlled trial. *BMC Public Health 9*:1186–1471.

22. Wantland, D. J., Portillo, C. J., Holzemer, W. L. et al. (2004). The effectiveness of web-based vs. non-web-based interventions: A meta-analysis of behavior change outcomes. *Journal of Medical Internet Research 6*:4.

23. Neve, M., Morgan, P. J., Jones, P. R., & Collins, C. E. (2009). Effectiveness of web-based interventions in achieving weight loss and weight loss maintenance in overweight and obese adults: A systematic review with meta-analysis. *Obesity Reviews.* Published online.

24. Booth, A. O., Nowson, C. A., & Matters, H. (2008). Evaluation of an interactive, Internet-based weight loss program: A pilot study. Health Education Research, published online.

25. Morgan, P. J., Lubans, D. R., Collins, C. E., et al. (2009). The SHED-IT randomized controlled trial: Evaluation of an Internet-based weight-loss program for men. *Obesity (Silver Spring) 17*(11):2025–2031.

26. Harvey-Berino, J., Pintauro, S., Buzzell, P., et al. (2002). Does using the Internet facilitate the maintenance of weight loss? *International Journal of Obesity 26*(9):1254–1260.

27. Stevens, V. J., Funk, Brantley, P. J., et al. (2008). Design and implementation of an interactive website to support long-term maintenance of weight loss. *Journal of Medical Internet Research 10*(1):e1.

28. Svetkey, L. D., Stevens, V. J., Brantley, B, et al. (2008). Comparison of strategies for sustained weight loss: The weight loss maintenance randomized control. *Journal of the American Medical Association 299*:1139–1148.

29. Hurling, R., Catt, M., De Boni, M., et al. (2007). Using Internet and mobile phone technology to deliver an automated physical activity program: randomized control trial. *Journal of Medical Internet Research 9*:e7.

30. Van den Berg, M., Schoones, J. W., Vliet Vlieland, T. (2007). Internet-based physical activity interventions: A systematic review of the literature. *Journal of Medical Internet Research 9*:e26.

31. Vandelanotte, C., Spathonis, K. M., Eakin, E. G., & Owen, N. (2007). Website-delivered physical activity interventions: A review of the literature. *American Journal of Preventive Medicine 33*:54–64.

32. Harvey-Berino, J., Pintauro, S., Buzzell, P. & Gold, E. C. (2004). Effect of Internet support on the long-term maintenance of weight loss. *Obesity Research 112*:320–329.

CHAPTER NOTES

Chapter 1

1. The National Health and Nutrition Examinations Surveys, or NHANES, is a program of studies designed to assess the health and nutritional statues of adults and children in the United States. The survey is unique in that it combines interviews and physical examinations. NHANES is a major program or the National Center of Health Statistics and is part of the Centers for Disease Control and Prevention. The NHANES program began in the early 1960s and has been conducted as a series of surveys focusing on different population groups or health topics. NHANES continues today.

2. See www.cdc.gov/nccdphd/dnpa/obesity/trend/index.htm.

3. Palmer, S. "Normal weight, but obese. (September 2010). *Environmental Nutrition 33*(9):2.

4. Svendsen, O. L. (2003). Should measurement of body composition influence therapy for obesity? *Acta Diabetol 40(Suppl 1)*:S250–S253.

5. Prentice, A. M. (2001). Beyond body mass index. *Obesity Review 2*:141–147.

6. Razak, R., et al. (2007). Defining obesity cut points in a multiethnic population. *Circulation 115*(16):2111–2118.

7. To calculate your exact BMI, multiply your weight in pounds by 700. Then divide your answer by your height in inches. Take that result and divide it again by your height in inches. The resulting figure is your BMI.

8. See http://blue.regence.com/trgmedpol/radiology/rad41.html.

9. ACSM. (2005). *ACSM Guidelines for exercise testing and prescription,* 7th ed. New York: Lippincott, Williams, and Wilkins, 61.

10. See www.cdc.gov/nccdphd/dnpa/obesity/defining.html.

11. Type 2 diabetes is also known as adult-onset diabetes or non-insulin-dependent diabetes. It is a disorder with a gradual onset, usually in obese individuals. It is characterized by insulin resistance or insensitivity, rather than a lack of insulin production.

12. Go to www.cdc.gov/healthyweight/assessing/bmi/childrens_bmi to calculate BMI in percentages for any given child or adolescent.

13. Munsey, C. & Meyers, L. (2007). U.S. children: overweight and oversexed? *APA Monitor 38*(9):58–59.

14. Peeke, P. (2005). *Body-for-LIFE for Women: A Woman's Plan for Physical and Mental Transformation.* Emmaus, PA: Rodale Press.

15. McCarthy, W. J., and Kuo, T. (2009). Support for benefit of physical activity on satiety, weight control and diabetes risk. *Archives of Internal Medicine 169*(6):635.

16. Kessler, D. A. (July/August 2009). Why we overeat. *Nutrition Action Healthletter 32*:3–6, Center for Science in the Public Interest.

17. See www.mayoclinic.org/news2008-rst/4738.html.

18. Ibid.

19. Ibid.

20. Ibid.

21. Beydoun, M. A., Beydoun, H. A., and Wang, Y. (2008). Obesity and central obesity as risk factors for incident dementia and its subtypes: a systematic review. *Obesity Reviews 9*(3):204–218.

22.   Somers, V. K., White, D. P., Amin, R., et al. (2008). Sleep apnea and cardiovascular disease. *Journal of the American College of Cardiology Foundation 52*:686–717.

23.   Young, T., Finn, L., Peppard, P. et al. (2008). Sleep-disordered-breathing and mortality: Eighteen-year follow-up of the Wisconsin Sleep Cohort. *Sleep 31*:1071–1078.

24.   Fontaine, K. R., et al. (2003). Years of life lost due to obesity. *Journal of the American Medical Association, 289*:187–193.

25.   Adams, K. F., et al. (2006). Overweight, obesity, and mortality in a large prospective cohort of persons 50 to 71 years old. *The New England Journal of Medicine 355*:763–778.

26.   Bender, R., et al. (1999). Effect of age on excess mortality in obesity. *Journal of the American Medical Association 281*:1498–1504.

27.   Strine, T. W., et al. (2008). The association of depression and anxiety with obesity and unhealthy behaviors among community-dwelling US adults. *General Hospital Psychiatry 30*(2):127–137.

Chapter 2

1.   Locke, E., A., & Latham, G. P. (1990). *A Theory of Goal Setting and Task Performance.* Englewood Cliffs, NJ: Prentice Hall.

2.   Dahl, J. C., Wilson, K. G., Luciano, C., & Hayes, S. C. (2005). *Acceptance and Commitment Therapy for Chronic Pain.* Reno, NV: Context Press.

3.   Forsyth, J. P., & Eifert, G. H. (2007). *The Mindfulness & Acceptance Workbook for Anxiety.* Oakland, CA: New Harbinger.

4.   Prochaska, J. O., DiClemente, C. C., & Norcross, J. C. (1992). In search of how people change. *American Psychologist 47*:1102–1104.

Chapter 3

1.   Lally, P., van Jaarsveld, C. H. M., Potts, H. W. W. & Wardle, J. (2010). How are habits formed? Modelling habit formation in the real world. *European Journal of Social Psychology 40(6)*:999–1009.

2.   Thoreson, C. E., & Mahoney, M. J. (1974). *Self-Control: Power to the Person.* Monterey, CA: Brooks/Cole.

3.   See http://gurusoftware.com/Gurunet/Personal/Topics/Values.htm.

4.   Boutelle, K. N., & Kirschenbaum. (1998). Further support for consistent self-monitoring as a vital component of successful weight control. *Obesity Research 6*:219–224.

5.   Deci, E. L., & Ryan, R. M. (1985). *Intrinsic Motivation and Self-Determination in Human Behavior.* New York: Plenum Press.

6.   Tribole, R., & Resch, E. (1995, 2003). *Intuitive Eating: A Revolutionary Program That Works.* New York: St. Martin's Griffin.

7.   Kabat-Zinn, J. (1990). *Full Catastrophe Living.* New York: Bantam Dell.

8.   See www.eatingmindfully.com/bookoverview/3.htm.

9.   See www.tcme.org.

10.   See www.divinecaroline.com/22177/33557-rules-normal-eating/2.

Chapter 4

1.   See http://www.nutritiondata.com/topics/fullness-factor.

2.   Morris, M. C., Evans, D. A., Bienias, J. L., et al. (2003). Dietary fats and the risk of incident Alzheimer disease. *Archives of Neurology 60*:194–200.

3.   Palmer, S. (January 2010). The new science behind diet and weight loss—it's all about diversity. *Environmental Nutrition Newsletter 33*(1):1, 4.

4. See http://clinicaltrialsfeeds.org/clinical-trials/show/NCT00160108.
5. Barnard, N. D. (2003). *Breaking the Food Seduction.* New York: St. Martin's Press.
6. DesMaisons, K. (1998/2008). *Potatoes Not Prozac: Solutions for Sugar Sensitivity.* New York: Fireside.
7. See www.mendosa.com/gilists.htm and www.glycemicindex.com.
8. Webb, D. (December 2006). "Better blood sugar for better health: 10 diet tips that work wonders." *Environmental Nutrition Newsletter* 1, 4.
9. Staff writer. (July 2007). Glycemic load not key to long-term weight loss. *Tufts Health & Nutrition Letter* 1, 4.
10. See www.nutritiondata.com/topics/fullness-factor.
11. See www.ohsu.edu/healthyaging/caregiving/images/food_pyramid.gif.
12. See www.diabetes.org/nutrition-and-reipes/nutrition/foodpyramid.jsp.
13. See www.diabetesdiabeticdiet.com/food_pyramid.htm.
14. See www.vrg.ort/nutrition/adapyramid.htm.
15. Willett, W. C. (2001). *Eat, Drink, and Be Healthy.* New York: Simon & Schuster.

Chapter 5

1. Clark, H. H. (July 1971). Basic understanding of physical fitness. *Physical Fitness Research Digest, Series 1,* p. 1.
2. http://wiki.answers.com/Q/What_is_the_definition_of_physical_fitness.
3. Caspersen, C. J., & Merrit, R. K. (1995). Physical activity trends among 26 states, 1986–1990. *Medicine and Science in Sports and Exercise* (27):713–720.
4. Clark, J. (2009). *Best iPhone Apps: The Guide for Discriminating Downloaders.* Sebastopol, CA: O'Reilly Media.
5. *Nutrition Action Healthletter.* (April 2009). You must remember this: How to keep your brain young. pp. 1, 4.
6. Clark, J. (2009). *Best iPhone Apps: The Guide for Discriminating Downloaders.* Sebastopol, CA: O'Reilly Media.
7. Ibid.
8. LeVitus, B. (2010). *Incredible iPhone Apps for Dummies.* Hoboken, NJ: Wiley.
9. Borg, G. A. (1982). Psychophysical bases of perceived exertion. *Medicine and Science in Sports and Exercise* (14):377–381.
10. LeVitus, B. (2010). *Incredible iPhone Apps for Dummies.* Hoboken, NJ: Wiley.
11. Lee, I., Djousse, L., Sesso, H. D., et al. (2010) Physical activity and weight gain prevention. *Journal of the American Medical Association* 303(12):1173–1179.
12. See www.sport-fitness-advisor.com/fitt-principle.html.
13. Ibid.
14. Ibid.
15. Hill, J. O., Peters, J. C., & Jortberg, B. T. (2004). *The Step Diet Book: Count Steps, Not Calories, to Lose Weight and Keep It Off Forever,* New York: Workman.

Chapter 6

1. Roemer, L., & Orsillo, S. M. (2009). *Mindfulness- and Acceptance-Based Behavioral Therapies in Practice.* New York: Guilford.
2. Hayes, S. C., Strosahl, K. D., & Wilson, K. G. (1999). *Acceptance and Commitment Therapy: An Experiential Approach to Behavior Change.* New York: Guilford.

3. See http://gurusoftware.com/Gurunet/Personal/Topics/Values.htm.

4. Schwartz, R. M. (1986). The internal dialogue: On the asymmetry between positive and negative coping thoughts. *Cognitive Therapy and Research 10*:591–605.

5. Schwartz, R. M., & Garamoni, G. L. (1986). A structural model of positive and negative states of mind: Asymmetry in the internal dialogue. In P. C. Kendall (Ed.), *Advances in Cognitive-Behavioral Research and Therapy 5*, 1–62. New York: Academic Press.

6. Schwartz, R. M. (1986). The internal dialogue: On the asymmetry between positive and negative coping thoughts. *Cognitive Therapy and Research 10*:591–605.

7. Nash, J. D. (1993). *Self-talk of dieters and maintainers: States-of-mind, stimulus situations, binge eating, weight cycling, and severity of weight problem.* Unpublished dissertation. Pacific Graduate School of Psychology, Palo Alto, CA.

8. Ibid.

9. Ibid.

10. Kreitler, S., & Chemerinski, A. (1988). The cognitive orientation of obesity. *International Journal of Obesity 12*:403–415.

11. Luoma, J. B., Hayes, S. C., & Walser, R. D. (2007). *Learning ACT.* Oakland, CA: New Harbinger.

Chapter 7

1. Stone, H., & Stone, S. (1989). *Embracing Ourselves: The Voice Dialogue Manual.* Novato, CA: New World Library.

2. See www.delos-inc.com/articles/Voice_Dialogue-_An_Introduction.htm.

3. See www.voicedialogue.com/voicedialogue.htm.

4. See www.delos-inc.com/articles/Embracing_All_Our_Selves.pdf.

5. Zitek, E. M., Jordan, A. H., Monin, B., & Leach, F. R. (2010). Victim entitlement to behave selfishly. *Journal of Personality and Social Psychology 98*:245–255.

6. Seigman, M. P. (1991, 1998). *Learned Optimism: How to Change Your Mind and Your Life.* New York: Knopff/Pocket Books.

Chapter 8

1. See http://www.psy.cmu.edu/~scohen/.

2. Nauthton, F. O. (1997). In R. R. Cornelius (Ed.), *The Science of Emotion.* New York: Prentice Hall. Seminar at California State Northridge on Emotion and Motivation.

3. www.csun.edu/~vcpsy00h/students/coping.htm.

4. Lazarus, R. S., & Folkman, S. (1984). *Stress, Appraisal and Coping.* New York: Springer.

5. Peterson, C., Maier, S. F., & Seligman, M. E. P. (1995). *Learned Helplessness: A Theory for the Age of Personal Control.* New York: Oxford University Press USA.

6. Coyne, J., Aldwin, C., & Lazarus, R. S. (1981). Depression and coping in stressful episodes. *Journal of Abnormal Psychology 90*:439–447.

7. Van Eck, M., Berkhof, H., Nicolson, N., & Sulon, J. (1996). The effects of perceived stress, traits, mood states, and stressful daily events on salivary cortisol. *Psychosomatic Medicine 58*:447–458.

8. McCann, U. D., Rossiter, E. M., King, R., & Agras, W. S. (1991). Nonpurging bulimia: A distinct subtype of bulimia. *International Journal of Eating Disorders 10*:679–689.

9. Devlin, M. J., Goldfein, J. A., & Dobrow, I. (2003). What is this thing called BED? Current status of binge eating nosology. *International Journal of Eating Disorders 34*: Supplement: S2–S18.

10. Black, A. E., Prentice, A. M., Goldberg, G. R., Jebb, S. A., Bingham, S. A., Livingstone, M. B., Coward, W. A. (1993). Measurements of total energy expenditure provide insights into the validity of dietary measurements of energy intake. *Journal of the American Dietetic Association 93*(5):572–579.

Chapter 9

1. Grilo, C. M., Hrabosky, J. I., White M. A., Allison, K. C., Stunkard, A. J. (2008). Overvaluation of shape and weight in binge eating disorder and overweight controls: Refinement of a diagnostic construct. *Journal of Abnormal Psychology 117*:414–419.
2. Didie, E. R., & Fitzgibbon, M. (2004). Binge eating and psychological distress: Is the degree of obesity a factor? *Eating Behaviors 6*:35–41.
3. Mond, J. M., Hay, P. J., Rodgers, B., & Owen, C. (2007). Recurrent binge eating with and without the "undue influence of weight or shape on self-evaluation": Implications for the diagnosis of binge eating disorder. *Behaviour Research and Therapy 45*:929–938.
4. Hudson, J. I., Hiripi, E., Pope, H. G., & Kessler, R. C. (2007). The prevalence and correlates of eating disorders in the National Comorbidity Survey Replication. *Biological Psychiatry 61*:348–358.
5. Those who rise again after falling asleep in order to eat and do so without recollection of the event may be suffering from a sleep disorder known as night eating syndrome, rather than an eating disorder per se.
6. Luskin, F. (2002). *Forgive for Good.* New York: HarperCollins.
7. Enright, R. D., & Fitzgibbons, R. P. (2000). *Helping Clients Forgive: An Empirical Guide for Resolving Anger and Restoring Hope.* Washington, DC: American Psychological Association.

Chapter 10

1. Marlatt, G. A., & Gordon, J. R. (1985). *Relapse Prevention.* New York: The Guilford Press.
2. See http://findarticles.com/p/articles/mi_m0CXH/is_2_23/ai_59246580/.
3. Schlundt, D. G., Sbrocco, T., Bell, C. (1989) Identification of high-risk situations in a behavioral weight loss program: application of the response prevention model. *International Journal of Obesity 13*:223–234.
4. Luszczynska, A., Sobczyk, A., & Abraham, C. (2007). Planning to lose weight: Randomize controlled trial of an implementation intervention prompt to enhance weight reduction among overweight and obese women. *Health Psychology 26*:507–512.
5. Ajzen, I. (2001). Nature and operation of attitudes. *Annual Review of Psychology 52*:27–58.
6. Bach, R. (1977). *Illusions: The Adventures of a Reluctant Messiah.* New York: Dell.
7. See www.relaxationexpert.co.uk/using-prayer-coping-stress.html.

Chapter 11

1. See http://www.sparkpeople.com/resource/wellness_articles.asp?id=1063.
2. Anderson, J., Kanz, E., Fredrick, R., & Wood, C. (2001). Long-term weight-loss maintenance: A meta-analysis of U.S. studies. *American Journal of Clinical Nutrition 74*:579–584.

Chapter 12

1. Ogden, C. L., Carol, M. D., & Flegal, K. M. (2003). Epidemiological trends in overweight and obesity. *Endocrinology and Metabolism Clinics of North America 32*:741–760.
2. Apple, R. F., Lock, J., & Peebles, R. (2006). *Is Weight Loss Surgery Right for You?* New York: Oxford.
3. Ibid.
4. Ibid.
5. See www.lap-bandsandiego.com/surgery-compared.html.
6. De Zwaan, J., Mitchell, J. E., Howell, L. M., et al. (2002). Two measures of health-related quality of life in morbid obesity. *Obesity Research 10*:1143–1151.
7. Yanovski, S. Z., Nelson, J. E., Dubbert, B. K., & Spitzer, R. L. (1993). Association of binge eating disorder and psychiatric comorbidity in obese subjects. *American Journal of Psychiatry 150*:1472–1479.

8.   Adami, G. F., Gandolfo, P., Bauer, B., & Scopinaro, N. (1995). Binge eating in massively obese patients undergoing bariatric surgery. *International Journal of Eating Disorders 7*:45–50.

9.   Kolotkin, R. L., Meter, K., & Williams, G. R. (2001). Quality of life and obesity. *Obesity Reviews 2*(4):219–229.

10.   Mitchell, J. & de Zwann, M. (2005). Overview of bariatric surgery procedures. Mitchell & de Zwann (Eds.). *Bariatric Surgery: A Guide for Mental Health Professionals.* New York: Routledge.

11.   MacLean, L.D., Rhode, B. M., & Nohr, C. W. (2000). Late outcome of isolated gastric bypass. *Annals of Surgery 231*:524–528.

12.   See www.bariatric-surgery.info.

RESOURCES

ACSM Guidelines for Exercise Testing and Prescription (7th ed). (2005). Philadelphia: Lippincott, Williams, and Wilkins.

Apple, R. F., Lock, J., & Peebles, R. (2006). *Is Weight Loss Surgery Right for You?* New York: Oxford.

Barnard, N. D. (2003). *Breaking the Food Seduction.* New York: St. Martin's Press.

Clark, J. (2009). *Best iPhone Apps: The Guide for Discriminating Downloaders.* Sebastopol, CA: O'Reilly Media.

Deci, E. L., & Ryan, R. M. (1985). *Intrinsic Motivation and Self-Determination in Human Behavior.* New York: Plenum Press.

DesMaisons, K. (1998/2008). *Potatoes Not Prozac: Solutions for Sugar Sensitivity.* New York: Fireside.

Enright, R. D., & Fitzgibbons, R. P. (2000). *Helping Clients Forgive: An Empirical Guide for Resolving Anger and Restoring Hope.* Washington, DC: American Psychological Association.

Forsyth, J. P., & Eifert, G. H. (2007). *The Mindfulness and Acceptance Workbook for Anxiety.* Oakland, CA: New Harbinger.

Hayes, S. C., Strosahl, K. D., & Wilson, K. G. (1999). *Acceptance and Commitment Therapy: An Experiential Approach to Behavior Change.* New York: Guilford.

Hill, J. O., Peters, J. C., & Jortberg, B. T. (2004). *The Step Diet Book: Count Steps, Not Calories, to Lose Weight and Keep It Off Forever.* New York: Workman.

Kabat-Zinn, J. (1990). *Full Catastrophe Living.* New York: Bantam Dell.

Lazarus, R. S., & Folkman, S. (1984). *Stress, Appraisal and Coping.* New York: Springer.

LeVitus, B. (2010). *Incredible iPhone Apps for Dummies.* Hoboken, NJ: Wiley.

Locke, E. A., & Latham, G. P. (1990). *A Theory of Goal Setting and Task Performance.* Englewood Cliffs, NJ: Prentice Hall.

Luoma, J. B., Hayes, S. C., & Walser, R. D. (2007). *Learning ACT.* Oakland, CA: New Harbinger.

Luskin, F. (2002). *Forgive for Good.* New York: HarperCollins.

Marlatt, G. A., & Gordon, J. R. (1985). *Relapse Prevention.* New York: The Guilford Press.

Mitchell, J. E., & de Zwann, M. (Eds.) (2005). *Bariatric Surgery: A Guide for Mental Health Professionals.* New York: Routledge.

Peeke, P. (2005). *Body-for-LIFE for Women: A Woman's Plan for Physical and Mental Transformation.* Emmaus, PA: Rodale Press.

Peterson, C., Maier, S. F., & Seligman, M. E. P. (1995). *Learned Helplessness: A Theory for the Age of Personal Control.* New York: Oxford University Press USA.

Roemer, L., & Orsillo, S. M. (2009). *Mindfulness- and Acceptance-Based Behavioral Therapies in Practice.* New York: Guilford.

Seligman, M. P. (1991, 1998). *Learned Optimism: How to Change Your Mind and Your Life.* New York: Knopff: Pocket Books.

Stone, H., & Stone, S. (1989). *Embracing Ourselves: The Voice Dialogue Manual.* Novato, CA: New World Library.

Tribole, E., & Resch, E. (1995, 2003). *Intuitive Eating: A Revolutionary Program That Works.* New York: St. Martin's Griffin.

Willett, W. C. (2001). *Eat, Drink, and Be Healthy.* New York: Simon & Schuster.

Index

Note: tables are indicated by a *t*; self-tests, by an *s*; figures, by an *f*.

A

ABCs of behavior, 54–55
ACT (Acceptance and Commitment Therapy)
    acceptance, 153–154
    choose, 154–155
    observing self, 155–156
    overview, 153
    take action, 155
Adjustable gastric band (AGB), 304–306, 305*f*
Aerobic exercise, 130–131
AGB. *See* Adjustable gastric band (AGB)
Age and obesity, 15
Alcoholics Anonymous, 237
Anaerobic exercise, 120
Anxiety and obesity, 25
Assertiveness
    with "I" statements, 224–225
    lack of, and weight problems, 222
    and managing interpersonal conflict, 225, 226*t*
    overview, 218–219
    and personal rights, 223*t*
    with refusal, 223, 224*t*
    and weight management, 222

B

Backsliding
    causes of 254–255
    changes to limit
        behavior, 270–271, 271*t*, 272*t*
        environment, 268
        interpersonal effectiveness, 268
        limitations, 269
        overview, 267–270
        with spiritual support, 270
    and cognitive distortions, 263, 265
    coping with, 259–261, 264–265*f*, 266*f*
    emotional hazards of, 255–256
    in high-risk situations, 256–257
        interpersonal determinants, 257–258

intrapersonal/environmental determinants, 257
        triggers, 258
    Implementation Intervention Plans, 261, 262*f*, 263
        and motivation, 255
        overview, 253–254
        triggers for, 258
Bariatric surgery
    and binge eating, 235
    challenges, post-surgery
        addictions, 319
        caretaking others, 321
        cheating, 318–319
        converting to solid food, 316
        eating habits, changing, 317–318
        giving up, 319–320
        honeymoon phase, 316
        hunger, 316–317
        loose skin, 320
        overview, 316
        regaining weight, 320
    and digestive process, 301, 302*f*, 303
    emotional reactions to, 313
    failure of, 315
    improvement after, 315
    lifestyle transition needed, 321–322
    open versus laparoscopic, 303
    options for
        adjustable gastric band (AGB), 304–306, 305*f*
        biliopancreatic diversion with duodenal
    switch (BPD-DS), 307–309, 308*f*
        Roux-en-Y gastric bypass (RYGB), 306, 307*f*
        vertical sleeve gastrectomy (VSG), 309–310, 309*f*
    physical activity, 312
    pre-surgery weight loss, 310
    quality of life issues, 311
    results of, 313–314
    risks associated with, 310–311
    and weight loss, 303
    weight regain, 312
Barnard, Dr. Neil D., 91